Post-viral Fatigue Syndrome

Post-viral Fatigue Syndrome

Edited by

Rachel Jenkins MA, MBBChir MD(Cantab), MRCPsych
*Principal Medical Officer, Department of Health
and Honorary Senior Lecturer, Institute of Psychiatry
London, UK*

and

James F. Mowbray MBBChir(Cantab), FRCP
*Professor of Immunopathology in the Department of Experimental Pathology
St Mary's Hospital Medical School
London, UK*

JOHN WILEY & SONS
Chichester · New York · Brisbane · Toronto · Singapore

Other Wiley Editorial Offices

John Wiley & Sons, Inc., 605 Third Avenue,
New York, NY 10158-0012, USA

Jacaranda Wiley Ltd, G.P.O. Box 859, Brisbane,
Queensland 4001, Australia

John Wiley & Sons (Canada) Ltd, 22 Worcester Road,
Rexdale, Ontario M9W 1L1, Canada

John Wiley & Sons (SEA) Pte Ltd, 37 Jalan Pemimpin 05-04,
Block B, Union Industrial Building, Singapore 2057

Library of Congress Cataloging-in-Publication Data

Post-viral fatigue syndrome / edited by Rachel Jenkins and James F.
  Mowbray.
     p. cm.
  Includes bibliographical references and index.
  ISBN 0 471 92846 1
  1. Myalgic encephalomyelitis.   2. Chronic fatigue syndrome.
I. Jenkins, Rachel.   II. Mowbray, James F.
  [DNLM: 1. Fatigue Syndrome, Chronic.   WC 500 P857]
  RC370.P67   1991
  616.7'4—dc20
  DNLM/DLC
  for Library of Congress   90-13138
                                                                  CIP

     A catalogue record for this book is
     available from the British Library

  ISBN 0 471 92846 1

Phototypeset by Inforum Typesetting, Portsmouth
Printed and bound by Biddles Ltd, Guildford and King's Lynn

Contents

Contributors

Dr Leonard C. Archard BSc, PhD
Senior Lecturer in Biochemistry, Charing Cross and Westminster Medical School, Charing Cross Hospital, Fulham Palace Road, London W6, UK

Research interests include molecular aspects of pathology in infectious disease. Current projects involve virus-related heart and muscle diseases, mechanisms of virus persistence and tissue tropism, virus-coded growth factors, structure and expression of bacterial toxin genes and mechanisms of antigenic variation in spirochaetes.

Dr Sverrir Bergmann MD
Consultant Neurologist, Department of Neurology, University Hospital, and Senior Reader in Neurology, Faculty of Medicine, University of Iceland, Reykjavik, Iceland

Research interests include clinical and epidemiological aspects of various neurological diseases in Iceland, including multiple sclerosis, motor neurone disease and Parkinson's disease.

Dr Neil E. Bowles BSc, PhD
Maître Assistant, Département de Biologie Moléculaire, Université de Genève, CH-1211 Genève, Switzerland

Research interests include the role of enteroviruses in the pathogenesis of acute and chronic diseases of cardiac and skeletal muscle, the molecular basis of enterovirus tissue tropism, and the role of the GAG gene of Rous sarcoma virus in the recognition and maturation of virus genomic RNA during virus particle assembly and in the correct localization of the transfer RNA primer of reverse transcription.

Professor Dedra Buchwald MD
Assistant Professor of Medicine, University of Washington, and Chronic Fatigue Clinic, Harborview Medical Center, Seattle, Washington, USA

Research interests include humoral immunity to viral infections.

Dr Richard Budgett MB BS, MA, MRCGP, Dip Sports Med, DRCDG, DCH
Part time partner in general practice and a clinical assistant five sessions a week at the British Olympic Medical Centre, Northwick Park Hospital, Harrow, Middlesex, UK

He is a specialist in sports medicine and orthopaedic medicine, with a special interest in chronic fatigue in athletes. He was awarded a Gold Medal for rowing at the Los Angeles Olympics.

Sue Butler RMN, SRN
Senior Behaviour Therapist at the National Hospital for Nervous Diseases, Queen's
Square, London, UK

Research interests include the management of chronic fatigue syndrome.

Trudie Chalder SRN, RMN, MSc
Behaviour Therapist, National Hospital for Nervous Diseases, Queen's Square,
London, UK

*Research interests include chronic fatigue syndrome, cognitive processing and post-viral
fatigue syndrome, and the relationship between infection and the development of fatigue.*

Dr Jeremy Chase MB ChB, DCH, MRCPsych
Consultant Psychiatrist, Watford General Hospital, UK

*Research interests include the relationship between psychological stress and immunity, un-
dertaken in the Academic Department of Immunology at the Middlesex Hospital, London.*

Dr Anthony David MB ChB, MRCPsych
Lecturer, Institute of Psychiatry, De Crespigny Park, Denmark Hill, SE5 8AF,
London, UK

*Current research interests include epidemiology of fatigue and the neuropsychology of
schizophrenia.*

Dr Leo Galland MD, FACP, FACN
Dr Galland is in private practice, and is Senior Research Consultant, Great Smokies
Diagnostic Laboratory, Asheville, North Carolina, USA

*Research interests include altered microbial ecology as a cause of disease, and the effects of
nutrition on immune function.*

Dr R. G. Gold MBBS (Adelaide), FRACP, FRCP
Consultant Cardiologist, Regional Cardiothoracic Unit, Freeman Hospital,
Newcastle-upon-Tyne, NE7 7DN, UK. Consultant in Administrative Charge, North-
ern Regional Pacing Service, Freeman Hospital, and Clinical Lecturer in Cardiology,
University of Newcastle-upon-Tyne, UK

*Research interests since 1965 include the effects of virus infections on the heart and
pericardium.*

Professor Jaap Goudsmit, MD, PhD
Professor of Virology, Department of Virology, Academisch Ziekenhuis, Bij de Universiteit van Amsterdam, Academisch Medisch Centrum, Heibergd neef, 1105 AZ Amsterdam, The Netherlands. Chief of the Human Retrovirus Laboratory, University of Amsterdam, and formerly Visiting Scientist, Laboratory of Central Nervous System Studies, NINCDS, National Institutes of Health, Bethesda, Maryland, USA

Research interests include antigenic variation of HIV-1 and the role of neutralizing antibodies in protection against infection and disease.

Dr David F. Horrobin MA, DPhil, BM, BChir(Oxon)
Scotia Pharmaceuticals Ltd, Woodbridge Meadows, Guildford, Surrey GU1 1BA, UK. Director of Research, Efamol Research Institute in Nova Scotia and Visiting Professor of Pharmaceutical Medicine, Wolverhampton Polytechnic. Previously Professor of Medical Physiology, Nairobi University, Reader in Physiology, Newcastle University, and Professor of Medicine, University of Montreal, Canada

Main research interests are therapeutics, essential fatty acids and eicosanoids.

Dr Byron Hyde
The Nightingale Research Foundation, 382 Danforth Avenue, Ottawa, Canada K2A 0E1

Research interests include the long-term sequelae of post-viral fatigue syndrome.

Dr Goran A. Jamal MB ChB(Hons), MD(Glasgow), PhD(Glasgow), MRCP
Consultant and Senior Lecturer in Neurology, University of Glasgow, Institute of Neurological Sciences, Southern General Hospital, Glasgow G51 4TF, UK

Research interests include the assessment and investigation of pathophysiological mechanisms of peripheral neuromuscular diseases and post-viral fatigue syndrome, the pathogenesis and treatment of diabetic neuropathy, assessment of selective small or large fibre neuropathies, quantitative evaluation of sensation, the evolution and pathophysiological mechanisms of the Guillain–Barre syndrome and its variants.

Dr Rachel Jenkins MA, MB BChir, MD(Cantab), MRCPsych
Principal Medical Officer, Department of Health, and Honorary Senior Lecturer, Institute of Psychiatry, London, UK. Formerly consultant and senior lecturer, St Bartholomew's Hospital Medical School, London, UK

Research interests include epidemiology of mental illness, primary care of mental illness, sex differences in mental illness, the multiaxial classification of illness, the consequences of mental illness in employed populations, the relationship of alcohol consumption to sickness absence, the institutional care of the elderly, and the development of a system of outcome indicators in mental health.

Dr Anthony L. Komaroff AB, MD
Director, Division of General Medicine and Primary Care, Department of Medicine, Brigham and Women's Hospital, 75 Francis Street, Boston, Massachusetts 02115, USA, and Associate Professor of Medicine, Harvard Medical School

Research interests include the management of common medical problems, and the aetiology, diagnosis and treatment of chronic fatigue syndrome.

Professor Anthony Mann MD, MPhil, FRCP, FRCPsych
Professor of Epidemiological Psychiatry, Institute of Psychiatry and Royal Free Hospital School of Medicine, London, UK. Formerly Senior Lecturer at Royal Free Hospital School of Medicine

Main research interests include epidemiology of mental disorders of old age, psychiatric aspects of cardiovascular disease and psychiatry in primary care settings.

Dr Harvey Marcovitch MA(Cantab), FRCP, DCH, DObst, RCOG
Consultant Paediatrician, Oxfordshire Health Authority and Clinical Lecturer in Paediatrics, University of Oxford, UK. Formerly Deputy Director of the MSD Foundation for Medical Education

Interests include parent/patient/doctor communication skills.

Dr Elizabeth M. McDonald MB BCh, BAO, MRCPsych
Research worker, section of epidemiology and general practice, Institute of Psychiatry, De Crespigny Park, Denmark Hill, London SE5 8AF. Also Honorary Senior Registrar, Maudsley Hospital, London, UK

Main research interests include the psychological effects of interferon treatment and the epidemiological study of fatigue.

Dr Peter H. Merry BM, BCh(Oxon), MRCS, LRCP, DPhys Med, DObst, RCOG, FRCP
Consultant in Rheumatology and Rehabilitation to the Burnley, Pendle and Rossendale Health Authority, and Consultant in charge of Rakehead House, the Younger Disabled Unit, Burnley General Hospital, UK

Research interests include neurological sequelae of trauma.

Professor James F. Mowbray MB BChir(Cantab), FRCP
Professor of Immunopathology in the Department of Experimental Pathology, St Mary's Hospital Medical School, Norfolk Place, London W2 1PG, UK

Research interests include transplantation immunology, foetal/maternal immunology and its relationship to infertility (he has developed a large service for couples with infertility associated with recurrent abortion), viral myocarditis, and post-viral fatigue occurring in patients with viral myocarditis. (With Dr Yousef, he has shown that the majority of ME patients have enteroviruses.) He is currently very interested in chronic enteroviral infection, and its importance in causing other diseases, including viral myocarditis, adult myositis, chronic central nervous system disease, motor neurone disease, etc.) and in the pathogenesis and the elimination of such chronic viral infections.

Dr Linda M. Parsons MBChB, MD(Sheffield), MRCP
Senior Research Fellow, Department of Neurovirology and Neurology, The Rayne Institute, St Thomas' Hospital, London SE1 7EH, UK. Also holds posts in clinical neurology at St Thomas' Hospital, Luton Hospital and Dunstable Hospital.

Research interests include the immune response in the CNS to virus infections, the effect of virus infections on the thymus, and the immune response to virus infections in multiple sclerosis.

Dr Michael Peel MB, BS, MRCGP, MFOM
Senior Lecturer in Occupational Health at the United Medical and Dental Schools of St Thomas' and Guy's Hospitals, Honorary Consultant in Occupational Health at St Thomas' Hospital, and Medical Advisor to the Houses of Parliament and Balfour Beatty plc.

Dr Peel has worked for a number of companies including British Airways and British Telecom, and has a particular interest in the interrelationships between work and health in the modern commercial environment.

Professor Timothy J. Peters MBChB, PhD, FRCP, FRCPath, DScx
Professor of Clinical Biochemistry, King's College Hospital, Denmark Hill, London SE5, UK

Research interests include alcohol abuse and toxicity with special interest in muscle damage and nutritional deficiency.

Dr P. Portegies MD
Staff Neurologist, Departments of Neurology and Virology, Academisch Ziekenhuis, Bij de Universiteit van Amsterdam, Academisch Medisch Centrum, Heibergd neef, 1105 AZ Amsterdam, The Netherlands

Research interests include AIDS and viral infections of the nervous system.

Dr V. R. Preedy BSc(Hons), PhD
Lecturer in the Department of Clinical Biochemistry, King's College School of Medicine and Dentistry, King's College Hospital, Denmark Hill, London SE5, UK

Current research interests include muscle protein metabolism and tissue protein synthesis.

Dr Colette Ray PhD, CClinPsychol
Senior Lecturer in Psychology, Department of Human Sciences, Brunel University, Uxbridge, Middlesex UB8 3PH, UK

Besides post-viral fatigue syndrome, her research interests include stress and coping within the context of physical health and disability.

Dr Andrew Smith BSc, PhD, CPsychol, FBPS
Director of the Health Psychology Research Unit, University of Wales College of Cardiff, UK. Formerly a post-doctoral fellow in the Department of Experimental Psychology, University of Oxford 1976–1982, lecturer in the MRC, Perceptual and Cogniture Performance Unit, University of Sussex 1982–1988, and Charles Hunnisett Research Fellow 1988–1990.

Dr Smith leads teams working on the behavioural effects of viral infections, and on the relationship between nutrition and behaviour.

Dr David Smith MBChB(Edin), BSc(Hons), PhD
High Road, Horndon on the Hill, Essex SS17 0EZ, UK

Main interest is diagnosis and clinical management of post-viral fatigue syndrome and research into its causes.

Dr Alan Stewart MB, BS, MRCP(UK)
Works in private practice at the Biolab Medical Unit, 9 Weymouth Street, London W1N 3FF, UK. He is Medical Advisor to the Women's Nutritional Advisory Service

Research interests are in clinical nutrition.

Dr Richard Stone MA(Juris), BM, MRCGP
2 Garway Road, London W2 4NH, UK

Senior partner in a five doctor group practice in Inner London. Previous activities include member of the District Health Authority, Chair of Area Review Committee on Non-accidental Injury, Founder of Bayswater Project for Hotel Homeless Families, Chair of Pensioners' Link.

Professor Hugh E. Webb MA, BMBCh, DM(Oxon), DSc, FRCP, FRCPath(Lond)
Professor of Neurovirology, Rayne Institute, St Thomas' Hospital, and Consultant Neurologist, St Thomas' Hospital, London SE1 7EH, UK, with responsibility for inpatients, outpatients, and teaching medical students. He also runs a daily general practice clinic for hospital staff

Research interests include the pathogenesis of virus infections of the nervous system.

Dr W. R. C. Weir MBChB, MRCP
Consultant Physician, Department of Infectious Diseases, The Royal Free Hospital at Coppets Wood Hospital, Coppetts Road, Muswell Hill, London N10 1JN, UK. Honorary Senior Lecturer in Infectious Diseases, Royal Free Hospital, and Honorary Senior Lecturer in Clinical Tropical Medicine, London School of Hygiene and Tropical Medicine

Research interests include post-viral fatigue syndrome, the pathogenesis of tuberculosis and the pathophysiology of Falciparum *malaria.*

Dr S. Wessely MA(Cantab), BM BCh(Oxon), MSc, MRCP, MRCPsych
Institute of Psychiatry, De Crespigny Park, Denmark Hill, London, SE5 8AF, UK.
Senior Lecturer in Liaison Psychiatry, King's College Hospital Medical School and
Institute of Psychiatry, Honorary Consultant in Psychiatry, King's College Hospital
and Maudsley Hospital, London

Research interests include chronic fatigue syndrome, schizophrenia, and psychiatric aspects of skin disease, and of low blood pressure.

Foreword

Anthony Clare
St Patrick's Hospital, Dublin, Eire

A particularly challenging problem for contemporary medicine is how its practitioners can cope with those puzzling clinical entities which are defined purely in terms of symptoms, which are accompanied by little in the way of consistent physical signs, which affect quite large numbers of patients and for which no specific treatment appears effective. 'The very success of bio-medicine', Leon Eisenberg recently wrote, 'has exacted a price in the way it has narrowed the physician's focus exclusively to the biology of disease.' (Eisenberg, 1988). Confronted by chronic fatigue states, many such narrowly focused physicians respond to their own diagnostic and therapeutic frustrations by regarding sufferers as hysterics or malingerers and their symptoms as 'all in the mind' or by concluding, somewhat prematurely, that the symptoms are entirely due to abnormal immune, muscle, viral or hormonal function.

The post-viral fatigue syndrome is just such a condition. There are doctors who, irritated by the failure to establish a consistent aetiology and pathogenesis, consider the condition a chimera. Others with a matching dogmatism insist on an organic basis and regard any argument suggesting a psychological component as tantamount to classifying sufferers as frauds. In the midst of such fractious debates, there is a small but growing body of researchers and clinicians painstakingly sifting through the evidence to establish a fragile foundation for more substantial research.

The heterogeneity of patients with chronic fatigue is matched only by the diversity of laboratory abnormalities, particularly those involving the immune system. The research questions multiply. Is myalgic encephalomyelitis a chronic viral infection, perhaps of enteroviruses replicating in the gut, muscle fibres and the brain with physical symptoms such as recurrent fever, lymphadenopathy, muscle pains, paraesthesia, and psychological symptoms including depression, irritability and anxiety? Does a patient's emotional status determine the distress produced by biological disturbances and the duration of such changes and, if it does, how does it do it? How might changes in immune function influence mood, cognition and behaviour and in turn how might such effects feed back and influence immune function? How can such questions be answered without a genuinely multidisciplinary research approach?

They cannot, which is why Rachel Jenkins and James Mowbray have assembled an impressive array of clinicians and researchers, biochemists, neurologists, immunologists, virologists, psychologists and psychiatrists who have followed Eisenberg's exhortation not to abandon reductionism but to incorporate it within a larger social framework 'to enable the physician to attend to the patient as well as to the disease'. It is entirely appropriate that the collection should open with a contribution from clinical epidemiology spanning as it does the divide which still exists between so much of biology and the behavioural and social sciences. Given the state of knowledge and research, it is inevitable that contributors do not always agree. It is a measure of the value of this volume that it quite deliberately refuses to impose certainty where there is none and struggles instead to provide the reader with an accurate picture of the state of our thinking concerning post-viral fatigue.

The volume embraces a very definite strategy aimed at breaking away from the fossilized dichotomy of organic versus functional which threatens to paralyse clinicians and patients alike. 'Can we not acknowledge that there is never one cause for a patient getting ill?' asks Gill (1970) a trifle dispairingly. We not only can but we will the more we involve in the growing research effort not merely the basic scientist but also the clinical investigator, that 'bridge tender', as described by a distinguished American academic surgeon (Moore, 1984), standing between the research scientist and the practising clinician. There is an understandable temptation on the part of the busy clinician to throw up the hands at the confusing terminology (ME, neurasthenia, fatigue syndrome, fibromyalgia), to despair at the multiplicity and contrary nature of organic and psychological findings, to view with scepticism the many and varied claims concerning the plethora of remedies. Given the severity of the illness, its impact on patients and the demand it places on family, friends and services, the temptation must be resisted. Instead, we must continue to struggle to make sense of the confusion, the activity that in Medawar's view most reliably distinguishes the true scientist (Medawar, 1986); and the labours undertaken by the contributions in this book should serve further to focus our enthusiasm, stimulate our energies and curb that nihilism in the face of uncertainty which is the occupational hazard of the busy physician.

REFERENCES

Eisenberg, L. (1988) Science in medicine: Too much or too little or too limited in scope? In: *The Task of Medicine* (Edited by Kerr L. White), pp. 190–217. The Henry J. Kaiser Family Foundation, Menlo Park, California.

Gill, C. H. (1970) *British Medical Journal*, 299.

Medawar, P. (1986) *Memoir of a Thinking Radish*. Oxford University Press, Oxford.

Moore, F. D. (1984) In: *Conversations in Medicine* (Edited by Allen B. Weisse). New York University Press, New York.

Preface

A puzzling, disabling illness, variously called epidemic neuromyasthesia, benign myalgic encephalomyelitis, Icelandic disease, or Royal Free Hospital disease, has occurred in sporadic form and in more than 20 outbreaks over the past 35 years, in association with chronic nonspecific symptoms of muscle fatigue, mental fatigue weakness, myalgias, low grade fevers, lymphadenopathy, paraesthesias, memory loss and depression. The illness usually begins abruptly and recovery usually ensues within several months, but some patients have continuing relapses or persistent symptoms for years.

Over the last two or three decades there has been debate concerning the cause of this condition. Routine laboratory tests are almost always normal, and yet the observations that outbreaks usually occur in the summer months and often affect hospital staff have been taken to suggest a viral causation. However, other observers noting the apparently greater incidence in women have suggested that it is a psychological illness, akin to hysteria, pointing to the high prevalence of psychological symptoms associated with the syndrome.

More recently, as virological techniques have advanced, there has been further research on this curious illness, with attempts to demonstrate that the prolonged course represents a continuing viral infection and that there is impaired host response to the virus. There has also been an ever-growing demand for medical recognition and effective treatment by the sufferers. Recent years have witnessed a huge increase in media coverage of the condition and the growth of the ME Association and the ME Action Campaign. As general practitioners and other specialists are often understandably confused by the syndrome, are reluctant to diagnose a chronic disabling illness in people who were apparently perfectly fit until recently, do not wish to miss some other more treatable condition, and do not have effective treatments to offer, many sufferers find it hard to obtain a clear diagnosis or medical advice. At a time when alternative medicine is growing in popularity, it is perhaps therefore not surprising that sufferers are trying a variety of 'alternative' approaches to their illness, with varying reports of success. However, we are also now beginning to see the publication of trials of treatments such as the antiviral agent acyclovir, and gamma-globulin.

This book is written mainly for primary care physicians, but also for hospital specialists such as cardiologists, endocrinologists, infectious diseases specialists and neurologists, to any of whom people with ME may present for assessment, diagnosis and treatment.

The book contains a historical account of the early literature on ME; current expert reviews from the research disciplines of virology, biochemistry, immunology, psychology and psychiatry on both sides of the Atlantic; descriptions of presentation, investigation, diagnosis and management in the wide range of settings in which patients may present, including general practice, general medicine, cardiology, rheumatology, psychiatry, neurology, paediatrics, and sports medicine. The book includes up-to-date reviews of physical and psychological factors which may influence immunity, and concludes with a clear review of future research directions.

Glossary

In this section are explanations of some of the terms used in this book. It is not intended as an exhaustive 'dictionary', but to define the use of some of the terms with which the reader may be unfamiliar.

Affective disorders

These refer to mental illness where the predominant abnormality is a disturbance of affect or mood; they include various forms of depression, and mania. Affective disorders may be either neurotic or psychotic.

Chronic fatigue syndrome

This term was coined in the US to represent the chronic fatigue states, mental and muscular, which were the subject of the Holmes criteria. There was no attempt in the latter to define an aetiological cause, infectious or other. A recent UK consensus document has been agreed as a result of a multidisciplinary meeting in Oxford, chaired by Antony Clare. The consensus document is intended to lay down the criteria for inclusion of patients and control subjects in studies in the whole area (ref BMJ, until the full document is published ? this year).

Creatine kinase

There are enzymes which are found in particular tissues of the body, and creatine kinase (CK) is one of them. Muscles use creatine phosphate as the high-energy phosphate source of energy for contraction. Thus the enzyme creatine kinase, which is used to transfer the high-energy phosphate from ATP to creatine, is found in smooth or striated muscle. When damage to the muscle cells occurs, the enzyme leaks from the cytoplasm and may be detected in the blood. The presence of elevated CK levels in the blood indicates damage to muscle cells, but does not say which are involved. Thus levels of hundreds of units/ml are found in myocardial infarction, and of tens of thousands in generalised skeletal muscle damage. The very high levels in the latter are related to the large mass of muscle cells which may have cell membranes which are damaged and leaking CK.

In acute myositis there is obvious muscle damage on histopathological examination, and it is not surprising that levels are high. Although there is no demonstrable lack of muscle power, or true muscle cell fatigue, in ME, there is indeed demonstrable virus infection of scattered muscle cells. The normal finding in the established case is of normal CK levels, but in the acute onset ME patients raised CK levels have been found in the first three months or so. In contrast, in chronic myositis there is a continued high level of CK, indicating continuing muscle damage to a large number of muscle fibres. The 'down-regulated' enteroviruses seen in one in 500 myocytes, by *in situ* hybridisation with enteroviral probes, either do not cause leakage of enzyme, or are too few in number for that amount to be detectable. The lack of inflammatory changes related to the infected fibres suggests that the former explanation is more likely to be the reason for normal levels.

The lack of elevated CK in the blood, and the absence of inflammatory changes in the muscle in ME, contrast with the conditions in chronic viral myositis. In the latter, muscle weakness and gross muscle wasting occur, neither of which are features of ME.

Cytokines

Cytokines are chemical messengers between cells. They represent a part of the overall endocrine system, but are peptide in nature, rather than simple chemicals such as hydrocortisone. Obviously some 'ordinary hormones' such as ACTH or insulin are also peptide hormones.

Cytokines are produced from a cell surface and diffuse to other cells. Cells are affected if they have receptors on their cell surface for the peptide. The effects produced are of two kinds, binding to a receptor and stimulating it, or binding *without* stimulating, but blocking stimulation of the receptor by another cytokine. The overall action of cytokines can then be very complex.

The best known cytokines are the ones which have immunological and viral interest, although many are now known as growth factors for particular cell types. The best known are the interferons, of which the alpha- and beta-interferons (INF-α and INF-β) are released from virus-infected cells, and INF-γ by stimulated lymphocytes. INF secreted by a virus-infected cell can protect other cells from virus infection by the same or unrelated viruses. It can also prevent cell division, a property which has been used in anticancer therapy. These interferons are now available in quantity thanks to molecular cloning techniques, and have been used to treat patients. The side effects include cognitive difficulties, muscle aches and a set of symptoms described by the patient as a cold without the blocked nose. They have obviously become of interest as possible mediators of at least some of the symptoms of fatigue syndromes associated with infections, or immunological responses. The other well-known cytokines are those which are produced during immune responses, interleukin-1 and interleukin-2 (Il-1 and Il-2). The former, in tiny doses, injected into the lateral ventricle will produce fever, and is the substance which in the past was shown to be released by macrophages exposed to bacterial endotoxin. It was at that time usually called intrinsic pyrogen. When Il-1 is released from stimulated macrophages fever is *inter alia* the usual consequence. In ME fever is not usual after the onset, but recurrent fevers are a characteristic of the related fatigue syndrome, glandular fever. The latter, caused by Epstein–Barr virus, may have a subacute febrile course for many weeks, but is clinically somewhat different from ME.

Il-2 is a key cytokine in immune responses. The division of lymphocytes producing a specific response is mediated by Il-2, and cells which release it and have receptors for it may demonstrate the autocrine effect, that is be stimulated by their own cytokine to divide. The receptors for Il-2 on lymphocytes are induced by exposure to Il-1 release, as stated above, from macrophages. Exposure to antigen then leads to fever, production of Il-2 receptors on lymphocytes, presentation of the antigen to lymphocytes and their clonal multiplication under the influence of Il-2 to increase the number of cells taking part in the response.

Many of the other cytokines have been found controlling division of specific cell types, particularly in the bone marrow, where differentiation and multiplication of stem cell sources controls the production of the different bone marrow cellular elements in the blood. The members of this group of cytokines are usually called 'growth factors', but Il-2 is of course a growth factor for lymphocytes. Some other cytokines with the ability to damage cells are known, such as tumour necrosis factor or TNFα. This produces some innate protection against tumour cells, some of which have a surface receptor for it. Produced by macrophages, it can then lead to the death of tumour cells to which it can bind, without affecting the normal cells that do not express this surface marker. TNFα has been shown to be present in high levels during septicaemic shock, and may be an important mediator of many of the problems therein.

Cytokines can be seen to be important components of immune responses and infections, and their role in producing untoward side effects in acute or chronic infections is now being unravelled. Their actual mediator role in ME is just beginning to be explored.

Depression

The term 'depression' is potentially confusing as it may refer either to the symptom of depression (i.e. low, depressed mood) or the syndrome of depression (i.e. depressive disorder).

Depressive illness

The range of depressive illness stretches from sporadic, lowered mood, associated with a few other neurotic symptoms (e.g. poor concentration, fatigue and irritability), through severe continuous low mood associated with a full house of associated neurotic symptoms (e.g. not only poor concentration, fatigue and irritability but also anxiety, phobias, obsessional thoughts and activities, and impaired sleep, appetite and libido) causing severe impairment of occupational, domestic and family relationships, to psychotic depression which is accompanied by delusions, hallucinations and retardation. The delusions (false, irrational, fixed beliefs which are not culturally held) may be hypochondriacal, self-condemnatory or ritualistic and are in keeping with the depressive affect. The hallucinations (false perceptions which occur without the sensory stimuli which characterise illusions) may be hypochondriacal, self-condemnatory or ritualistic. The hallucinations, when present, are also in keeping with the depressed mood.

They may be auditory (e.g. hearing voices mocking him or telling him to kill himself), or olfactory (e.g. perceiving foul odours emanating from him). Retardation is a general slowing of mental and motor activity which tends to occur only in psychotic depression; when extreme it is called stupor. Physiological sluggishness such as bradycardia, low blood pressure, dryness of mucous membranes and constipation, is more commonly associated with psychotic depression.

Most depressive illness, whether neurotic or psychotic, is preceded by acute or chronic physical or psychological trauma. In the literature, acute psychological trauma is often termed 'life events' and chronic psychological trauma 'chronic social stress'. The commoner precipitants include:

(a) Physical—infections, particularly viral, such as influenza, infective hepatitis, glandular fever and others; operations, accidents, pregnancy and childbirth; some drugs, for example reserpine, oestrogens, corticosteroids, and contraceptive pills.

(b) Psychological—withdrawal of affection, damage to self-esteem or disappointment, bereavement and moving house. There is also evidence that there is some genetic predisposition to psychotic depressive illness. There is little or no genetic predisposition to non-psychotic or neurotic depression, and although this condition sometimes runs in families, this is not because of heredity, but because of environmental and subcultural influences.

Not everyone who experiences acute or chronic stresses becomes depressed, and a major factor which seems to protect people from depression is social support which may be derived from family, friends and colleagues.

Enteroviruses

The enteroviruses are small RNA viruses. They are part of the larger group of picornaviruses (*pico* + RNA = little RNA viruses). Their genetic material, RNA, is protected by capsid protein composed of four polypeptides (VP1, VP2, VP3 and VP4). Among the larger group of picornaviruses are several animal viruses such as foot and mouth disease virus. The human enteroviruses comprise about 70 different serotypes, with some degree of antigenic cross-reaction between them, and thus to some extent shared immunity. There are several different groups of them, echoviruses, polio viruses, Coxsackie viruses and ones just known as enterovirus, followed by a number, e.g. enterovirus 71 (e.g. echo 9, Coxsackie A3). The viruses are very prevalent in temperate climates in the summer, May to October in the UK. They infect the gastrointestinal tract and are sewage and water borne. The initial infection, usually acute and lasting for only a few days, presents as a flu-like illness, with sore throat and painful, enlarged cervical lymph nodes. There may be diarrhoea and vomiting, but this is usually mild. They represent the great majority of all 'summer colds'. The importance of the group was originally because of the three polio virus strains, which spread in the summer widely through the population; the paralytic strains infected the CNS of non-immune patients, causing destruction of anterior horn cells in some territories, leading to lower motor neurone paralysis. It is of some interest that the muscle groups which tended to be most affected were those which were subject to exercise. Much care was taken to avoid active muscle movement in the early stages of the disease to prevent this, but it was not uncommon to find that a careful, full, neurological examination of an area might be followed by the development of paralysis in that area. Unlike fatiguability *qv*, the affected territory was usually associatedwith the exercised muscle groups.

The enteroviruses are extremely infectious and when they are present in a community virtually all the people will be infected. Since there is such a large number of serotypes, cross-immunity is not very effective, and few people in a community escape infection. In the UK the average expectation is about one infection per year per individual, but in warmer climates, where the viruses are perennially endemic, there may be four or five infections per year.

The viruses produce well-defined epidemics of infection, but there is a background of infection continuously apart from detectable epidemics. The importance of the latter is that when such occur, there is evidence that nearly everyone may have IgM antibodies to the virus, indicating recent exposure, but only a small number go on to a chronic persistent infection and develop the features of a chronic post-viral fatigue syndrome.

Epstein–Barr virus

The Epstein–Barr virus (EBV) is one of the herpes viruses, and hence is a DNA virus. It infects only those cell types in the body for which there is a receptor, and this limits the infection very largely to B lymphocytes. The acute or subacute infection presents as a pharyngeal infection with enlarged painful cervical lymph nodes, largely in teenagers and young adults. The condition clinically described as glandular fever is at onset very similar to the onset of enteroviral infections or indeed quite a few other viruses (see Interferon). The infection is associated with a considerable degree of debility, and if it persists for more than a few days is usually diagnosed as glandular fever, or if the EBV is detected by specific serological responses, infectious mononucleosis. This latter is the usual US term for the condition, and glandular fever is not a term often used there.

EBV infects B lymphocytes, and results in some immunosuppression while it is present in the active form. Some strains of the virus are oncogenic, particularly those of African origin, and are the cause of Burkitt's lymphoma, or nasopharyngeal carcinoma in Asia. Fortunately most of the EBV in the UK only produces glandular fever, and rarely neoplasia.

Spread is by droplet and saliva; hence the name of 'kissing disease'. The onset of such osculatory activity in teenagers results in a rapid rise in the presence of detectable antibodies in sera between ages 12 and 18. By the latter age about 80% of the population appear to have met the virus. As with other herpes viruses, dormancy and integration occur, so that, once infection has taken place, the virus survives, usually dormant, in everyone infected. Thus it is possible to recover virus from the lymphocytes of the majority of healthy adults in the country. To determine active infection then requires other markers, and in reactivation the immune responses to the viral capsid (VCA) and 'early antigen' (EA) are used to show this. Such serological techniques are tedious, and hence not widely available. At present they have been used very largely for research purposes. Unlike some other viruses, where measurement of the virus protein can be used to measure persisting infection, e.g. hepatitis B and hepatitis B surface antigen (HB_5Ag) and enteroviruses and VP1, there is no simple measure of viral protein production which indicates an active EBV infection.

EBV is also useful in the laboratory, causing transformation of normal human B lymphocytes in tissue culture into a permanently dividing malignant transformed population. This is used for 'immortalisation' of B lymphocytes for a number of research and routine tissue-typing procedures.

Fatiguability

This condition, considered a hallmark of ME, consists of the delayed recovery from exhaustion. As an example, when a healthy but not particularly fit adult runs unexpectedly for a bus, and just makes it, gasping, into his or her seat, there is a short period of dyspnoea, muscle pain and discomfort, lasting for a few minutes only. At the end of that brief recovery period the subject could run again the same way for another bus. Fatiguability, as seen in ME, means that having gone to the point of exhaustion, although some improvement may occur in the next few minutes, mostly in dyspnoea, tachycardia etc., there is a long-term effect, carried on for days or weeks, in which further exertion is extremely limited.

Exercise to the point of exhaustion results in prolonged exacerbation of fatigue not only in the function which produced the fatigue. Thus if running to the point of exhaustion, the prolonged fatigue would apply to other muscle groups, such as the arms, and also impairment of cognitive functions. This kind of fatiguability is thus a systemic manifestation of local exhaustion. (Mental 'activity', to the point of exhaustion, may also produce prolonged muscle fatigue.) It is likely that the mediators are common to both, and production of cytokines which can act in many territories will prove to be the underlying cause. As shown in Figure 1, the local symptoms produced are not likely to be of a single cause. Virus infection of muscles or brain may be able to produce the local changes, but cytokines produced elsewhere, possibly in lymphoid tissues or muscle, may affect the brain.

The polyarthropathy experienced by 20% of ME patients, in our large series, is probably mediated by immune complexes, which are detectable in the circulation of about two-thirds of ME patients. The circulating immune complexes, predominantly with IgM antibody, are often composed of enteroviral antigens and antibody to them (Al Kadiry *et al.*, 1983).

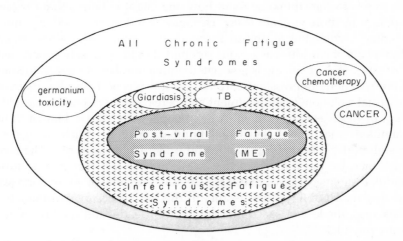

Figure 1 Mediators of symptoms of ME. Local virus infection may cause local changes in muscle and CNS, but cytokines produced elsewhere, in infected tissues of lymphoid, may pass to the CNS and produce remote effects

Fatigue

The dictionary definition of fatigue is concerned with muscles. The concept of psychological or central fatigue is one of psychiatric origin. In either case it means that after physical or mental exercise, the patient tires abnormally early during prolonged activity, or cannot sustain the same level of activity as normal.

Low, depressed mood

Feeling low may range from one or two spells of low mood a week lasting an hour or two at a time, through to a persistently lowered mood which is impossible to snap out of. The person may feel like crying, or may in fact be tearful, particularly when shown a little sympathy. Upsetting items on television may elicit tears. (For cultural reasons, men on the whole tend to cry less easily than women, but will report on questioning about feeling close to tears.)

Rather than admit to feeling low, the person may simply describe feeling flat, feeling no pleasure in life, family or work. This is known as 'anhedonia'. Whether experiencing anhedonia, or low mood, life may be described as empty, bleak or even hopeless. The person may start to feel that he would not mind going to sleep and never waking up, or being run over by a bus, or catching a fatal illness. This is the start of suicidal 'ideation', which may proceed to a feeling that one would rather be dead, and then to a wish to kill oneself, prevented only by the desire not to upset family and friends. The next step is to start thinking about how one might kill oneself, for example by pills or by more violent means. This may be followed by active planning, including buying the means to kill oneself. Anyone who is entertaining actual plans of suicide is at serious risk and should be closely supervised.

Increased risk of suicide is associated with a number of factors, including severe psychotic depression, chronic, painful physical disease, increasing age, social isolation, unemployment and bereavement. Men are more likely to kill themselves than women. A few people with ME are known to have committed suicide and the actual numbers may be much higher, both through under-reporting of suicide and underdiagnosis of ME. The factors which increase the risk of suicide in ME are the fact that it is a chronic, painful, disabling disease, that it is sometimes accompanied by depression, and that the disability often results in the loss of occupation (and hence colleagues), the loss of social life (and hence friends) and the loss of active leisure pursuits.

Lowered mood or depression may sometimes be accompanied by feelings of guilt or self-blame. These are usually exaggerated or even completely unjustified, and may concern events years ago, such as a family death. The person frequently sees the future as empty or non-existent, and feels that there is nothing to look forward to.

Useful questions to elicit lowered mood include:

Have you had spells of feeling sad or miserable?
How bad does it get?
Do you feel like crying?
Do you ever find yourself crying without reason?
Can you snap out of it?
Do you sometimes feel hopeless?
Have you felt like making an end of it all?
Have you thought how you might do it?
Have you made actual plans?
Do you ever blame yourself for being like this?
Do you even find yourself feeling guilty?
Do you sometimes feel inferior to other people?
How do you feel about the future?

Other psychological symptoms which may be associated with depressed mood are poor concentration, fatigue, irritability, anxiety, impaired sleep, appetite and libido, phobias and obsessional thoughts and activities, and somatic symptoms, such as headache, backache and abdominal pains where there is a clear relationship with psychological stress.

ME

ME was derived as a short form of myalgic encephalomyelitis, which was far too much of a mouthful for medicine, let alone the patient! It implies a problem of an inflammatory nature in the brain, associated with painful muscles. This is not really what is encompassed by ME, which has been defined as:

(a) Abnormal muscle fatigue on exercise, with very slow recovery from exercising to the point of exhaustion (fatiguability *qv*).
(b) Cognitive difficulties in concentration and short-term memory.
(c) Nominal dysphasia.
(d) In the majority of patients this is associated with an ongoing, persistent infection with an enterovirus, and in a minority with activation/ reactivation of Epstein–Barr virus (EBV).

In addition to the central, core features above there may be any of a large number of other, less characteristic, features. These include muscle pain at rest, tinnitus, feelings of heat or cold in the extremities, hyperacusis and hippus.

Mood, affect

These are terms used to describe the emotional or feeling aspects of mental life.

Mood disturbance in organic cerebral disorder

In acute organic cerebral disorder, anxiety and fear are especially common, sometimes developing to terror and panic with tachycardia, flushing and tremor. In addition, depression, elation, irritability, hostility and suspicion may all occur. The affective changes are often fleeting and change abruptly. The effect is partly determined by the physical insult to the cerebrum, partly by the stress of the physical illness, and partly by a vague awareness of the cognitive impairments. Vulnerable aspects of the patient's personality may be exaggerated, with the appearance of depressive, hypochondriacal, or phobic features. Some patients may become histrionic and importuning. A few patients can develop hysterical conversion symptoms, which are usually transient but sometimes persistent, and which may lead to mistakes in diagnosis. Paranoid developments are frequent, and a distinct schizophrenic colouring to the total picture may occur. With the progression of the cerebral disorder the true situation soon becomes obvious. However, mild self-limiting acute organic reactions can occasionally be misdiagnosed as functional psychiatric illness.

In chronic organic cerebral disorder, the picture is as above in the acute phases. Further deterioration produces emotional changes of a distinctive organic kind, with affective blunting and shallowness of affect which may progress to a state of apathy or empty euphoria. Emotions may become childlike, with petulant importuning and excessive anger at annoyances and frustrations. Emotional lability is common, and may be extreme. The 'catastrophic reaction' may be observed when the patient is taxed beyond his ability to cope, and may then explode with excessive anger, anxiety or tears.

Neuroses

These are mental disorders which are not organic, and which, although potentially particularly distressing and disabling, do not possess the qualities of very severe affective change and disturbance of thought, beliefs and perceptions which are associated with the psychoses, i.e. they are non-psychotic. They include depression and anxiety.

Post-infectious fatigue syndromes

There are many established infections which are associated with fatigue states, both of muscle to some extent, and of brain 'fatigue' to a more obvious extent. These may follow infection with a wide variety of agents, bacterial, viral, fungal or parasitic. The best known example is probably of tuberculosis, where it is readily seen that the fatigue follows the onset of infection, and persists through to its cure. There is a diminution in fatigue during recovery, so that it is not apparent before the infection has been cured, but this is somewhat variable. What is common between the different kinds of infection and the final common pathway of fatigue generation is probably that the mediators of fatigue are produced predominantly by the immune response to the infection. Thus only the cytokines generated by the infection control the majority of the symptoms produced. Obviously with specific chronic infections there may be specific local effects producing signs and symptoms characteristic of a particular agent, but there will be an overlap, for the most part, of the common symptoms. Thus although pulmonary damage in TB may lead to cough and sputum, and in chronic giardiasis gastrointestinal symptoms are usual, both may, and usually do, exhibit features of moderate to severe central fatigue. The chronic infection with enteroviruses found most frequently with ME also produces a local effect of muscle fatigue and myalgia not found with the other two.

The prerequisite for a chronic infectious fatigue syndrome is a chronic infection. The idea that an infection sets up a fatigue state which persists after recovery is not borne out by follow-up of the chronic infectious states, where recovery from infection is associated with recovery of symptoms, although a degree of 'institutionalisation' may cause some delay in loss of all nonspecific central symptoms as the patient returns towards the normal activities of the active individual.

There is only a limited number of chronic infections which remain active and can cause one of the syndromes. They consist of some bacteria such as mycobacteria producing chronic tuberculosis and leprosy, chronic intestinal parasitic infections, and a few viruses. Each must have a way of escaping the rapid elimination from the body which would prevent chronic active or persistent infection.

Post-viral fatigue syndrome

This is a subset of chronic fatigue syndromes, in which there is evidence that the fatigue state followed the onset of a virus infection. The demonstration of persistent virus infections in patients with this subset removes the need for the old idea that the process was self-supporting when established and was 'triggered' by a virus infection. That concept was related to the failure to find evidence of viral infection in established fatigue states, because (a) the appropriate viruses were not sought, or (b) the techniques for showing viral persistence in chronic states were developed only recently. It is now clear for many such virus infections that the persistence of the infection is required for persistence of symptoms, and the disease state disappears when the virus infection is eliminated.

Psychoses

These are major mental redisorders in which impairment of mental function has developed to a degree that interferes grossly with insight, ability to meet some ordinary demands of life, or ability to maintain adequate contact with reality. It is not an exact or well-defined term. Mental retardation is excluded. Psychoses may be organic or functional. Organic psychoses are associated with physical disease or injury to the brain, and include dementia, delirium, alcohol psychoses, drug psychoses, and encephalitides, e.g. encephalitis lethargia, tertiary syphilis, subacute sclerosing panencephialitis, and HIV. Functional psychoses include schizophrenia, the affective psychoses (manic, manic-depression and depressive psychosis) and paranoid states.

REFERENCES

Al Kadiry, W., Gold, R. G., Behan, P. O. and Mowbray, J. F. (1983) Analysis of antigens in the circulating immune complexes of patients with Coxsackie infections. In P. O. Behan, V. TerMeulen and C. F. Rose (eds) *Progress in Brain Research*, Vol. 59, pp. 61–67. Elsevier Science Publishers, Amsterdam.

Lishman, W. A. (1987) *Organic Psychiatry: The Psychological Consequences of Cerebral Disorder*, 2nd edn, Blackwell Scientific Publications, Oxford.

World Health Organization (1978) *Mental Disorders: International Classification of Diseases*, 9th revision, WHO, Geneva.

Part I

History, Epidemiology and Aetiology

1

Introduction

Rachel Jenkins

Institute of Psychiatry, London, UK

This chapter aims to introduce the reader to the recorded history of ME, including the early epidemics, the development of the concept, and the realisation that endemic cases also existed; to the debate about whether it is an 'organic' or 'hysterical' illness and to the importance of placing all diseases within a multiaxial framework of aetiology and host response; and to the development of present-day nomenclature and diagnostic criteria. It is not exhaustive, which would have taken a whole book in itself, but I have tried to bring to the interested reader's attention some of the key literature on ME, between 1934 and 1978, and to set the scene for the other contributions in this book, which review the more recent research of the 1980s.

It has been said that nothing can now be learned from the early epidemics of ME; that they happened too long ago for us to be sure what really occurred. Nothing, of course, could be further from the truth. Some of the epidemics are brilliantly described in careful clinical and epidemiological terms which we would do well to emulate today. The men who described them raised questions which we have yet to answer and, in their thoughtful discussions, anticipated much of the ensuing debate on the aetiology of the condition.

It is more than half a century since the first descriptions of a puzzling new clinical entity began to emerge in the medical literature, under the names of 'abortive poliomyelitis' or a 'disease resembling or simulating poliomyelitis'. The illness generally occurred in both epidemic and endemic forms, although it was the epidemics which were easiest to recognise and which caught most medical attention.

Post-viral Fatigue Syndrome. Edited by R. Jenkins and J. Mowbray
© 1991 John Wiley & Sons Ltd

THE EARLY EPIDEMICS

The first recorded epidemic occurred among the doctors and nurses of several hospitals in Los Angeles, USA in 1934. On 12 June 1935, two orthopaedic surgeons, John Wilson and Pierre Walker, read a paper before the Joint Meeting of the American Medical Association and the Canadian Medical Association, Atlantic City, where they reported an outbreak of supposed poliomyelitis in Los Angeles which was not only more extensive but also milder than any previous outbreak of poliomyelitis in California. Peculiar features of this epidemic which Wilson and Walker noted were the unusual communicability of the disease, the early peak (in June) and the large number of adults infected. In children the disease followed the usual clinical course of poliomyelitis, but amongst the adults, an atypical form of the disease was observed, in which sensory, vasomotor and arthritic symptoms predominated, and recurrent exacerbation of acute symptoms occurred over the following 12 months. Out of 100 cases, 35 still had muscle weakness after a year.

Wilson and Walker suggested that the mildness of the attack, the marked degree of muscle weakness without proportionate atrophy and without loss of tendon reflexes, and the recurrences, all suggested that this was, at the very least, atypical poliomyelitis, rather than the usual form of acute anterior poliomyelitis. They also considered the possibility that many of the later symptoms complained of by the adult patients may have been of 'functional', i.e. of psychological, origin. However, they argued that the striking uniformity of the clinical picture presented by the patients, and the prostrating severity of the symptoms, led most observers to believe that an organic basis for the complaints was present in virtually every case.

Wilson and Walker carefully described the symptoms of the illness in 100 of the patients they saw in the orthopaedic department of the Los Angeles General Hospital. These symptoms included muscle weakness, involuntary muscle contractions and twitching, clonic movements and cramps in the affected muscles, and muscular inco-ordination. However, sensory symptoms predominated, with pain in the back and extremities which was often intractable, excruciating and persistent for weeks or even months, and which only responded to opiates. There was also local tenderness of muscles, hyperaesthesia, paraesthesia, and areas of anaesthesia, sometimes following the distribution of a nerve trunk and sometimes involving a whole extremity. Vasomotor and trophic disturbances were almost constant findings. There was excessive sweating or abnormal dryness of the skin, coldness, cyanosis and brittle nails. The authors wrote 'It was the impression of many observers that a generalised disturbance of vasomotor control occurred in these patients, which best explained the emotional instability'. Inflammation of the joints occurred in a third of adult cases, with a third of these being transitory and the remaining two-thirds developing permanent arthritic changes in the joints.

The authors acknowledged that their 100 reported cases cannot serve to give a true cross-sectional picture of the epidemic because of the selection factors which influence the process of admission to an orthopaedic ward, and they commented that many patients are included in the lists of public health reports at the time who presented the picture of a mild and rapidly vanishing illness.

The same epidemic was described by A. G. Gilliam in more detail and covering the whole of the hospital, as it occurred among the personnel of Los Angeles County General Hospital in that same year, 1934 (Gilliam, 1938). Dr Gilliam, writing from the Office of Epidemiological Studies, US Public Health Service, balanced the epidemiological facts with the clinical features, and he noted that the timing of the epidemic in the personnel of the Los Angeles General Hospital was similar to the time distribution of the epidemic in Los Angeles City and County combined. The epidemic in the community in 1934, when compared with other epidemics of poliomyelitis, was characterised epidemiologically by a relatively high attack rate and high communicability, a low case fatality rate and a low paralytic rate, relative age selection of adults over children, and coincident institutional epidemics in the personnel of the Los Angeles County General Hospital, the Children's Hospital, the Ross-Loos Clinic, the Pasadena Hospital, the Glendale Medical Group and the Orthopaedic Hospital. There was also an outbreak among nurses in the Orange County Hospital. None of these other institutional outbreaks were reported in detail, and no other institutional outbreak was reported elsewhere in California in 1934.

Gilliam obtained his clinical data by painstaking personal interviews of the patients, together with examination of the hospital case notes. The main features of the illness in hospital staff as described by Gilliam were:

(a) Fever characterised by daily fluctuations in temperature from 97°F to 99°F (36.0–37.2°C) was more characteristic than an elevation of temperature above 100°F (37–38°C).

(b) Pain which was described as rheumatoid or influenzal in character, an ache in the muscles or bones, but often of sufficient intensity to awaken the patient from sleep, and, in most instances, it was aggravated by exercise. It was not confined to any particular part of the body, and characteristically varied from day to day in its distribution. However, common sites were the muscles at the back of the neck, between the shoulders, and in the lumbar region of the back. Pain in the muscles of the limbs was also common. Abdominal cramps, associated with tender and painful abdominal muscles, were not infrequent.

(c) Headaches.

(d) Muscle tenderness (Gilliam reported that it was the impression of some clinicians that the muscles found to be tender early in the illness were those that were later involved in weakness).

(e) Muscle twitching, which consisted of fibrillar twitching of muscle fibres, individual muscles or whole groups; tremors.

(f) Nausea, and, occasionally, vomiting.

(g) Irritability and drowsiness.

(h) Stiff neck and back.

(i) Vertigo.

(j) Photophobia accompanied by severe ocular pain.

(k) Sore throat, coryza, or cough and chills and diarrhoea were usual pro-dromal symptoms.

(l) Sensory symptoms included skin hyperaesthesia, paraesthesia, and anaesthesia, and varied from day to day.

(m) Easy fatiguability.

(n) Menstrual disturbances (increase or decrease in flow, or change in cycle).

(o) Emotional upsets, including irritability and crying spells.

(p) Memory difficulty, difficulty in concentration.

(q) Transient personality changes of varying degree of severity.

(r) Urinary difficulties giving a clinical picture of cystitis.

(s) Insomnia.

(t) Localised muscle weakness, obtained from records of the hospital physiotherapists, orthopaedic surgeons and personal interview of the patients.

Gilliam noted that, in general, it was more frequent to find a patient stating that no localised weakness was present while the hospital history recorded it, than it was to find the reverse. Six months after the onset 43 patients (28%) still had demonstrable localised muscular weakness which was severe in five cases. One hundred and four patients (55%) were still absent from duty.

Among all employees of the General Hospital, the groups most severely attacked were nurses and doctors, with attack rates of 10.7% and 5.4%. The picture was similar in the County Hospital, 11.4% of nurses and 6.2% of doctors being attacked. Those most closely associated with the patients seemed to be the ones to succumb, particularly those on duty in the communicable diseases wards or in the main admitting office, and those living inside rather than outside the hospital grounds.

Gilliam deduced that the observed distribution of the disease was similar to that of scarlet fever, spread by direct personal contact with cases and carriers. It is quite different from what one would have expected in an epidemic such as typhoid fever, spread by contamination of the hospital water, milk or food supply. He and other observers thought that the illness may have resulted from modification of the disease prevailing in the community, poliomyelitis, or from another central nervous system infection of unknown aetiology. Emotional disturbance was recognised as a symptom of the illness, but was not considered to be an aetiological factor and Gilliam pointed out that 'from an epidemiological point of view the disease was distributed as an infectious disease would be expected to be distributed'. Subsequent epidemics of this mysterious illness displayed the basic features of the Los Angeles outbreak, and revealed further information about the epidemiology of the disease.

In the late 1930s there were several epidemics in Switzerland with similar symptoms, in both military and community hospitals, affecting both patients and staff (Gsell, 1958). The prolonged convalescent period was noted to be characterised by relapses, marked fatiguability and autonomic disturbances (Gsell, 1949, 1958). There was also a small epidemic among young nurses at Harefield Sanatorium in England at the same time in 1939 (Houghton and Jones, 1942). Pyrexia and muscle pains persisted for up to five months, with accompanying menstrual disturbances and spontaneous epistaxis. The authors suggested that the condition was due to an unidentified myotropic strain of virus.

In the early months of the winter 1948 to 1949, an extensive epidemic of a disease apparently involving the central nervous system (CNS) broke out in the town of Akureyri, on the northern coast of Iceland. This epidemic, which was again at first thought to be poliomyelitis, presented such peculiar features that the authors decided it justified a detailed clinical description (Sigurdsson *et al.*, 1950). Epidemiologically, women were affected more than men, although the sex ratio was equal below the age of 20. There was a low incidence in childhood and the elderly, with maximal incidence in the 15–19 years age range (15% of males and 18% of females). The incidence was exceptionally high in the schools. The illness spread rapidly, but was confined to the town. It did not appear to be spread by water or milk or food or sewage, but by close contact with other cases, and there were multiple cases in families as well as schools. The incubation period was between five and ten days.

Clinically, the onset could be sudden or gradual, with pain in the back of the neck and the back, accompanied by a low fever, rarely exceeding 38°C, and a tachycardia of 90–94/min. The back pain often radiated to the limbs, was sometimes accompanied by numbness and paraesthesia, and became worse on exertion. Patients displayed nervousness, and were tired out of all proportion to their illness, and they perspired easily. The muscles were tender to the touch, and there was muscle twitching and muscle weakness. Patients reported that the affected limbs felt heavy and that certain movements could not be performed with normal force. Subacute arthritis was noted in the convalescent period, during which multiple relapses occurred in some patients, with renewal of fever, muscle tenderness and weakness.

The cerebrospinal fluid (CSF) was examined in eight patients, four of whom had slightly raised cell and protein readings. Viral studies at the time failed to demonstrate poliomyelitis, Coxsackie or known encephalitic viruses.

In 1955, 39 patients affected by the 1948 epidemic in Akureyri were re-examined (Sigurdsson and Gudmundsson, 1956) and it was found that of those more severely affected in 1948, only 25% had completely recovered, 52% had residual muscle tenderness, and 65% had objective neurological signs. Many patients still complained of nervousness, abnormal fatiguability of muscles, muscle pain, sleeplessness and loss of memory. Of those mildly affected in 1948, only 44% had fully recovered, 50% had muscular tenderness, and 19% had residual objective neurological signs.

In that same year, 1955, there was an epidemic of true type 1 poliomyelitis in Iceland, which spread around the relatively more inhabited coast. It failed to become established in Akureyri, and the neighbouring town of Sandárkrókurn. Antibody to type 1 poliomyelitis was found in 50–95% of schoolchildren in areas affected by poliomyelitis, and no antibody was found in children in areas affected by the 1948 epidemic in Akureyri, subsequently called epidemic neuromyasthenia or benign myalgic encephalomyelitis. However, children in areas affected by the 1948 epidemic responded to poliomyelitis vaccination with higher antibody titres than in other areas not affected by the poliomyelitis epidemic, as if these children had already been exposed to an agent immunologically similar to poliomyelitis virus (Sigurdsson et al., 1958). Thus the agent responsible for the 1948 epidemic would appear to be able to inhibit the pathological effects of poliomyelitis.

A few months after the 1948 Akureyri epidemic in Iceland, an epidemic of poliomyelitis started in May 1949 in Adelaide, Australia. By August, cases of epidemic neuromyasthenia, as it was then called, had begun to appear and continued to spread until, by 1951, 800 patients had been admitted to Northfield Infectious Diseases Hospital (Pellew, 1951). Most cases were again adults and the male : female ratio was 1 : 1. The condition in the early stages was indistinguishable from poliomyelitis; the patients complained of bursting headache, stiff back, aching limbs, pain behind the eyes, upper respiratory tract infection, mild muscle weakness and fever. The persistent aching of limbs and mild muscle weakness continued, together with the psychological sequelae of irritability, depression, lack of concentration and emotional instability for up to two years after the initial illness. Material from each of five cases was inoculated into a pair of monkeys. The monkeys inoculated from three cases remained well, but the four monkeys inoculated from two of the cases became ill and one died of the illness. At postmortem examination, minute red spots were observed along the course of the sciatic nerves. Microscopically, infiltration of nerve roots with lymphocytes and mononuclear cells was seen and some of the nerve fibres showed patchy damage to the myelin sheaths and axon swellings. In the sciatic nerves there were small localised infiltrations with inflammatory cells associated with exudation of a few red blood cells. The only abnormality in the skeletal muscle was the presence of sarcosporidiosis in all sections from one animal. However, examination of the heart muscle of the monkey which had died showed severe myocarditis with widespread infiltration mainly with lymphocytes and mononuclear cells. The authors reported that passage of affected tissue from these monkeys to other monkeys did not lead to any evidence of ill-health. A repeat inoculation with the original human material caused similar symptoms in two of four monkeys, but again passage was unsuccessful (Pellow and Miles, 1955).

In the late summer and early autumn of 1950, a widespread epidemic of poliomyelitis occurred in New York State. Most cases were diagnosed as acute anterior poliomyelitis, abortive poliomyelitis or 'poliomyelitis suspect'. However, two physicians, White and Burtch (1954), noted that certain definite distinctive features distinguished many of the cases from poliomyelitis, and they became increasingly convinced that the disease they were seeing was not poliomyelitis. They described 19 cases drawn from a single practice. Their cases differed from poliomyelitis in that muscle aching, pain and tenderness were the prominent features throughout the course of the illness, whereas the extreme muscle weakness and wasting seen in poliomyelitis were rare, and they concluded that the illness was similar to that reported in Iceland in 1949. The most consistent symptom was muscle aching and tenderness. Mild fever, lymphadenopathy, neck tenderness, photophobia, paraesthesia, numbness, and impaired touch sensation and joint position sense were frequent. Eleven of the 19 patients had marked mental depression. Ten of them were easily moved to tears and the authors wrote 'it is perhaps significant that eight of these ten were normally stoic individuals for whom such exhibitions were quite unusual'. Laboratory tests did not isolate the presence of poliomyelitis or Coxsackie virus. Fifteen months later, eight of the original 19 presented themselves for a follow-up examination and, of the eight, not one was symptom-free. Patients complained of continuing muscular aches after exertion and in damp weather, fatigue, persistent paraesthesiae, and emotional upsets.

Many subsequent epidemics occurred in the ensuing decade in Denmark (Fog, 1953; Pederson, 1956), Rockville USA (Shelokov *et al.*, 1957) and elsewhere (Parish, 1978). Detailed descriptions of outbreaks in this country also exist for this period. In 1953, 'towards the end of a busy poliomyelitis season', 13 nurses in a Coventry hospital became ill with symptoms involving the CNS, and were described by the medical superintendent J. F. Galpine at Whitley Hospital, Coventry and the bacteriologist of the Virus Reference Laboratory at Colindale (Macrae and Galpine, 1954). The authors wrote:

It was hard to be sure that any individual patient had not got mild atypical poliomyelitis; but the cumulative picture, with various degrees of paresis in 12 cases, the preservation of tendon reflexes with only slight occasional disturbance, the sensory phenomena, the consistently normal findings in the CSF and the tendency to early and complete recovery, differed from classical poliomyelitis.

And, indeed, the subsequent failure to isolate a poliomyelitis virus or to demonstrate a rise of serum antibodies to poliomyelitis made this diagnosis unlikely. It was felt that the clinical findings indicated an organic infectious disorder. However, in some of the patients, psychological symptoms were also present, but the authors felt it improbable that the psychological features alone could explain an illness in 13 of the staff, including senior and experienced members, within a short period. In addition a similar illness was prevalent in Coventry and a wide area of Warwickshire at the same time.

In 1954 Acheson published an account of an outbreak of an infection of the CNS accompanied by intense myalgia in 14 nurses resident at the Middlesex Hospital, describing its unusual features and its resemblance to other atypical epidemics such as those in Iceland, Adelaide and New York (Acheson, 1954). Acheson drew evidence about the nature of the epidemic from the clinical pattern, the epidemiology and the results of viral studies. The characteristic clinical features were mild fever, severe muscular pain, neck stiffness, diffuse mild involvement of the CNS, paraesthesia and a normal CSF. None had the residual flaccid paralysis of poliomyelitis, fever was milder than in poliomyelitis and bladder symptoms were much more common than in poliomyelitis. In poliomyelitis the CSF is abnormal in most cases. Similarities were noted with Bornholm disease (epidemic myalgia) but benign aseptic meningitis, which is a recognised complication of Bornholm disease, was not seen in these cases. Virological tests for poliomyelitis were inconclusive and tests for Coxsackie, mumps and lymphocytic choriomeningitic viruses were negative.

Acheson concluded that either the characteristics of poliomyelitis were changing due to a milder strain of the virus or that these cases were caused by an unidentified virus similar to that causing the epidemic in Iceland, Adelaide, Coventry and New York.

During the summer of 1955, the Royal Free Hospital Teaching Group, with a total staff of about 3500, experienced an epidemic of encephalomyelitis simulating poliomyelitis which affected more than 300 people. By late November, 255 cases had been admitted to the Royal Free Hospital, while the remainder were either nursed at home or admitted elsewhere. The epidemic was described by the consultant physician, Melvin Ramsay, and E. O'Sullivan, the senior registrar at the time (Ramsay and O'Sullivan, 1956), and subsequently by Richardson (1956), Medical Staff of the Royal Free Hospital (1957), and Crowley et al. (1957). A diagnosis of poliomyelitis was held to be untenable because the pareses were unaccompanied by wasting, tendon reflexes were generally unaffected or exaggerated, sensory disturbances were prominent, and CSF was normal. In addition, electromyographic studies failed to reveal any evidence of neuronal degeneration, although the weak muscles showed abnormalities of motor unit activity. Electroencephalograms in five patients were also abnormal.

The clinical picture varied in severity and in natural history. In some cases, characteristic symptoms appeared early and in others later. But, in general, the onset of the disease was marked by sore throat, headache, stiff neck, dizziness, blurred vision, bodily prostration and low-grade fevers and lymphadenopathy of posterior cervical glands. After a few days, the illness progressed to vertigo, diplopia, paraesthesia, pareses, aesthesia, myalgia, apathy and depression with tender glands, and a tender liver. The first few cases were labelled as glandular fever although it was appreciated from the start that they were not true cases of infectious mononucleosis. This term was used so as not to cause alarm.

It became clear early on in the outbreak that there was organic involvement of the CNS, but there were also abnormal signs outside, particularly lymphadenopathy and mild fever, accompanied by severe malaise. Nearly half the cases had cranial nerve palsies affecting mostly the oculomotor, facial and vestibular nerves. Occasional pupillary changes occurred, but the fundi and visual fields remained normal. Bulbar palsy occurred in 7% of cases.

Both motor and sensory disturbances occurred in the limbs. Painful muscle spasms were provoked by passive movement, and there was jerkiness of voluntary movement against resistance. This was matched by abnormal electromyogram (EMG) findings. There were also spontaneous involuntary movements. More than a quarter of all patients had bladder dysfunction with disturbances of micturition. Reflex changes were not pronounced, but were sometimes diminished and sometimes exaggerated. The plantar responses were often equivocal, and only in two cases clearly extensor. Muscle wasting was rare. There were varying degrees of paraesthesiae. To summarise, the limbs exhibited a combination of both irritative and paretic phenomena.

Richardson (1956) reported the EMG findings of 28 cases. There were no signs of lower motor neurone degeneration except in one case. Electromyograms were normal in four, but in the remainder showed profound disturbances of volition characterised in severe cases by a reduction in the number of motor unit potentials even to discrete motor unit activity, the individual potentials often being polyphasic and in the less severely involved muscles and, particularly during recovery, by groupings of these motor unit potentials.

As Crowley *et al.* (1957) argued, the failure to isolate the infectious agent does not mean it was not an infectious disease. The course of the illness was wholly consistent with changing phases of a host–parasite relationship which are reflected in the clinical picture. Firstly, during the period of invasion, the parasite left traces of its passing in the pharynx and the regional lymphatic filter. Secondly, until the sudden onset of neurological disorder after several days, the disease was often silent, except in those who displayed tenderness of muscles, glands, liver or spleen. This interval allowed time for an organism to disseminate, to pass the reticuloendothelial defence barrier with greater or lesser ease in different hosts, and to multiply in the susceptible tissue before the pathogenic effect became clinically observable in the CNS. Thirdly, the morphological changes in mature lymphocytes and altered ratio of immature to mature mononuclear cells in the blood was additional evidence of activity in the antibody-forming cells of the host.

Acheson (1959) reviewed 14 outbreaks, including those described in this chapter. He made a number of telling points, some of which will be commented upon here. Firstly, he drew attention to the difficulties inherent in defining a disorder from which no deaths have occurred, and for which no causative infective or toxic agent has been discovered. He stated 'recognition has to depend on the clinical and epidemiological pattern. These features must be sufficiently characteristic to separate the disorder from other conditions'. He drew two helpful parallels, one with the diagnosis of encephalitis lethargica which is made on the basis of the clinical triad of fever, stupor and ophthalmoplegia in the absence of specific pathology or specific diagnostic testing; and the other with Bornholm disease (epidemic myalgia or epidemic pleurodynia) where the disease became established as a clinical entity on clinical grounds long before the discovery of the Coxsackie viruses. Clinically, all the outbreaks he reviewed displayed the following characteristics of (1) headache, (2) myalgia, (3) paresis, (4) symptoms or signs other than paresis suggestive of damage to the brain, spinal cord or peripheral nerves, (5) mental symptoms, (6) low or absent fever, and (7) no mortality. In addition, (1) a higher frequency in women, (2) a predominantly normal CSF, and (3) relapses, have occurred in almost all outbreaks. In 11 of the 14 epidemics which he reviewed, symptoms which suggest activity and chronicity of the disease have persisted for months or even years in a few cases. In eight instances, there was an apparent predilection for the nursing or medical profession. The case for a clinical entity depends on the distinctiveness of these findings.

Secondly, he thoroughly reviewed the common epidemiological and clinical features. Epidemiologically, the common features of these outbreaks are: (1) the high attack rate as compared with poliomyelitis, (2) the predilection for residential communities, (3) a higher attack rate in women than in men, (4) a tendency to occur more commonly in young adults, and (5) the commencement of most outbreaks in the summer months.

The evidence is consistent with the hypothesis that the disorder is an infection spread by personal contact.

Clinically, the characteristic picture is that of an acute or subacute onset with headache, symptoms of a gastrointestinal or upper respiratory upset, muscular pains and low or absent fever, followed by muscle weakness which is rarely associated with the classic signs of lower motor neurone or pyramidal tract involvement. This is often accompanied by paraesthesiae, sometimes by sensory loss, and occasionally by painful muscular spasms, myoclonus or other types of involuntary movement. As the paresis recovers, a curious jerky muscular contraction on volition has been noted in some instances. Involvement of the crucial nerves and bladder may occur. Convalescence is prolonged by fatigue and recurring myalgia but recovery usually occurs within three months. In a proportion, which varies from outbreak to outbreak, a well-defined state of chronic ill-health has developed, characterised by fluctuating myalgia and paresis, partial remissions and exacerbations, and depression, emotional lability and lack of concentration.

Thirdly, he confronted the issue that it might be argued that at least some of the apparent clinical similarities are due to unconscious bias or undue emphasis on the part of observers familiar with the features of previous epidemics. Acheson points out that such bias cannot have contributed towards the striking reported similarities between the Los Angeles and Royal Free outbreaks because Gilliam's paper was then unknown to the British authors. He writes that these similarities are even more impressive when it is appreciated that bias was probably operating in the opposite direction. In the Los Angeles outbreak the initial diagnosis was poliomyelitis, and the patients were cared for by orthopaedic surgeons. In the Royal Free Hospital epidemic, the initial diagnosis was infectious mononucleosis and the patients were treated by general physicians and neurologists. Acheson concluded that it cannot therefore be held that the syndrome is simply a self-perpetuating medical concept.

Fourthly, Acheson carefully examined the question of hysteria as a cause of illness. The question of hysteria had been raised in several epidemics, including the Los Angeles outbreak, and most authors agreed that hysterical. manifestations occurred in a few patients, particularly in the later stages, but none felt that it contributed significantly to the pattern of the disease. However, illness with a selectivity for young women and few positive laboratory findings often raises the uneasy spectre of hysteria. Epidemic hysteria has been recognised for many centuries as a particular hazard in institutions containing women or female adolescents. However, as Acheson points out, no-one can seriously contend that every patient in all the outbreaks has been hysterical. The presence of definite ocular, facial and palatal paresis, nystagmus and, rarely, of extensor plantar responses, indicates organic disease of the nervous system in a minority of patients at least. A more reasonable viewpoint would be that the majority of cases were a hysterical reaction to a small number of cases of poliomyelitis among the staff. Thus an epidemic of poliomyelitis, as occurred in Los Angeles in 1934, would produce overwork and emotional strain in the nursing staff of the hospital and many nurses would become apprehensive about catching it themselves. When a few genuine cases of poliomyelitis did occur, it is possible to envisage the occurrence of an epidemic of hysterical paralysis. Such a hypothesis would explain the epidemiological findings of high attack rates in women, particularly nurses, and the association with preceding or concurrent outbreaks of poliomyelitis. It might also explain the clinical findings of absent fever, the prominence of sensory phenomena which are often of bizarre distribution and content, the daily fluctuation of symptoms and signs, the high incidence of negative CSF findings and the peculiar nature of the paresis (i.e. weakness without disappearance of tone, deep reflexes or subsequent atrophy on the one hand or true spasticity and extensor plantar responses on the other.)

Acheson then presented the arguments against the idea that the syndrome constitutes a mass hysterical reaction to a few cases of poliomyelitis. Firstly, the minority with undoubted objective physical signs did not have the clinical picture of poliomyelitis. Nystagmus, opthalmoplegia, facial palsy, palatal paresis and extensor plantar responses were recorded, but true flaccid paralysis with absent reflexes did not occur, and subsequent atrophy was unusual. Furthermore, the patients with these objective findings also shared the other characteristic features of the illness, namely myalgia, sensory changes, low pyrexia, mental symptoms, and a chronic or relapsing course, which were experienced by the majority of patients who had no truly objective physical signs. 'Thus we would be forced to the conclusion, on this hypothesis, that even the patients with objective findings were also suffering from hysteria. This seems unlikely.'

Secondly, the relationship of outbreaks of the illness with outbreaks of poliomyelitis is not constant.

At the Royal Free Hospital, no patient with poliomyelitis had been admitted to the hospital prior to the outbreak, nor was the diagnosis entertained in the initial cases. There was no undue apprehension about poliomyelitis among this hospital staff, but rather about infectious mononucleosis which was the early diagnosis. In spite of this, the course of the disease and the type of neurological involvement was similar to that found in Los Angeles. In the Coventry outbreak six of the twelve patients had been nursing poliomyelitis cases for several years, and it is difficult to imagine why such experienced persons should suddenly manifest a hysterical reaction to the fear of this disease. In the Middlesex Hospital, Berlin and Bethseda cases there was no known poliomyelitis and, in the early cases at least, no reason for anxiety about it in the communities concerned.

Thirdly, Acheson pointed out that mental symptoms which are a constant feature of all the outbreaks are not typical of hysteria.

Disorders of consciousness and convulsions such as may be seen in hysteria have been extremely rare. A single grand mal seizure was reported in a small child in Alaska. Shallowness of affect and 'belle indifference' have not been seen. On the contrary, depression and undue emotional lability have been the rule. In the acute stage, terrifying dreams, panic states, uncontrollable weeping and hypersomnia occur. In the convalescent stage the prominent features are impairment of memory, difficulty in concentration and depression. These symptoms are more consistent with cerebral damage than with hysteria. Many years ago Von Economo stressed the ease with which the mental symptoms of encephalitis may be confused with those of psychoneurosis. The slight lymphocytosis in the CSF in two outbreaks which shared many other features with the remainder, and the presence of a characteristic electromyogram in cases from three separate localities are further strong arguments in favour of an organic aetiology.

Acheson's final points against mass hysteria as a major factor in the syndrome were the consistency of the course of illness, and the similarities in the symptoms described, in spite of a wide variation in the types of community affected, from hospital staffs on the one hand to semi-rural and urban populations on the other.

A further description of an outbreak, which, like Acheson's review, is well worth reading in the original and which was not known to Acheson at the time he wrote his review, is a general practitioner's careful analytical description of the epidemiological and clinical features of an epidemic in his practice in Dalston, Cumbria in 1955 (Wallis, 1957). It preceded the Royal Free epidemic, starting in January of that year and continued until July, by which time 233 cases had been recorded out of the practice population of 1675, a case incidence of 14%. The male : female ratio was 1 : 1. While all age groups were affected, the peak incidence was in children and adolescents, particularly in closed communities. The illness was thought to be transmitted by person to person contact, with an incubation period of five to seven days. The severity of the illness varied, with some recovering within a month, and others suffering a protracted course with frequent relapses. Residual psychological sequelae and minor physical complaints proved remarkably persistent in the postinfective period. ECT was required in several cases of severe depression following the illness.

Wallis felt there was sufficient clinical difference between cases of acute onset and those of insidious onset to give separate descriptions for each. Abrupt onset cases presented with exhaustion sleepiness, severe headaches, myalgia, dizziness, sore throat, lymphadenopathy, sore eyes and blurred vision. The fatigue and weariness were extreme, and the effort of climbing stairs left patients feeling exhausted with aching, tender legs. The aching muscle pains affected the back of the neck, the lower limbs, the back, the shoulders and the upper limbs in that order of frequency. Patients also complained of pain along the costal margin and fairly frequently in the right iliac fossa, extending into the groin and the right thigh. Muscle pains were accompanied by hyperaesthesia of the skin overlying the affected muscle. Eyes were sore with retro-orbital pain, photophobia, conjunctivitis, blepharitis and watering. Patients told Dr Wallis that it needed a conscious effort to bring objects into focus. Eyelids were puffy and the upper lid tended to droop. Abnormal perceptions of taste and smell were common. Paraesthesiae were also common, consisting of feelings of numbness, 'pins and needles' and other abnormal cutaneous sensations.

Four cases complained of a feeling as if a worm was crawling in their legs, under the skin. In one case where I was present at the time of the complaint, a slow wave of contraction was seen to travel along a bunch of muscle fibres in the gastrocremius muscle at the site of the complaint.

Drenching sweats were common, often occurring at night.

On examination, patients were pale and apathetic. Temperatures were either moderately raised or subnormal, and the pulse was raised to 100/min (more rarely to 150/min). The tongue was dry and coated with a yellowish fur, and the nasophoynx was also dry and injected, occasionally accompanied by a few clusters of petechiae on the palate and two or three ulcers.

The abdomen showed some degree of flatulent distension. Palpation of the abdominal wall revealed occasional tender nodes especially in the recti. Tenderness without muscular guarding was always present on palpation at the subcostal margins, and was also frequently present over the right iliac fossa, the zone of tenderness extending down, over the inguinal ligament, to a point an inch or so distal to the saphenous opening. The liver and spleen were very tender in the more severe cases, and in a few instances the spleen was enlarged. No enlargement was noted in the case of the liver.

Cases of insidious onset presented with a several-week history of feelings of being off-colour, excessive tiredness, sudden sweats, cold hands and feet, difficulty in keeping warm, dizziness and unsteadiness, headaches and neuralgic pains, insomnia, poor concentration, aching in the legs and back, a feeling of heaviness in the legs, pins and needles in the hands and feet, a hard, dry cough, hoarseness or partial aphonia, and blurred vision. These patients usually told Dr Wallis that they thought they had got a 'chill' or 'a touch of flu' which they had tried to work off, but the symptoms had persisted. A few cases had been frightened by their inability to walk any distance.

On examination, cases of insidious onset were tired and anxious. The temperature was often subnormal, and the pulse rate was only slightly raised to 80/90 per min. Larynx and trachea were inflamed, but the lungs were clear. Tender enlarged glands were found in the cervical chain, inguinal, saphenous and axillary groups, and there were tender nodes in the muscles of the abdominal wall. Liver and spleen were tender (and three cases had an enlarged spleen), and there was tenderness on deep palpation in the right ileac fossa, extending over the inguinal ligament and distal to the saphenous opening. Vision was blurred, and conjunctivitis and blepharitis were common.

Generalised muscular weakness was frequent, and patients complained that walking, lifting and carrying were particularly limited. Some patients showed particular loss of power particularly in the tibialis anterior, the flexors, abductors and adductor of the thigh, the deltoid, and the interosseous and hypothenar muscles of the hand. A few cases showed muscle atrophy which recovered within six months in all but one case. Ataxia (with a positive Romberg's test) and tremor were common, and impaired coordination occurred in all cases showing neurological disturbances (patients complained of dropping crockery, spilling tea or colliding with doorways).

Reflexes were at first normal or diminished but in the later stages of protracted illness became brisk with occasional knee and ankle clonus. Abdominal reflexes were often diminished or absent but plantar reflexes were normal except for two cases where a unilateral plantar extensor response was elicited which lasted for six and eight weeks respectively. Pupils were often sluggish in their light accommodation.

Objective evidence of sensory disturbance was less common than subjective complaints of sensory disturbance, but it included hyperaesthesia in the skin overlying the painful muscles, diminished sensitivity to light touch with cotton wool and to pinprick, impaired position sense and joint sense, a positive Romberg's test and impaired vibration sense.

Abnormal findings in the mental state of these patients included depression (four cases requiring inpatient care and one committing suicide), loss of energy persisting long after the original infection, retardation of thought processes, with difficulty in abstract thought, difficulty in finding the right word (with marked nominal aphasia in two cases), difficulty with mental arithmetic, impairment of concentration, and impairment of recent memory. These cognitive problems often interfered with schooling, business activities or even domestic activities such as knitting where frequent errors would be made. The sleep rhythm was often inverted, and nightmares and night terrors were common in children, with vivid dreams in adults. Affected children showed behavioural disturbances, including nocturnal enuresis, disobedience, unmotivated acts of aggression, directed at other children, wilful damage to property, unsociability, facile lying, rapid changes of mood, and weeping. Most returned to their normal preinfective behaviour over the ensuing months, but in several children these traits persisted for longer than 18 months.

The most prominent complication was the recurrence of symptoms, over the ensuing months and even years. Other complications included a frank pneumococcal pneumonia, shortly after the onset, three cases of bronchitis, myocarditis (the tachycardia was raised out of proportion to the degree of pyrexia, and four cases developed a persistent tachycardia with dyspnoea on slight effort, cyanosis of the lips, oedema of the ankles, soft heart sound and lowered blood pressure; the heart was not enlarged), a persistent rise in blood pressure, returning to normal over many months, jaundice, orchitis, and rashes.

Wallis, like the other early observers of this condition, made the diagnosis on clinical grounds in the absence of any specific test and without the isolation of a causative organism. His clinical criteria were dizziness; headache and extreme lassitude; drowsiness and lethargy by day and restlessness by night; blurred vision, diplopia on upward and lateral gaze, and a mild conjunctival reaction; spontaneous severe pain in the back of the neck and the lower limbs, and frequently also in the back and upper limbs; muscle tenderness and some loss of muscle power; paraesthesia and some degree of sensory impairment; tender enlargement of lymph glands in the neck, inguinal region and axillae, splenic and hepatic tenderness and subcostal pain; depression, with feelings of foreboding and a labile emotional state; and low-grade fever or subnormal temperature with mild tachycardia.

The illnesses which he considered in the differential diagnosis were glandular fever, influenza, poliomyelitis, adenoviruses, Coxsackie virus, echoviruses, psittacosis, Q fever, mumps, toxoplasmosis, viral encephalitides and encephalitis lethargica. Most were excluded by laboratory means. The clinical picture was thought to be suggestive of Coxsackie virus or echovirus infection but virological evidence did not confirm this.

ENDEMIC CASES

During these same years, endemic cases also appeared but received less publicity for obvious reasons. Innes, writing from the Neurological Unit in Edinburgh in 1970, reported four cases which presented at intervals of some months, did not arise in a closed community, and were all males; there was no poliomyelitis 'scare' at the time. His case histories resembled the descriptions of benign ME but seemed to follow an initial enteroviral infection. In one case enterovirus was isolated from CSF in the fourth month of the illness. He suggests that there is either a persistent enteroviral infection or that the infection, in predisposed or previously sensitised subjects, sets in train some process, say of an allergic nature, which accounts for the similarity of symptoms and the chronic relapsing course, analogous to the Guillain–Barre syndrome (Innes, 1970).

Innes warns that

cases such as these are in some danger of being dismissed as 'functional'. The initial influenza-like illness may be forgotten or the patient may not think to mention it, believing it irrelevant to his present complaints. They are depressed, profoundly so, and volunteer this information. Their complaints of bizarre patches of scalp pain and stabbing head pains might reasonably reinforce suspicions of a functional illness. Motor weakness may not be confirmed on formal testing since it appears to take the form of an incapacity for sustained muscular effort. The muscle twitchings of which they complain may only be evident after exercise.

Lewis-Price (1961) reported the cases of two patients, who had no contact with any known case of myalgic encephalitis or with any other well-defined virus illness, who developed symptoms of benign ME. He concludes that 'this illness is probably commoner than is usually realised and mild sporadic cases may easily be labelled as hysteria, glandular fever or myalgia, and muscle spasm should lead one to suspect this disease.'

Kendall (1967) described two endemic cases of epidemic ME with severe psychological sequelae persisting over many years. One developed temporal lobe epilepsy and had recurring bouts of depression for eight years, with histrionic, attention-seeking behaviour, hysterical fits and frequent suicide attempts; and the other had similar recurrent depressions, with a striking restlessness and inability to concentrate, and frequent aggressive and self-destructive outbursts which showed no signs of improvement five years after the original illness. He sifted the evidence carefully to assess how far the psychiatric disturbances subsequently displayed in these two patients were the result of damage to the cerebral mechanisms subserving emotional and behavioural control, or whether they were simply the neurotic reactions of previously vulnerable personalities to a distressing and frightening disease. Kendall argued that, in general, if a high proportion of patients develop, either after or during an encephalitic illness, psychiatric symptoms which are rarely seen in the course of other encephalitides, there are strong grounds for assuming that the illness is responsible for those symptoms. He gave the example of the delinquent behaviour which followed the epidemics of encephalitis lethargica in the 1920s. Kendall took the view that the psychiatric disturbances occurring during the acute phase of epidemics of ME were so widespread and so similar from one epidemic to another that the presence of a specific underlying disturbance of cerebral function can hardly be doubted. He points out that, after all, neurotic unstable young women must frequently have been affected in outbreaks of poliomyelitis or acute infective polyneuritis, and yet these comparable illnesses, both involving more serious risk of death or permanent paralysis, have never been accompanied by such striking psychological disturbances. In the specific instance of the two cases he described, both were young women with some evidence of neurotic predisposition before the original illness. They both developed such severe and longstanding changes in mood and behaviour afterwards that Kendall argued that damage to cerebral mechanisms underlying the control of mood and behaviour must underlie such severe and prolonged disturbances.

THE QUESTION OF HYSTERIA

In 1970, two young psychiatrists, McEvedy and Beard, re-examined the case notes of patients from the Royal Free epidemic of 1955, and suggested that epidemic hysteria was a much more likely explanation of the illness than an organic disease for the same reasons which had made earlier writers (ranging from Gilliam (1938) to Acheson (1959) at first consider a psychological aetiology, namely the high attack rate in females compared with males, the intensity of the malaise compared with the slight pyrexia, the presence of subjective symptoms similar to those produced by overbreathing, the glove and stocking distribution of the anaesthesia, and the normal findings on special investigations (McEvedy and Beard, 1970a). However, they unfortunately did not go on to examine the reasons which had led earlier observers ultimately to reject the hysteria hypothesis, and which have been discussed earlier in this chapter. McEvedy and Beard (1970b) then reexamined the reports of the other epidemics reviewed by Acheson (1959) and suggested that those had been caused by hysteria as well.

Their papers elicited a storm of protest in the *British Medical Journal*. One writer with postgraduate experience in psychiatry and infectious diseases had been a clinical student at the time of the Royal Free epidemic (Gosling, 1970). She made a number of telling points. Firstly, as psychiatrists, McEvedy and Beard should have been aware that the diagnosis of hysterical illness should be made on positive grounds of finding evidence of both primary and secondary gain, and not just on negative grounds of not being able to explain the symptoms in another way. Secondly, in 1955, a very high proportion of the staff and student population and all the nurses at the Royal Free Hospital were females. Most of the male students were at that time preclinical and were away, as it was the long vacation. Even in term time, there was minimal contact between clinical and preclinical students. However, there was contact between male and female clinical students and between male and female staff. These factors would have contributed to the lower frequency of affected male students, and should be considered in any epidemiological assessment of the relative risk to each sex. Thirdly, disproportionate depression and emotional lability are common concomitants of most viral infections (for example, the well-known post-influenzal depression), especially those affecting the CNS.

In the same issue of the *British Medical Journal*, a general practitioner wrote in to point out that

Most astute general practitioners have observed diseases which were not described in the textbooks. However, the clinical features of some of these, such as 'drop attacks', epidemic myalgia, and hand, foot and mouth disease have now become clear and well-known, and I would agree that one should hesitate before attributing any unaccountable bizarre syndrome to hysteria because the entity does not fit any disease mentioned in present medical books. (Hopkins, 1970)

This advice is as important today as it was then.

Galpine, who had reported the Coventry outbreak, wrote to remind McEvedy and Beard that the question of mass hysteria had indeed been carefully considered in the Coventry cases, but had ultimately seemed unacceptable for much the same reasons, clinical and epidemiological, as in the other outbreaks (Galpine, 1970).

A north London general practitioner Scott (1970), wrote to report an epidemic, between 1964 and 1966, of 370 patients. She made the diagnosis of benign ME on the basis of low-grade pyrexia, headache, blurred vision and/or diplopia, occipital pain, stiff neck, vertigo with positive Romberg test, nausea and/or vomiting, lymphadenitis, pharyngitis, lower costal pain, generalised weakness and depression, emotional instability in previously stable personality, loss of memory, profound fatigue unrelieved by rest, insomnia and/or vivid dreams, often in colour, impaired perception to sound, frequency or retention of urine, diarrhoea or constipation, areas of muscle tenderness, and neuritis with or without paresis. She refuted McEvedy and Beard's suggestion that the diagnosis was more likely to be made by a practitioner familiar with the disease, as she had not previously seen the illness before encountering the epidemic in her own practice. She pointed out that recognition of the organic nature of the disease is crucial so that patients recognise the limitations which the disease has imposed upon them and thereby avoid recurrences or permanent incapacity. She wrote

It is my hope that the views expressed by Drs McEvedy and Beard will not be taken seriously, especially as the implied diagnosis of 'hysteria' to a seriously ill patient can cause acute distress and prolong the illness indefinitely. Inability to concentrate, fumbling and lack of co-ordination in fine movements, as well as disturbances in the autonomic nervous system are constant features in the aftermath, and if a diagnosis of 'hysteria' is even hinted, the patient experiences a profound loss of confidence in his medical advisers. Restoration of confidence may take months. It is essential to treat this disease seriously, and to give strong reassurance and encouragement in the difficult period when the patient is learning to 'come to terms with his disability'.

Mayne (1970) wrote briefly to point out that

studies of virus antibody titres have shown that infection occurs before the patients or relatives notice anything, temperatures do not need to rise, and the doctor doesn't see the patient until long after the infecting organism has entered the host. To consider Paul–Bunnell tests, liver function tests, electrocardiograms, or white cell counts as evidence of absence of infection or organic aetiology is not satisfactory, and hysteria needs more than the points offered if it is to be an acceptable psychiatric diagnosis.

On the other hand, a medical officer of health (Baines, 1970) made the unarguable statement that

psychological origins for illness must obviously be borne in mind when considering a multitude of incidents ascribed to food poisoning, gassing by boiler fumes, explosive outbreaks of diarrhoea, over exposure to swimming baths chlorine, winter vomiting disease, and hitch hiker's paralysis.

Unfortunately, he then went on to make the mistaken assertion that 'hysteria would seem to be essentially a diagnosis of exclusion'. This issue is taken up later in this chapter.

Another ex-clinical student from the Royal Free Hospital (Howells, 1970) wrote

I think that a consideration of the nurses and students who did not get the Royal Free Disease would have been of pertinent interest. I was a clinical student at the time of the outbreak, and looking back on myself then I rather feel if any hysteria was around I would have succumbed. However, I remained disgustingly healthy, though my flat mate (a very level headed girl) was a sufferer from the disease!

Gill (1970) wrote

Can we not acknowledge that there is never one cause for a patient getting ill? Virus and hysteria are with us always, and the wise doctor never thinks in terms of 'either or'. Whether the patient has hepatitis or a slipped disc, the timing and severity of the illnesses are always affected by emotional factors to some degree.

THE 1978 SYMPOSIUM

In 1978, a symposium was held at the Royal Society of Medicine (RSM) to discuss the disease and plan research. There was clear agreement that ME is a distinct nosological entity. The other names for it were variously rejected as unsatisfactory: 'Iceland disease' is not specific enough, and 'neuromyasthenia' suggests a relationship to myasthenia gravis whereas the muscle fatiguability is different, as are the electrophysiological findings. From the patient's point of view, the adjective 'benign' is also misleading, because the illness may be devastating even though it is not fatal. A *British Medical Journal* leader at the time concluded that the organic basis of the illness was now clear from the finding that the putative agent can be transferred to monkeys (Pellow and Miles, 1955), the detection of an increased output of creatine (White and Burtch, 1954; Albrecht *et al.*, 1964), the persistent finding of abnormal lymphocytes in peripheral blood (Wallis, 1957), the presence of lymphocytes and an increased protein concentration in some patients (Acheson, 1959) and the neurological findings. At the RSM symposium, more new evidence was produced to support the organic nature of the disease. Increased serum concentrations of lactic dehydrogenases and transaminases have been found in several patients in the acute phase. Immunological studies in the outbreak at Great Ormond Street Hospital showed a high incidence of anti-complementary activity and the presence of ill-defined aggregates on electron microscopy of acute phase. A perplexing finding, suggesting the possibility of a persistent virus infection, was the ability of lymphocytes from patients to proliferate and survive *in vitro* for up to 19 weeks (Editorial, 1978).

During the symposium, N. D. Compston summarised the points against the 'hysteria' hypothesis (Compston, 1978):

(a) The Royal Free outbreak occurred in the middle of a more sporadic outbreak in northwest London which had started before the Royal Free outbreak and continued after it.
(b) Case to case contact between patients and relatives occurred.
(c) There was objective fever, lymphadenopathy, cranial palsies and abnormal limb signs.
(d) There are many infective disorders in which malaise and fever are not correlated.
(e) Overbreathing produces only transient sensory and motor phenomena.
(f) A glove and stocking distribution of the anaesthesia occurs in a number of organic diseases of the CNS, e.g. in the peripheral neuropathies.
(g) Normal findings in the CSF are not incompatible with organic disease of the CNS, and a normal ESR is frequently found in infectious mononucleosis.

Compston concluded:

Those of the medical staff of the Royal Free Hospital who witnessed the epidemic in 1955 are firmly of the conclusion that they were dealing with an organic disease complicated by encephalomyelitis in which myalgia was a dominant feature. Objective evidence of brain stem and spinal cord involvement was observed.

At the same symposium, Dr Dillon reviewed a further outbreak of what was called 'epidemic neuromyasthenia' which occurred at the Hospital for Sick

Children, Great Ormond Street, between August 1970 and January 1971 (Dillon *et al.*, 1974). One hundred and forty-five staff out of a total of about 1900 were affected, mostly nurses, although a few doctors and other staff were affected. At least four men were affected (two doctors and two administrators); the rest were women. None of the inpatients (all children) were affected during this period. Overall, 15% of nurses were affected, 3% of the medical staff, and 2% of the remainder. There were two distinct waves, with 33 cases in the first wave, most of whom were student nurses. During the second wave, all levels of nursing staff were affected together with some doctors, domestic staff and others.

The symptoms were similar to those reported in other outbreaks, namely rapid fatigue on exercise, headache, sore throat, nausea, back pain, malaise, vomiting, neck pain, tiredness, limb pains, depression, dizziness, giddiness, sore eyes, cough and chest pain. A few patients also reported abdominal pain, diarrhoea, photophobia, diplopia, blurred vision, earache, laryngitis, paraesthesia, faintness, jaw pain, bladder symptoms, anorexia, subjective limb weakness and painful joints. Examination of the patients revealed pharyngeal infection, enlarged cervical lymph nodes, neck stiffness, pyrexia and photophobia. Six patients had a rash, two had slight splenomegaly and two had distended retinal veins. Papilloedema, sluggish pupillary reactions to light and arthritis were also seen. Objective neurological findings were less prominent than in some other outbreaks.

The question of a functional disorder was considered early on in the 'epidemic' in the light of the suggestions by McEvedy and Beard (1970a) that such epidemics were likely to be due to hysteria. However, the undoubted physical signs in many patients, the biphasic pattern of the disease, the anti-complementary activity in sear, the presence of ill-defined aggregates in some acute sera on immune electron microscopy, and the ability of some patients' lymphocytes to proliferate *in vitro*, all pointed to an infective agent, despite the inability to isolate such an agent. It was felt that the anti-complementary activity plus the immune electron microscopy findings suggest the presence of circulating immune complexes in the serum. A substantial proportion of patients (28 out of 145) suffered symptomatic relapses for several years after the initial illness, while some were fully recovered within 12 months. Dr Dillon recorded that treatment was generally unsatisfactory. The headaches and back pain did not respond to simple analgesics but were more responsive to pentazocine, dihydrocodeine and dextropropoxyphene. Antiemetics were useful for the nausea, but antidepressants were 'of little value'.

During the years 1976–1978, several children were referred to the Hospital for Sick Children with symptoms similar to those recorded in the adult patients seen in 1970. The main symptoms were headache, back and limb pains, lethargy and rapid fatiguability on exercise. Some also complained of nausea, abdominal pains and sore throat. On examination there was little to find except slight pharyngeal injection, moderate cervical lymphadenopathy and, in some, slight pyrexia. The illness in the children also ran a protracted course and over half continued to have symptomatic relapses up to two years or more after the onset. Dr Dillon concluded that epidemic neuromyasthenia may be more common in the community than is generally realised, but may be more difficult to recognise in sporadic cases than in epidemics, and may be mistakenly labelled as psychiatric disturbance.

Thomas (1978) pointed out some general epidemiological principles which need to be borne in mind when examining the literature. Cases of epidemic disease are more readily recognised in institutions than elsewhere, partly because close and repeated contacts convey infection and partly because the inconvenience of multiple illnesses within a short time span comes to administrative attention. In the community, however, epidemic infection may not be recognised unless a search is made, either because the condition does not have distinctive symptomatology like the vesicles of chicken pox, or the colour of jaundice; or because the attack rate is low, as among a population that is largely immune.

The results of following up an institutional outbreak of a communicable disease can differ from those obtained by studying either hospital admissions or cases in the community because the family doctor will tend to send his most ill patients into hospital and those least affected by the illness may not even consult him; whereas the captive population in an institution would be expected to include a higher proportion of cases with minimal symptoms.

Thomas proposed setting up an advisory panel for the study of future epidemics, consisting of co-ordinator, an epidemiologist and a virologist, with an infectious disease physician, a psychiatrist and a neurologist.

HYSTERIA RECONSIDERED

As we have seen, right from the early epidemics, the question of hysteria was considered by observers, who nonetheless decided that the evidence pointed to an organic aetiology. However, since the McEvedy and Beard papers were published, the standard psychiatric teaching, and indeed often the standard medical teaching, has been that ME is primarily a functional illness, namely hysteria. Before reassessing this viewpoint, it is important to establish precisely what we mean by hysteria. The term has been used in many different ways.

Inappropriate uses of the term include the following:

(a) Hysterical is sometimes used by both lay people and occasionally doctors to describe inappropriate dramatic or histrionic behaviour.

(b) 'Hysterical' personality is the old-fashioned term for histrionic personality, which is characterised by attention-seeking or histrionic behaviour, demanding interpersonal behaviour, and displays of emotion which are easily aroused and are more intense than the circumstances require. The concept arose as a way of describing those thought to be at high risk for hysteria. However, it is now recognised that the majority of people with hysterical illnesses do not have hysterical (histrionic) personalities. People with histrionic personalities are at high risk for manipulative and attention-seeking behaviour such as drug overdoses. It is important to remember that personality disorders are, by definition, life-long tendencies. If someone suddenly starts to behave in this way for the first time in adult life, the diagnosis cannot be a histrionic personality, and is much more likely to be an illness of some kind, probably affective in nature.

Appropriate uses of the term include the following:

(a) Hysterical symptoms which are unconscious simulations of the signs of disease, and involve a disruption of normal voluntary functions. Common examples include the ability to stand and walk (astasia abasia), fits, tremor, anaesthesia, paralysis, amnesia and dysphonia. For the interested reader, an excellent account of the various syndromes which are traditionally subsumed under the term hysterical is given by Kendall (1983).

Conversion is the psychological defence mechanism thought to be responsible for the production of simulated 'physical' symptoms, which are therefore called conversion symptoms (e.g. anaesthesias or pareses), and dissociation is the defence mechanism thought to result in the simulation of 'mental' symptoms (e.g. amnesia) and these are termed dissociative symptoms.

Hysterical symptoms can be identified on the basis of two criteria. Firstly, they mimic the phenomena of neurological and psychiatric disorders, but reflect the patient's concept of how such disorders present, and secondly the function that appears to be lost can often be demonstrated to be intact in conditions which the patient does not associate with the symptom. Hysterical symptoms can occur in almost any diagnostic setting, particularly in the affective disorders and schizophrenia. They also have an important association with organic brain disease, which results in the selective loss of normal inhibitory functions and the release of an underlying hysterical predisposition. When hysterical symptoms appear for the first time in a mature adult, they are particularly suggestive of a neurological disorder such as multiple sclerosis (MS), and this requires careful investigation. It is a common error to suppose that hysterical symptom are incompatible with organic disease.

Marsden (1986) emphasises that people with hysterical symptoms may have underlying recognised physical or psychiatric illness, and they could well have unrecognised physical or psychiatric illness in addition to exhibiting abnormal illness behaviour. He stresses that they always require further neurological and psychiatric exploration. 'In this way, mistakes can be avoided and hysterical symptoms can be respected.'

(b) Hysteria is a syndrome characterised by the presence of hysterical symptoms in the absence of any other demonstrable physical or psychiatric disorder. It should be possible to demonstrate that the symptoms have some adaptive value to the patient, for example in relieving anxiety when the symptom effectively removes the patient from conflict. This relief of anxiety is the primary gain of the illness. Because of the value of the primary gain to the patient, patients are surprisingly undistressed by their symptoms, hence the description 'la belle indifference'. Subsequent use of the symptom to manipulate others, for example to be inappropriately cared for and financially supported, is called secondary gain, which is of course not confined to hysteria, and may be a consequence of any physical or mental disorder. Ideally the diagnosis of hysteria should not be made in the presence of other conditions that might account for the hysterical symptoms, such as organic disease of the brain, or depressive illness.

In practice, hysteria should only ever be regarded as a first stage in the diagnostic process (Lloyd, 1986). This maxim is reinforced by the findings of follow-up studies of patients given a diagnosis of hysteria. For example, Slater (1965) studied patients given a diagnosis of hysteria by neurologists at the National Hospital, Queen Square. There were 85 patients in the study, a third of whom also had recognised physical disease at the start of the study. At follow-up nine years later, in a third, the diagnosis of hysteria had been replaced by a diagnosis of organic disease (e.g. hysterical pain had been rediagnosed as trigeminal neuralgia or basilar artery migraine, hysterical fits as epilepsy, and bizarre paraesthesiae and weakness as Takayashu's disease). Only 39% had no significant organic disease nine years later, and of these four had committed suicide, two had become schizophrenic and seven had developed recurrent endogenous depression. As Kendall (1982) pointed out, although at the time some psychiatrists were tempted to regard these findings as evidence of the inability of neurologists to recognise hysteria, rather than as evidence of the inherent defects of the concept, a similar follow-up study of 113 patients diagnosed as hysterical by psychiatrists (Reed, 1975) produced similar results.

Lloyd (1986) has emphasised that in every diagnosis of hysteria, doctors should proceed to look carefully for neurological and psychiatric illness, and remain alert to the possible presence of physical disease. Furthermore, there may be factors in the patient's social orbit that will be rewarding the sick role.

(c) Mass hysteria involves the epidemic spread of hysterical symptoms and is usually due to the combined effects of suggestion and shared apprehension which may occur amongst adolescents and young adults who are in close proximity.

(d) Briquet's syndrome is the other main variant of hysteria. It is characterised by multiple and recurrent somatic complaints, over many years or decades, for which medical attention is repeatedly sought, particularly surgical interventions. It is a diagnosis made much more commonly in the US than in the UK, possibly because Americans have easier access than Britons to specialists, so they may more easily acquire numerous diagnoses or be offered surgery. Cultural and iatrogenic factors may therefore play a prominent part in starting the condition (Lloyd, 1986) although a strong familial pattern has also been identified (Guze *et al.*, 1986).

HYSTERIA AND ME

Hysteria has been considered in the differential diagnosis of ME because of:

(a) The bizarre presentation of the illness, involving many systems of the body.
(b) The preponderance of affected women (although this has not always been so in every epidemic, e.g. those in military establishments).
(c) The emotional upsets, including irritability and crying spells.
(d) The prominence of sensory symptoms, often of bizarre distribution and content.
(e) The peculiar nature of the paresis (i.e. weakness without loss of tone, deep reflexes or subsequent atrophy on the one hand, or true spasticity and extensor plantar responses on the other).
(f) The daily fluctuation of symptoms and signs.

However, if we take each of these points in turn:

(a) The bizarre presentation, affecting many systems of the body. This is not in itself a diagnostic criterion for hysteria. Chronic bacterial infections may become systemic, e.g. TB, leprosy or septicaemia, and can affect many systems of the body, and the same may well be true for many chronic viral infections, including AIDS.
(b) The preponderance of affected women. Sex ratios in illness are a fascinating study, and can provide important epidemiological clues to the origin of disease. But it is nonsensical to suggest that any disease which is more common in women is therefore likely to be hysteria on those grounds alone. Many physical diseases are more common in one sex than another, and sex ratios often change, reflecting changes in the frequency of important aetiological factors. Peptic ulcer was more common in women in the nineteenth century, and was thought to be partially due to the constricting clothes which were then the fashion for women. In this century, with looser clothing, peptic ulcer has been more common in men, reflecting their more stressful lifestyles, although women may

again now be catching up. MS is more common in women and its cause is unknown, although the organic pathology is well documented.

(c) The emotional upsets, including crying spells. In depressive illness, mood is lowered, usually in proportion to the severity of the illness. In severe depression mood is consistently extremely low although there may be some diurnal variation, while in mild depression mood may fluctuate more easily. However, in ME the quality of the depressed mood is different in that it is generally much more labile, mild frequent elation is common, it is associated with irritability, and is in general much more reminiscent of the mental symptoms of encephalitis. In hysterical, or more properly histrionic, personality, the emotional displays are life-long traits, not symptoms which arise suddenly in the context of an illness such as ME. In hysteria, emotional displays are not generally seen; more usually the patient displays 'la belle indifference', and is not distressed by his or her motor or sensory symptoms.

(d) The prominence of sensory phenomena, often of bizarre distribution and content, not corresponding with precise dermatoses. The glove and stocking distribution of some of the paraesthesia led McEvedy and Beard, and more recently others to suggest that the paraesthesiae were simply caused by overbreathing due to anxiety. However, such paraesthesiae associated with overbreathing are transitory, whereas the paraesthesiae of ME usually last for months or even years. Furthermore, attempts to demonstrate that patients with ME are overbreathing are not usually successful. Similar sensory phenomena, not corresponding with precise dermatoses, may occur in some vitamin deficiencies, and other peripheral neuropathies.

(e) The peculiar nature of the paresis, i.e. not corresponding with either an upper or lower motor neurone lesion. This requires an explanation, and the reader is referred to Chapters 7 and 8.

(f) The daily fluctuation of symptoms and signs, like the other phenomena, requires an explanation, but is not a feature of either the conversion or dissociative symptoms of hysteria.

ILLNESS BEHAVIOUR AND A MULTIAXIAL APPROACH TO DIAGNOSIS

The concept of illness behaviour has been developed by sociologists in order to understand better the relationships between physical and psychological illness (Parsons, 1951; Mechanic and Volkart, 1961; Segall, 1976a, b). Illness behaviour has been defined as the ways in which given symptoms may be differentially perceived, evaluated, and acted upon (e.g. taking over-the-counter medication, consulting a doctor, taking prescribed medication, taking time off work, going to bed, avoiding customary activities and roles). In general, people have a habitual pattern of illness behaviour, a life-long tendency to have a low or a high threshold for consulting doctors, taking time off work etc., on which may be superimposed a temporary change in pattern related to current physical, social and psychological factors. Illness behaviour may be viewed as appropriate or inappropriate (either excessive or insufficient or taking an unusual form). Abnormal illness behaviour is used to refer to illness behaviours which are regarded as inappropriate, and would include hysteria. The presence of abnormal illness behaviour does not indicate that there is no physical or psychological illness present. It simply indicates that, in the clinician's view, the illness behaviour seems disproportionate to the physical or psychological illness.

What is crucial to realise is that none of these categories of psychological illness, physical illness, mental illness, social difficulties, and abnormal illness behaviour, are mutually exclusive. They frequently coexist, and abnormalities in one domain may lead to or be associated with abnormalities in another. Some research psychiatrists have already faced up to these issues, and have realised for some decades that the most sensible solution is to develop a multiaxial system of diagnosis, using axes for physical illness, psychological illness, social difficulties, personality and illness behaviour. Every patient can be diagnosed on such a system, which does not require that all the patient's symptoms are made to fit a single diagnosis. A patient may have abnormalities on each axis. Information is often lost by using a category such as 'hypochondriasis', when real physical pathology, a depressive illness, abnormal illness behaviour, and abnormal personality traits may all be present in one patient.

Many doctors tend to oscillate uneasily in the 'either or' framework, i.e. either there is an organic disease present, or the patient is psychologically ill. McEvedy and Beard (1973) regrettably only proposed the two alternatives of definite physical illness or definite psychiatric illness, without taking a more coherent multiaxial approach to the Royal Free patients, and this fruitless dichotomy of organic versus functional has greatly hampered research on ME (David et al., 1988). Abnormality may of course be present or absent on any of the physical, psychological, social, personality and illness behaviour axes, and the presence or absence of abnormality in one axis does not preclude its presence or absence on another axis (Balla, 1985). Thus there is a major logical fallacy in the diagnostic approach, unfortunately all too common, that takes the view that a constellation of symptoms, where no physical abnormality has been demonstrated, must be psychological in origin. It may or may not be so. Physical abnormalities may be present but undetected. For example, several conditions previously regarded as hysteria are now thought to have an organic basis, including spasmodic torticollis, blepharospasm and writers' cramp (Lloyd, 1986).

Therefore it is vital to diagnose psychological abnormality, not on the negative grounds of absent physical abnormality, but on the positive grounds of the presence of psychological phenomena, and to place the psychological phenomena in their multiaxial framework (Jenkins *et al.*, 1988a). Such a scheme has been proposed for use in general practice (Jenkins *et al.*, 1988b).

Having recorded the presence or absence of abnormality on each of the five axes, to complete the descriptive picture of the patient's clinical state, the next step in the diagnostic process is, where possible, to elucidate aetiological and maintaining factors. Because many diagnostic terms carry causal implications, and because opinion varies as to the strength of these aetiological assumptions, there is a powerful argument that all diagnoses should be stripped of their aetiological implications and be regarded simply as operational definitions (e.g. Stengel, 1959; Boyd *et al.*, 1984; Edlund, 1986). The advantages of separating the clinical syndrome (which is always present and may always be assessed) from aetiology (which may not be obvious or proven in the individual case) are substantial and have obvious relevance to research on aetiology. This realisation led Essen-Moller (1961) 30 years ago to propose the radical solution of one axis for symptomatology and another for aetiology. These issues are discussed further in the final chapter of this book.

Using such a multiaxial framework in patients with ME, it is possible that, on the physical axis, there is a chronic viral infection, perhaps of enterovirus replicating in the gut (see Chapter 3), but affecting other sites, including muscle fibres (see Chapter 8) and the brain (see Chapter 4); on the psychological axis there are psychological symptoms of abnormal mood and abnormal cognition (see Chapter 10), some of which may be a primary result of the viral infection of the brain (see Chapter 4), and some of which may be a result of secondary depression, following the viral illness (see Chapter 5); and some may indeed antedate the onset of the viral infection, and perhaps have been a contributory factor to the host susceptibility (see Chapter 25); on the social axis there may be any number of antecedent and consequent acute and chronic social problems and lack of support; on the personality axis, there may or may not be pre-existing abnormal personality traits; and on the illness behaviour axis there may be normal and abnormal illness behaviours. It is essential that research is planned and interpreted on such a multiaxial framework if we are not to make erroneous deductions from observed associations. This issue will be discussed in more detail in the final chapter of this book.

It may be instructive for the reader first of all to place our knowledge of chronic bacterial infections such as TB and leprosy in such a framework, remembering that although the bacillus is the direct cause, there are many physical, social and even psychological predisposing factors, including malnutrition, poverty, damp housing, poor sanitation etc. Indeed, much was

Table 1 A multiaxial framework of disease

	Physical	Psychological	Social	Personality	Illness behaviour
I Antecedent predisposing factors					
II Direct causes					
III Pathogenic processes caused by the aetiological agent					
IV Manifestations of the disease					
V Treatment					
VI Factors affecting prognosis					

written in the nineteenth century about personality and TB. Similarly, successful treatment involves more than eradicating the bacillus. A multifactorial and holistic approach works better than chemotherapy alone.

Having seen how it is possible to organise our knowledge in this way, the reader may then begin to compare those diseases with the knowledge we have of ME, described in the following chapters.

NOMENCLATURE

The first names appearing in the literature were geographical, relating to the outbreak in Iceland, and were the illness Iceland disease (White and Burtch, 1954) or Akureyri disease (Sigurdsson and Gudmundsson, 1956). In this country the illness has been called Royal Free disease, following the outbreak at the Royal Free Hospital. As with all eponyms, these names give no clues as to the nature of the disease, and they are also historically incorrect since the Los Angeles outbreak described by Gilliam (1938) is the original account in the literature.

Others have sought to find a name which described the essential nature of the illness. Fog (1953) suggested 'neuritis vegetativa' in the belief that the disease mainly affected the autonomic nervous system. A _Lancet_ editorial (1956) suggested 'benign myalgic encephalomyelitis, to emphasise the absent mortality, the severe muscular pain, the evidence of parenchyma damage to the nervous system, and the presumed inflammatory nature of the disorder.' The clinical impression that the lesion is central rather than peripheral is supported by the electromyogram and would seem to justify 'encephalomyelitis', and the epidemiological evidence that the disease is infectious makes the term 'encephalomyelitis' preferable to 'encephalopathy'. It has been pointed out that the term fails to describe the involvement of the lymph nodes and the liver, but a fully descriptive name such as 'benign ameningitic myalgic lymphoreticular encephalomyelitis' is impracticable.

Shelekov *et al.* (1957) and Poskanzer *et al.* (1957) have suggested 'epidemic neuromyasthenia', which has been used in several reviews and editorials (e.g. Ramsay, 1978), but this term is misleading because the disease is not confined to epidemics, and the term 'neuromyasthenia' suggests a disorder of the muscle end plate which is contrary to electromyographic evidence.

Acheson (1959) commented that 'It is unlikely that an adequate term will be found until fresh evidence is available. In the meantime, 'benign myalgic encephalomyelitis' may act provisionally as a rallying point in the current list of medical literature for patients with the clinical features already described.

Goodwin (1981) argued in the *Lancet* that as long as an aetiological agent could not be isolated from patients with this disease, it was important that the title 'myalgic encephalomyelitis' should be restricted to patients who show some of each of the three major features of the disease: firstly, symptoms and signs in relation to muscles, such as recurrent episodes of profound weakness and exhaustion, easy fatiguability, and marked muscle tenderness; secondly, neurological symptoms and signs—pyramidal or cranial nerve lesions, especially affecting the eyes, or weakness of peripheral muscles, as demonstrated by the voluntary muscle test, or some loss of peripheral sensation, or involvement of the autonomic nervous system (orthostatic tachycardia, abnormal coldness of the extremities, episodes of sweating or pallor, constipation and bladder disturbance); and thirdly, biochemical abnormalities, such as a raised urinary creatinine, low serum pyruvate, or raised serum myoglobulin, or an abnormal electrophoretic pattern with raised IgM.

The term 'post-viral fatigue syndrome' has been frequently used to describe fatigue syndromes following viral illnesses. It obviously covers the whole spectrum from mild fatigue lasting a few weeks to the overwhelming fatigue of many months or years duration of ME accompanied by the other symptoms of recurrent fever, lymphadenopathy, muscle pains, paraesthesiae etc. Thus it is a broad umbrella term for what is likely to prove to be more than one distinct syndrome and it excludes illnesses which are not post-viral in origin. In view of the accumulating virological evidence that ME is, at least in a substantial proportion of cases, caused by a continuing chronic active enteroviral infection (see Chapter 3), the adjective 'post' is a misnomer. Nonetheless the term is in widespread use, and is less cumbersome than myalgic encephalomyelitis.

The term 'chronic fatigue syndrome' is generally used by scientists in the US. It obviously makes no assumptions about whether or not the illness is virally induced. A research committee have laid down helpful diagnostic criteria (Holmes *et al.*, 1988), which are as follows.

CASE DEFINITION FOR THE CHRONIC FATIGUE SYNDROME

A case of the chronic fatigue syndrome must fulfil major criteria 1 and 2, and the following minor criteria: 6 or more of the 11 symptom criteria and 2 or more of the 3 physical criteria; or 8 or more of the 11 symptom criteria.

Major criteria

1. New onset of persistent or relapsing, debilitating fatigue or easy fatigability in a person who has no previous history of similar symptoms, that does not resolve with bedrest, and that is severe enough to reduce or impair average daily activity below 50% of the patient's premorbid activity level for a period of at least 6 months.

2. Other clinical conditions that may produce similar symptoms must be excluded by thorough evaluation, based on history, physical examination, and appropriate laboratory findings. These conditions include malignancy; autoimmune disease; localized infection (such as occult abscess); chronic or subacute bacterial disease (such as endocarditis, Lyme disease, or tuberculosis), fungal disease (such as histoplasmosis, blastomycosis, or coccidioidomycosis), and parasitic disease (such as toxoplasmosis, amebiasis, giardiasis, or helminthic infestation); disease related to human immunodeficiency virus (HIV) infection; chronic psychiatric disease, either newly diagnosed or by history (such as endogenous depression; hysterical personality disorder, anxiety neurosis; schizophrenia; or chronic use of major tranquilizers, lithium, or antidepressive medications); chronic inflammatory disease (such as sarcoidosis, Wegener granulomatosis, or chronic hepatitis); neuromuscular disease (such as multiple sclerosis or myasthenia gravis); endocrine disease (such as hypothyroidism, Addison disease, Cushing syndrome, or diabetes mellitus); drug dependency or abuse (such as alcohol, controlled prescription drugs, or illicit drugs); side effects of a chronic medication or other toxic agent (such as a chemical solvent, pesticide, or heavy metal); or other known or defined chronic pulmonary, cardiac, gastrointestinal, hepatic, renal or hematologic disease.

Specific laboratory tests or clinical measurements are not required to satisfy the definition of the chronic fatigue syndrome, but the recommended evaluation includes serial weight measurements (weight change of more than 10% in the absence of dieting suggests other diagnoses); serial morning and afternoon temperature measurements; complete blood count and differential; serum electrolytes; glucose; creatinine, blood urea nitrogen; calcium, phosphorus; total bilirubin, alkaline phosphatase, serum aspartate aminotransferase, serum alanine aminotransferase; creatine phosphokinase or aldolase; urinalysis; posteroanterior and lateral chest roentgenograms, detailed personal and family psychiatric history; erythrocyte sedimentation rate; antinulear antibody; thyroid-stimulating hormone level; HIV antibody measurement; and intermediate-strength purified protein derivative (PPD) skin test with controls.

If any of the results from these tests are abnormal, the physician should search for other conditions that may cause such a result. If no such conditions are detected by a reasonable evaluation, this criterion is satisfied.

Minor criteria

Symptom criteria

To fulfil a symptom criterion, a symptom must have begun at or after the time of onset of increased fatigability, and must have persisted or recurred over a period of at least 6 months (individual symptoms may or may not have occurred simultaneously). Symptoms include:

1. Mild fever—oral temperature between 37.5°C and 38.6°C, if measured by the patient—or chills. (Note: oral temperatures of greater than 38.6°C are less compatible with chronic fatigue syndrome and should prompt studies for other causes of illness.)
2. Sore throat.
3. Painful lymph nodes in the anterior or posterior cervical or axillary distribution.
4. Unexplained generalized muscle weakness.
5. Muscle discomfort or myalgia.
6. Prolonged (24 hours or greater) generalized fatigue after levels of exercise that would have been easily tolerated in the patient's premorbid state.
7. Generalized headaches (of a type, severity, or pattern that is different from headaches the patient may have had in the premorbid state).
8. Migratory arthralgia without joint swelling or redness.
9. Neuropsychologic complaints (one or more of the following: photophobia, transient visual scotomata, forgetfulness, excessive irritability, confusion, difficulty thinking, inability to concentrate, depression).
10. Sleep disturbance (hypersomnia or insomnia).

11. Description of the main symptom complex is initially developing over a few hours to a few days (this is not a true symptom, but may be considered as equivalent to the above symptoms in meeting the requirements of the case definition).

Physical criteria

Physical criteria must be documented by a physician on at least two occasions, at least 1 month apart.

1. Low-grade fever—oral temperature between 36.7°C and 38.6°C, or rectal temperature between 37.8°C and 38.8°C. (See note under Symptom Criterion 1).
2. Nonexudative pharyngitis.
3. Palpable or tender anterior or posterior cervical or axillary lymph nodes. (Note: lymph nodes greater than 2 cm in diameter suggest other causes. Further evaluation is warranted.)

Reproduced, with permission, from: Holmes, G. P., Kaplan, J. E., Gantz, N. M., Komaroff, A. L., Schonberger, L. B., Straus, S. E., Jones, J. F., Dubois, R. E., Cunningham-Rindles, C., Paliova, S., Tosato, G., Zegans, L. S., Purtilo, D. T., Brown, N., Schooley, R. T. and Bus, I., Chronic Fatigue Syndrome: A Working Case Definition. *Annals of Internal Medicine* 1988; **108**: 387–389.

REFERENCES

Acheson, E. D. (1954) Encephalomyelitis associated with poliomyelitis virua. An outbreak in a nurses' home. *Lancet*, **2**, 1044–1048.

Acheson, E. D. (1959) The clinical syndrome variously called benign myalgic encephalomyelitis, Iceland disease and epidemic neuromyasthenia. *American Journal of Medicine*, **26**, 569–695.

Albrecht, R. M., Oliver, V. L. and Poskanzer, D. C. (1964) Epidemic neuromyasthenia. Outbreak in a convent in New York State. *Journal of the American Medical Association*, **187**, 904–907.

Baines, J. H. E. (1970) Epidemic malaise. *British Medical Journal*, **1**, 170–171.

Balla, J. I. (1985) *The Diagnostic Process: A Model for Clinical Teachers*, Cambridge University Press, Cambridge.

Boyd, J. H., Burke, J. D., Greenberg, E., Holzer, C. E., Raes, D. S., George, L. K., Karno, M., Stottzman, R., McEvey, L. and Nestadt, G. (1984) Exclusion criteria of DSM—III. *Archives of General Psychiatry*, **41**, 983–989.

Editorial (1978) Epidemic myalgic encephalomyelitis. *British Medical Journal*, 1437.

Compston, N. D. (1978) An outbreak of encephalomyelitis in the Royal Free Hospital Group, London, in 1955. *Postgraduate Medical Journal*, **54**, 722–724.

Crowley, N., Nelson, M. and Stovin, S. (1957) Epidemiological aspects of an outbreak of encephalomyelitis at the Royal Free Hospital, London, in the summer of 1955. *Journal of Hygiene (Cambridge)*, **55**, 102–122.

David, A., Wessely, S. and Pelosi, A. (1988) Postviral fatigue: time for a new approach. *British Medical Journal*, **296**, 696–699.

Dillon, M. J., Marshall, W. C., Dudgeon, J. A. and Steigman, A. J. (1974) Epidemic neuromyasthenia: Outbreak among nurses at a children's hospital. *British Medical Journal*, **1**, 301–305.

Edlund, M. J. (1986) Causal models in psychiatric research. *British Journal of Psychiatry*, **148**, 713–717.

Essen-Moller, E. (1961) On classification of mental disorders. *Acta Psychiatrica Scandinavica*, **37**, 119–126.

Fog, T. (1953) Neuritis vegetative epidemica. *Ugeskrift for laeger*, **115**, 1244.

Galpine, J. F. (1970) Epidemic malaise. *British Medical Journal*, **1**, 501.

Gill, C. H. (1970) Epidemic medicine. *British Medical Journal*, **1**, 299.

Gilliam, A. G. (1938) *Epidemiological Study on an Epidemic, Diagnosed as Poliomyelitis, Occurring among the Personnel of Los Angeles County General Hospital during the Summer of 1934*, United States Treasury Department Public Health Service Public Health Bulletin, No. 240, pp. 1–90. Washington, DC, Government Printing Office.

Goodwin, C. S. (1981) Was it benign myalgic encephalomyelitis? *Lancet*, **i**, 37.

Gosling, P. (1970) Epidemic malaise. *British Medical Journal*, **1**, 499–500.

Gsell, O. (1938) *Abortive Poliomyelitis*, pp. 13–20. Verlag Thieme, Leipzig.

Gsell, O. (1949) Abortive poliomyelitis. *Helvetica Medica Acta*, **16**, 169.

Gsell, O. (1958) Encephalomyelitis myalgic epidemics, eine poliomyelitisahnliche Krankheit. *Schweizerische Medizinische Wochenschrift*, **88**, 488.

Guze, S. B., Cloninger, C. R., Martin, R. L. and Clayton, P. J. (1986) A follow up and family study of Briquet's Syndrome. *British Journal of Psychiatry*, **149**, 17–23.

Hardtke, E. F. (1955) Iceland disease in Indiana; a case report. *Journal of the Indiana State Medical Association*, **48**, 245–250.

Holmes, G. P., Kaplan, J. E., Gantz, N. M., Komaroff, A. L., Schonberger, L. B., Straus, S. E., Jones, J. F., Dubois, R. E., Cunningham-Rindles, C., Paliova, S., Tosato, G., Zegans, L. S., Purtilo, D. T., Brown, N., Schooley, R. T. and Bus, I. (1988) Chronic Fatigue syndrome: A working case definition. *Annals of Internal Medicine*, **108**, 387–389.

Hopkins, E. J. (1970) Epidemic malaise. *British Medical Journal*, **1**, 501.

Houghton, L. E. and Jones, E. I. (1942) Persistent myalgia following sore throat. *Lancet*, **i**, 196–198.

Howells, B. K. (1970) *British Medical Journal*, **1**, 300.

Innes, S. G. B. (1970) Encephalomyelitis resembling benign myalgic encephalomyelitis. *Lancet*, **i**, 969–971.

Jenkins, R., Aggett, P. and Newall, B. (1988a) *Teaching medical students and registrars: a multidisciplinary team approach to the management of chronic pain and abnormal illness behaviour*. Association of University Teachers of Psychiatry Newsletter, London.

Jenkins, R., Smeeton, N. and Shepherd, M. (1988b) *Classification of Mental Disorder in Primary Care*, Psychological Medicine Monograph No. 1, Cambridge University Press, Cambridge.

Kendall, R. E. (1967) The psychiatric sequelae of benign myalgic encephalomyelitis. *British Journal of Psychiatry*, **113**, 833–840.

Kendall, R. E. (1972) A new look at hysteria. *Medicine*, **30**, 1780–1783.

Kendall, R. E. (1982) A new look at hysteria. In A. Roy (ed) *Hysteria 1982*, pp. 27–36. Chichester, John Wiley.

Kendall, R. E. (1983) Hysteria. In G. F. M. Russell and L. A. Hersov (eds) *Handbook of Psychiatry No. 4. The Neuroses and Personality Disorders*. Cambridge, Cambridge University Press.

Lancet editorial (1956) A new clinical entity? *Lancet*, **i**, 789–790.

Lewis-Price, J. (1961) Myalgic encephalomyelitis. *Lancet*, **i**, 737–738.

Lloyd, G. G. (1986) Hysteria: A case for conservation. *British Medical Journal*, **293**, 1255–1256.

Macrae, A. D. and Galpine, J. F. (1984) An illness resembling poliomyelitis observed in nurses. *Lancet*, **ii**, 350–352.

Mann, A. H., Jenkins, R. and Belsey, E. (1981) The twelve month outcome of patients with neurotic illness in general practice. *Psychological Medicine*, **11**, 535–550.

Marsden, C. D. (1986) Hysteria—a neurologist's view. *Psychological Medicine*, **16**, 277–288.

Mayne, D. G. (1970) Epidemic malaise. *British Medical Journal*, **1**, 171.

McEvedy, C. P. and Beard, A. W. (1970a) Concept of benign myalgic encephalomyelitis. *British Medical Journal*, **1**, 11–15.

McEvedy, C. P. and Beard, A. W. (1970b) Royal Free epidemic of 1955: A reconsideration. *British Medical Journal*, **1**, 7–11.

McEvedy, C. P. and Beard, A. W. (1973) A controlled follow-up of cases involved in an epidemic of 'Benign Myalgic Encephalomyelitis'. *British Journal of Psychiatry*, **122**, 141–150.

Mechanic, D. and Volkart, E. H. (1961) Stress, illness behaviour and the sick role. *American Sociological Review*, **26**, 51–58.

Medical Staff of the Royal Free Hospital (1957) An outbreak of encephalomyelitis in the Royal Free Hospital Group, London in 1955. *British Medical Journal*, **1**, 895–904.

Ottoson, J. O. and Perris, C. (1973) Multidimensional classification of mental disorders. *Psychological Medicine*, **3**, 238–243.

Parish, J. G. (1978) Early outbreaks of epidemic neuromyasthenia. *Postgraduate Medical Journal*, **54**, 711–717.

Parsons, T. (1951) *Social Structure and Dynamic Process: The Case of Modern Medical Practice in 'The Social System'*, pp. 428–479. Free Press, New York.

Pederson, E. (1956) Epidemic encephalitis in Jutland. A clinical survey for the years 1952–54. *Danish Medical Bulletin*, **3**, 65–75.

Pellew, R. A. A. (1951) A clinical description of a disease resembling poliomyelitis seen in Adelaide 1949–1951. *Medical Journal of Australia*, Vol. 1, 1944–946.

Pellew, R. A. A. and Miles, J. A. R. (1955) Further investigations on a disease resembling poliomyelitis seen in Adelaide. *Medical Journal of Australia*, Vol. 1, 480–482.

Poskanzer, D. C. (1970) Epidemic malaise. *British Medical Journal*, **2**, 420–421.

Poskanzer, D. C., Henderson, D. A., Kunkle, E. C., Kalter, S. S., Clement, W. B. and Bond, J. O. (1957) Epidemic neuromyasthenia. An outbreak in Punta Gorda, Florida. *New England Journal of Medicine*, **257**, 356–364.

Ramsay, A. M. (1978) Epidemic neuromyasthenia 1955–1978. *Postgraduate Medical Journal*, **54**, 718–721.

Ramsay, A. M. and O'Sullivan, E. (1956) Encephalomyelitis simulating poliomyelitis. *Lancet*, **1**, 761–764.

Reed, J. L. (1975) The diagnosis of hysteria. *Psychological Medicine*, **5**, 13–17.

Richardson, A. T. (1956) Some aspects of the Royal Free Hospital epidemic. *Annals of Physical Medicine*, **3**, 81–89.

Rutter, M., Shaffer, D. and Shepherd, M. (1973) An evaluation of the proposal for a multiaxial classification of child psychiatric disorders. *Psychological Medicine*, **3**, 244–250.

Scott, B. D. (1970) Epidemic malaise. *British Medical Journal*, 170.

Segall, A. (1976a) The sick role concept: Understanding illness behaviour. *Journal of Health and Social Behaviour*, **17**, 163–170.

Segall, A. (1976b) Sociocultural variation in sick role behavioural expectations. *Social Science and Medicine*, **10**, 47–51.

Shelokov, A., Habel, K., Verder, E. and Welsh, W. (1957) Epidemic neuromyasthenia. An outbreak of poliomyelitis like illness in student nurses. *New England Journal of Medicine*, **257**, 345–355.

Sigurdsson, B. and Gudmundsson, K. R. (1956) Clinical findings six years after outbreak of Akureyri disease. *Lancet*, **1**, 766–767.

Sigurdsson, B., Sigurdsson, J., Sigurdsson, J. H., Thorkelsson, J. and Gudmundsson, K. R. (1950) A disease epidemic in Iceland simulating poliomyelitis. *American Journal of Hygiene*, **52**, 222–238.

Sigurdsson, B., Gudnadottir, M. and Petursson, G. (1958) Response to poliomyelitis vaccination. *Lancet*, **i**, 370–371.

Slater, E. (1965) Diagnosis of hysteria. *British Medical Journal*, **1**, 1395.

Stahel, H. (1938) Die poliomyelitis—Epidemie bei stats Geb I R37 und Geb Sch Bat 11 Erstfeld 18–30 Juli 1937. Die abortiv-poliomyelitis. *Schweizerische Medizinische Wochenschrift*, **68**, 86.

Stengel, E. (1959) Classification of mental disorders. *Bulletin of the World Health Organization*, **21**, 601–663.

Thomas, M. (1978) Epidemiological approaches to 'epidemic neuromyasthenia': syndromes of unknown aetiology (epidemic myalgic encephalopathies). *Postgraduate Medical Journal*, **54**, 768–770.

Wallis, A. L. (1957) 'An investigation into an unusual disease seen in epidemic and sporadic form in a general practice in Cumberland in 1955 and subsequent years.' MD Thesis, University of Edinburgh.

White, D. N. and Burtch, R. B. (1954) Iceland disease. A new infection simulating acute anterior poliomyelitis. *Neurology*, **4**, 506–516.

Wilson, J. C. and Walker, P. J. (1936) Acute anterior poliomyelitis: Orthopaedic aspects of the California epidemics of 1934. *Archives of Internal Medicine*, **57**, 477–492.

2

Post-viral Fatigue Syndrome: A Review of American Research and Practice

Anthony L. Komaroff

Harvard Medical School, Boston, USA

INTRODUCTION

The American medical literature makes scant reference to 'post-viral' fatigue syndrome or to myalgic encephalomyelitis (ME). Nevertheless, there was considerable discussion in the American literature (as in the British literature) of a very similar syndrome—neurocirculatory asthenia or neurasthenia—60–90 years ago. And, in the past decade, there has been rapidly growing interest in two illnesses which also go by other names but which have many similarities to ME: chronic fatigue syndrome and fibromyalgia or fibrositis.

Neursasthenia was studied primarily by cardiologists, because of the suspicion that some weakness of the cardiovascular system accounted for the symptoms. Chronic fatigue syndrome has been studied primarily by investigators with an interest in infectious diseases, because of a suspicion that the illness is triggered by infectious agents. Fibromyalgia has been investigated primarily by rheumatologists, because of the prominent musculoskeletal pain associated with the syndrome. Nevertheless, this is not entirely an example of the parable of the blind men feeling the elephant: cardiologists studying neurasthenia frequently remarked on a possible relationship with infectious disease, infectious disease investigators frequently remarked on the presence of cardiovascular symptoms, and rheumatologists also recognized that the illness they were studying bore little similarity to the objective findings in the majority of established rheumatologic diseases.

With each of these syndromes, chronic, debilitating fatigue is a prominent symptom. Of course, fatigue is also seen with many well-established

Post-viral Fatigue Syndrome. Edited by R. Jenkins and J. Mowbray
© 1991 John Wiley & Sons Ltd

'organic' and 'psychiatric' illnesses. We shall begin by considering the diversity of causes that may bring a patient to the doctor's office seeking help for the complaint of chronic fatigue.

FATIGUE IN GENERAL MEDICAL PRACTICE

Everyone experiences fatigue. Furthermore, nearly everyone occasionally experiences a fatigue which is felt to be 'unnatural', not clearly explained by the mental, emotional and physical stresses of the previous days. Usually, such fatigue is transient. However, some fraction of the population at large experiences chronic, debilitating fatigue. The size of that group is unknown.

It is known that chronic fatigue is a common problem in general medical practice (Allan, 1944; Morrison, 1980; Katerndahl, 1983; Nelson et al., 1987), accounting for 10–15 million office visits per year in the USA. Depression and anxiety with somatization (bodily complaints attributed primarily to psychological or social distress) is also common in general medical practice, and one of the more common complaints among somatizing patients is fatigue (Stoeckle et al., 1964; Reifler et al., 1979; Hoeper et al., 1979; Nielsen and Williams, 1980; Kessler et al., 1985; Barsky, 1981). Despite the commonly expressed opinion that the fast-paced life of modern industrial society is responsible for 'neurasthenia', the condition is seen even more frequently in agrarian societies such as mainland China (Kleinman, 1982).

While it is generally agreed that primary psychiatric disorders, particularly depression and anxiety, are the cause of most cases of chronic fatigue in a general medical practice, it is recognized that on occasion various 'organic' conditions can also produce fatigue—for example, occult malignancies, anemia, thyroid disorders, etc. In recent years, in the United States, there has been growing discussion of another illness that many believe has an 'organic' basis.

Recent interest was stirred by the description of a chronic fatiguing illness associated with serologic evidence of reactivated latent Epstein–Barr virus (EBV) infection. Now called 'chronic fatigue syndrome' (CFS) by most investigators, the syndrome was originally called 'chronic active EBV infection' (CEBV) or 'chronic mononucleosis', and is characterized by varying degrees of chronic fatigue, fever, pharyngitis, myalgias, headache, arthralgias, paresthesias, depression, and cognitive deficits. While the full syndrome has been described only in recent years (Tobi et al., 1982; Ballow et al., 1982; Edson et al., 1983; Hamblin et al., 1983; DuBois et al., 1984; Jones et al., 1985; Straus et al., 1985), earlier reports which may have been reporting the same phenomenon exist in the literature. A similar syndrome may follow infection with a variety of infectious agents (Benjamin and Hoyt, 1945; Lawton et *al.*, 1970; Rosene *et al.*, 1982; Cluff *et al.*, 1959; Imboden *et al.*, 1959; Hickson *et al.*, 1981; Salit, 1985).

The onset of the syndrome typically seems to be in late adolescence or young adulthood (Tobi *et al.*,1982; Ballow *et al.*, 1982; Edson *et al.*, 1983; Hamblin *et al.*, 1983; DuBois *et al.*, 1984; Jones *et al.*, 1985; Straus *et al.*, 1985), although it may also occur in childhood (Jones *et al.*, 1985). By definition, patients with this syndrome have been evaluated for a variety of chronic infectious, rheumatologic, endocrinologic and malignant diseases, and no chronic disease is apparent (Tobi *et al.*, 1982; DuBois *et al.*, 1984; Jones *et al.*, 1985; Straus *et al.*, 1985). The diagnosis has been made about twice as often in women as in men (Tobi *et al.*, 1982; Hamblin *et al.*, 1983; DuBois *et al.*, 1984; Jones *et al.*, 1985; Straus *et al.*, 1985). The illness may follow a documented episode of infectious mononucleosis, or an acute viral syndrome for which the patient has not sought medical attention, but also may appear spontaneously (Tobi *et al.*, 1982; DuBois *et al.*,1984; Jones *et al.*, 1985; Straus *et al.*, 1985). For most patients, the illness takes the form of a chronic, recurring 'flu-like' illness (DuBois *et al.*, 1984; Jones *et al.*, 1985; Straus *et al.*, 1985). Virtually all patients perceive themselves to be impaired in some way. Some patients are completely disabled by the fatigue, muscular weakness and pain. As will be discussed later, the role of EBV in this illness is uncertain.

The initial recent reports of this illness generated considerable public interest. Between early 1985 and late 1986, 10 000 individuals joined 'Chronic EBV' support groups around the United States (unpublished data, from National CEBV Syndrome Association, Portland, OR). Requests to perform EBV serologic testing increased greatly in many clinical laboratories.

POSSIBLY RELATED SYNDROMES

The illness called chronic fatigue syndrome bears a striking likeness to several other syndromes which have been described in the past.

The first of these is *neurasthenia* (or neurocirculatory asthenia). This illness was first described in the mid-nineteenth century (Paul, 1987). Typically an affliction of young adults, usually women, the illness was characterized by chronic malaise. Most investigators have been struck by how often the syndrome started with an acute infectious illness. In the early twentieth century, the illness was ascribed to 'weakness' of the nervous system and cardiovascular system, but no characteristic objective deficits were identified. For that reason, the illness slipped from favor, and has been rarely mentioned in the medical literature of the past 40 years.

Next, there is the illness I shall call *true chronic mononucleosis* (Komaroff, 1987; Straus, 1988). First described 40 years ago, this illness starts with classical acute infectious mononucleosis, as characterized by clinical, hematologic and serologic features (Isaacs, 1948). However, instead of recovering, these patients remain ill for years. Some of them have serologic evidence of persistently active EBV infection, although in our experience there are some patients who remain chronically ill but whose EBV serologic studies become unremarkable.

Another, much less frequent group of patients have apparent *severe chronic active EBV Infection* (Edson *et al.*, 1983; Schooley *et al.*, 1986). Often, but not always, these patients have a chronic illness which follows acute infectious mononucleosis. They all have strikingly abnormal serologic studies (EBV–viral capsid antigen (VCA)–IgG greater than or equal to 1 : 5120; or early antigen (EA)-Ab greater than or equal to 1 : 320). Most of them also have evidence of major organ involvement, such as recurrent interstitial pneumonia, persistent non-A, non-B hepatitis, splenomegaly and adenopathy, pancytopenia or selective cytopenia. Again, the parsimonious explanation is that these patients have an illness related to EBV infection, in which immunologic containment of EBV is impaired.

Myalgic encephalomyelitis (ME) is a very similar chronic fatiguing illness, variably called ME, epidemic neuromyasthenia, Akureyri disease or Icelandic disease (Sigurdsson *et al.*, 1950; Sigurdsson and Gudmundsson, 1956; Shelokov *et al.*, 1957; Poskanzer *et al.*, 1957; Medical Staff of the Royal Free Hospital, 1957; Acheson, 1959; Henderson and Shelokov, 1959). Most often, this illness strikes in mini-epidemics, affecting hundreds of individuals living in small towns, or large numbers of coworkers in a large institution. This lingering illness typically, if not always, is heralded by acute respiratory infection symptoms, followed by months or years of profound fatigue, muscular weakness and twitching, muscular pain (especially in the neck, shoulder girdle, low back and thighs), pharyngitis, nausea, vomiting, abdominal cramps, swelling in the fingers and feet, cognitive problems, emotional instability, depression, insomnia, paresthesias, and a tendency to transpose words. Not infrequently, these patients note that their symptoms worsen in damp weather, or in the premenstrual period. Physical examination is often entirely unremarkable, but a substantial number have been reported to suffer from low-grade fevers, adenopathy (especially in the posterior cervical chain), splenomegaly, and nystagmus. Past outbreaks have led to disability and work loss lasting many months or years. The few long-term follow-up studies which have been done suggest gradual improvement in the following years, although many patients continue to experience mild but similar episodes of illness. No particular viral agent has been definitively associated with these syndromes.

Fibromyalgia syndrome, also termed *fibrositis*, was first described in the nineteenth century and is now considered to be a very common cause of chronic musculoskeletal pain and fatigue (Goldenberg, 1987). Until recently, the syndrome of fibromyalgia has not been widely accepted as a specific medical condition, even though up to 5% of patients at a general medical clinic and 12% of new patients seen by rheumatologists may have fibromyalgia (Goldenberg, 1987; Yunus *et al.*, 1981; Wolfe *et al.*, 1984). Indeed, some rheumatologists believe that primary fibromyalgia is the most common rheumatologic condition seen in their practice, particularly in women under the age of 50 (Goldenberg, 1987; Yunus *et al.*, 1981; Wolfe *et al.*, 1984; Dinerman *et al.*, 1986; Felson and Goldenberg, 1986). Between 4% and 20% of new patients seen in ambulatory rheumatology clinics are diagnosed as having fibromyalgia; it has been estimated that 3–6 million people in the United States suffer from fibromyalgia (Yunus *et al.*, 1981; Wolfe and Cathey, 1983; Campbell *et al.*, 1983). Diagnostic criteria have been proposed and tested (Table 1).

The cardinal symptom of fibromyalgia is muscular pain, most commonly of the axial skeleton (Goldenberg, 1987; Yunus *et al.*, 1981; Wolfe *et al.*, 1984; Dinerman *et al.*, 1986; Felson and Goldenberg, 1986). The chronic pain is accompanied by stiffness, particularly in the mornings, and increased tenderness at specific sites known as 'tender points'. The disorder is frequently accompanied by poor sleep, headaches, irritable bowel syndrome, and major affective disorders. Patients with fibromyalgia also complain of fatigue. Indeed, Yunus has stated that 'one may question the diagnosis of primary fibromyalgia in the absence of tiredness' (Yunus *et al.*, 1931). Between 9% and 21% of patients are partially or totally work-disabled (Cathey *et al.*, 1986; Wolfe and Cathey, 1990).

On physical examination, fibromyalgia is characterized by 'tender points' at specific locations. These criteria differentiate patients with fibromyalgia from normals and from patients with other chronic rheumatic disorders (Goldenberg, 1987; Yunus *et al.*, 1981; Wolfe *et al.*, 1985). However, such

Table 1 Diagnostic criteria for fibromyalgia

Major (mandatory) criteria
1. Exclusion of any systemic condition that may cause similar symptoms
2. Generalized aches or stiffness involving three or more anatomic sites for at least three months
3. At least six typical and reproducible tender points

Minor criteria (must have at least four)
1. Generalized fatigue
2. Chronic headache
3. Sleep disturbance
4. Neuropsychiatric symptoms
5. Subjective joint swelling but no objective swelling
6. Numbness, tingling sensation
7. Irritable bowel syndrome
8. Modulation of symptoms by activity, weather or stress

Goldenberg (1987)

diagnostic criteria have not been tested in patients with other poorly understood chronic pain disorders such as chronic idiopathic low back pain.

The first pathophysiological abnormality reported in fibromyalgia was a disturbance in stage 4 or deep sleep, termed alpha wave intrusion in delta sleep (Moldofsky et al., 1975). Moldofsky and coworkers reproduced this sleep disturbance in normal controls and these normal subjects developed symptoms and signs consistent with fibromyalgia (Moldofsky and Searisbrick, 1976). More recent investigations have focused on the tissue changes in fibromyalgia. Such studies have described excessive cold sensitivity (Dinerman et al., 1986) and neurogenic hyperactivity (Littlejohn et al., 1987), type II muscle fiber atrophy (Kalyan-Raman et al., 1984), as well as alterations in muscle metabolism (Lund et al., 1986; Bengtsson et al., 1986; Bonfede et al., 1987). Preliminary reports have described abnormalities in T cell subpopulations and natural killer (NK) cell activity, as well as detectable cytokine levels in subsets of patients with fibromyalgia (Peter and Wallace, 1988; Russell et al., 1988). Furthermore, a subset of patients with fibromyalgia are reported to have positive antinuclear factor and immunoglobulin deposition at the dermal–epidermal junction (Dinerman et al., 1986; Caro et al., 1986).

CHRONIC FATIGUE SYNDROME

In 1988, the United States Centers for Disease Control led a group of investigators in developing a working case definition of an illness called chronic fatigue syndrome (Holmes et al., 1988). This case definition is summarized in Table 2. The definition relies entirely on a combination of symptoms and signs (not laboratory data), and on the exclusion of chronic active organic or psychiatric illnesses that can produce chronic fatigue. It is not yet clear whether the current case definition accomplishes the objectives of any case definition: the identification of a group of individuals with a common and characteristic pathological abnormality and/or a common and characteristic prognosis.

In the pages that follow, we summarize our experience with a group of 350 patients that we have been following over the past four years. All of them have been ill for at least six months. Most of them fully meet the working case definition of chronic fatigue syndrome. Those that do not fully meet the case definition are otherwise indistinguishable from those who do (Komaroff and Geiger, 1989). The findings in our group (which have not yet been published in detail) closely parallel those reported previously by others (DuBois et al., 1984; Jones et al., 1985; Straus et al., 1985).

In our series, the average patient is 37 years old, but the age at onset ranges from 11 years to 60 years. Approximately 70% of the patients are

Table 2 Working case definition of chronic fatigue syndrome

A case of chronic fatigue syndrome must fulfill major criteria 1 and 2, and the following minor criteria: 6 or more of the 11 symptom criteria and 2 or more of the 3 physical criteria; or 8 or more of the 11 symptom criteria.

Major criteria

1. New onset of persistent or relapsing, debilitating fatigue or easy fatigability in a person who has no previous history of similar symptoms, that does not resolve with bedrest, and that is severe enough to produce or impair average daily activity below 50% of the patient's premorbid activity level, for a period of at least 6 months.
2. Other clinical conditions that may produce similar symptoms must be excluded by thorough evaluation, based on history, physical examination, and appropriate laboratory findings. These conditions include malignancy; autoimmune disease; localized infection (such as occult abscess); chronic or subacute bacterial disease (such as endocarditis, Lyme disease, or tuberculosis), fungal disease (such as histoplasmosis, blastomycosis, or coccidioidomycosis), and parasitic disease (such as toxoplasmosis, amebiasis, giardiasis, or helminthic infestation); disease related to human immunodeficiency virus (HIV) infection; chronic psychiatric disease, either newly diagnosed by history (such as endogenous depression; hysterical personality disorder; anxiety neurosis; schizophrenia; or chronic use of major tranquilizers, lithium, or antidepressant medications); chronic inflammatory disease (such as sarcoidosis, Wegener granulomatosis, or chronic hepatitis); neuromuscular disease (such as multiple sclerosis or myasthenia gravis); endocrine disease (such as hypothyroidism, Addison disease, Cushing syndrome, or diabetes mellitus); drug dependency or abuse (such as alcohol, controlled prescription drugs, or illicit drugs); side effects of a chronic medication or other toxic agent (such as a chemical solvent, pesticide, or heavy metal); or other known or defined chronic pulmonary, cardiac, gastrointestinal, hepatic, renal, or hematologic disease.

Minor criteria

Symptom criteria

To fulfill a symptom criterion, a symptom must have begun at or after the time of onset of increased fatigability, and must have persisted or recurred over a period of at least 6 months (individual symptoms may or may not have occurred simultaneously). Symptoms include:

1. Mild fever—oral temperature between 37.5°C and 38.6°C, if measured by the patient—or chills. (Note: oral temperatures of greater than 38.6°C are less compatible with chronic fatigue syndrome and should prompt studies for other causes of illness.)
2. Sore throat.
3. Painful lymph nodes in the anterior or posterior cervical or axillary distribution.
4. Unexplained generalized muscle weakness.
5. Muscle discomfort or myalgia.
6. Prolonged (24 hours or greater) generalized fatigue after levels of exercise that would have been easily tolerated in the patient's premorbid state.
7. Generalized headaches (of a type, severity, or pattern that is different from headaches the patient may have had in the premorbid state).
8. Migratory arthralgia without joint swelling or redness.

continued

Table 2 (contd.)

9. Neuropsychologic complaints (one or more of the following: photophobia, transient visual scotomata, forgetfulness, excessive irritability, confusion, difficulty thinking, inability to concentrate, depression).
10. Sleep disturbance (hypersomnia or insomnia).
11. Description of the main symptom complex as initially developing over a few hours to a few days (this is not a true symptom, but may be considered as equivalent to the above symptoms in meeting the requirements of the case definition).

Physical criteria

Physical criteria must be documented by a physician on at least two occasions, at least one month apart.
1. Low-grade fever—oral temperature between 37.6°C and 38.6°C, or rectal temperature between 37.8°C and 38.8°C. (See note under Symptom Criterion 1.)
2. Nonexudative pharyngitis.
3. Palpable or tender anterior or posterior cervical or axillary lymph node. (Note: lymph nodes greater than 2 cm in diameter suggest other causes. Further evaluation is warranted.)

From Holmes *et al.* (1988).

women. The patients generally are middle-class, but all socio-economic groups are represented. The typical patient has been ill for over three years, and remains ill as of this writing. Approximately 25% describe themselves as regularly bedridden or shut-in, unable to work, something that had never occurred on a regular basis in the years prior to their illness. Approximately one-third can work only part-time. Before they became ill, the patients perceived that they typically were more energetic than most of their friends.

Symptoms

In contrast to most patients with chronic fatigue secondary to a primary depression, 85% of patients with CFS experience the *sudden onset* of an illness that then becomes chronic. Typically, the patients with chronic fatigue syndrome state that their chronic illness began on a particular day, with an acute 'infectious' illness characterized by fever, pharyngitis, adenopathy, myalgias and related symptoms. Unlike the usual such acute illness, the patients state that they have never fully recovered.

Along with the fatigue, patients typically complain of other *chronic* symptoms, as summarized in Table 3. Two particularly remarkable findings are worth highlighting: chronic post-exertional malaise and recurrent, often drenching night sweats. The post-exertional malaise is characterized not only by symptoms that could represent deconditioning—pain and weakness of the involved muscles—but also by exacerbation of 'systemic' symptoms, e.g. fever and adenopathy.

Table 3 Frequency of chronic symptoms and signs

Symptom/sign	Frequency
Fatigue	75–100%
Low-grade fever	60–95%
Myalgias	30–95%
Depression	70–85%
Headaches	35–85%
Pharyngitis	50–70%
Impaired cognition	50–70%
Sleep disorder	15–70%
Anxiety	50–70%
Adenopathy	40–60%
Nausea	50–60%
Arthralgias	40–60%
Diarrhea	30–40%
Cough	30–40%
Odd skin sensations	30–40%
Rash	30–40%
Weight loss	20–30%
Weight gain	50–70%
Low basal body temperature (95.0–97.6°F)	10–20%

Adapted from the experience of the author, plus others (DuBois *et al.*, 1984; Jones *et al.*, 1985; Straus *et al.*, 1985).

The patients state that these symptoms and others were typically *not* a chronic problem in the years before the onset of their illness, but became common after the illness began. For example, here are the frequencies of several common chronic symptoms *after* the illness began vs *before* the illness began: arthralgias (76% vs 6%); morning stiffness (62% vs 3%); distractibility (82% vs 4%); forgetfulness (71% vs 2%); dizziness (61% vs 4%); paresthesias (52% vs 2%); sleep disorder (90% vs 7%); irritability (68% vs 4%); depression (66% vs 7%). While all of these symptoms are surely nonspecific, and several are thought to be concomitant symptoms of depression, the fact that these symptoms typically started abruptly in the context of an acute 'infectious'-type illness makes it hard for us to attribute the symptoms exclusively to a psychiatric disorder.

A few of the patients that we have been following have had transient acute neurological events: primary seizures (7%), acute, profound ataxia (6%), focal weakness (5%), transient blindness (4%), and unilateral paresthesias (not in a dermatomal distribution). The clinical and laboratory findings in these relatively few patients with dramatic neurological events are very similar to those of the larger group of patients with chronic fatigue, except for the neurological events themselves. These acute and transient neurological events are also similar to the findings occasionally reported in outbreaks of ME.

Past medical history

The only clearly striking finding is a high frequency of atopic or allergic illness (in approximately 50%), as was first highlighted by Jones and his colleagues (Olson et al., 1986a,b), and confirmed by Straus et al. (1988).

Physical examination

Table 3 lists unusual and abnormal findings observed in 15–50% of our patients: fevers; unusually low basal body temperature (below 97°F); posterior cervical adenopathy; and abnormal tests of balance (Romberg and tandem gait). We are conducting physical examinations of patients and matched, asymptomatic control subjects, by observers blinded to the identity of the patients, to see if we can rigorously identify physical examination abnormalities that are seen more often in CFS than in healthy individuals.

Standard laboratory testing

On standard hematologic testing, it appears that results outside the normal range are seen in 15–50% of patients: leucocytosis; leucopenia; relative lymphocytosis; atypical lymphocytosis; monocytosis; elevated sedimentation rate; and unusually low sedimentation rates. These results have not yet been formally compared to results in a control group of healthy patients.

Standard serum chemistry testing is remarkable only for modestly elevated transaminases on one or more occasions in a quarter of the patients we have seen. None of these patients has had serologic evidence of active infection with hepatitis A, B or C virus.

Immunologic testing

We and others (DuBois et al., 1984; Jones et al., 1985; Straus et al., 1985; Peter and Wallace, 1988; Olson et al., 1986b; Wallace and Margolin, 1988; Cheney et al., 1989; Tosato et al., 1985; Caligiuri et al., 1987; Murdoch, 1988) have found evidence of subtle and diffuse dysfunction: partial hypogammaglobulinemia (25–80%); partial hypergammaglobulinemia (10–20%); low levels of autoantibodies, particularly antinuclear antibodies (15–35%); low levels of circulating immune complexes (30–50%); elevated ratios of helper/suppressor T cells (20–35%); reduced EBV-specific cytotoxic T cell activity; reduced in vitro synthesis of interleukin-2 and interferon by cultured lymphocytes; increased IgE-positive T and B cells; deficient functional activity of natural killer cells; anergy or hypoergy by skin testing; and elevated levels of various cytokines. Some investigators have found increased levels of circulating interferon, whereas others have not. Straus demonstrated a significant increase in levels of leukocyte 2',5'-oligoadenylate synthetase activity, an enzyme induced during acute viral infections (Straus *et al.*, 1985). In approximately half of the few patients who have had lumbar punctures there has been pleocytosis, predominantly lymphocytic, without other abnormalities.

Neurological evaluation

Formal neuropsychological tests of cognition performed by Bastien, Albert and their colleagues (unpublished data) suggest that one-third to one-half of our patients have cognitive impairment—particularly impairment of concentration and attention. It is the judgment of the neuropsychologists that the pattern of test performance suggests an 'organic' deficit, rather than cognitive dysfunction secondary to a mood disorder.

Because of the cognitive and neurological complaints, and because of the similarity of some of these symptoms to symptoms experienced by patients with multiple sclerosis, we obtained magnetic resonance images (MRI) of the brain. In the majority of over 100 patients studied in collaboration with our colleagues P. Cheney, R. Biddle, D. Peterson and F. Jolesz, there are multiple areas of high-intensity signal in the subcortical white matter (unpublished data). A comparison with MRI findings in healthy control subjects of the same age and sex is being conducted.

VIRUSES AND CHRONIC FATIGUE SYNDROME

As each of the chronic fatigue syndromes we have discussed has found its way into the medical literature, it has brought with it the speculation that the illness was initiated by an infectious agent. The speculation has centered most often on viruses, although non-viral infectious agents may also be able to trigger a similar postinfectious malaise (Rosene *et al.*, 1982; Salit, 1985).

ME was thought for some time to be produced by a less virulent strain of polio virus. Recently, Mowbray has reopened the possibility that enteroviral infection may indeed be associated with some cases of CFS, by demonstrating circulating enteroviral antigen more often in patients than in control subjects (Yousef *et al.*, 1988).

EBV has also been the subject of the investigation in the United States. Most studies of chronic fatigue syndrome patients have found higher levels of VCA-IgG and EA-Ab in patients than in matched, healthy control subjects; also, antibody to Epstein–Barr nuclear antigens (EBNA) is absent in 10–30% of patients, whereas this is thought to be quite unusual in seropositive healthy individuals (Tobi *et al.*, 1982; DuBois *et al.*, 1984; Jones *et al.*, 1985; Straus *et al.*, 1985). Moreover, it has been shown that antibody to EBNA-1 is absent in 10–30% of patients; it is absent more often in the more severely ill patients (Miller et al., 1987). Absence of antibody to EBNA-1 is thought to be quite unusual in healthy individuals, in patients convalescing from acute infectious mononucleosis, and in patients with cancer. It is, however, seen frequently in children with AIDS (Miller et al., 1987).

In our judgment, there is no strong evidence that EBV plays a *primary* role in the pathogenesis of most cases of chronic fatigue syndrome: there are substantial numbers of patients who have normal (or absent) antibody levels to EBV but who are clinically indistinguishable from the other patients; furthermore, one report cites evidence that other herpes viruses can also be reactivated in this illness and that antibody levels to measles virus may also be higher (Holmes et al., 1987). In those few patients who develop a chronic, debilitating condition directly following acute infectious mononucleosis, the parsimonious assumption is that EBV may be playing a role in the chronic illness, since it is very likely to have caused the acute illness. However, in most patients with CFS, the EBV serologic results in most patients probably represent *secondary* evidence of some immunologic perturbation, rather than a primary pathogenetic role for EBV. Nevertheless, secondary reactivation of EBV may not be just an epiphenomenon, as will be discussed shortly.

The recently discovered human herpes virus-6 (HHV-6) is an interesting candidate for a pathogenetic role in some cases of chronic fatigue syndrome, primarily because it is lymphotropic and gliotropic (Salahuddin et al., 1986; Josephs et al., 1986; Ablashi et al., 1987). There appears to be a serologic association of this virus with both chronic fatigue syndrome and fibromyalgia (Buchwald et al., 1988; Komaroff et al., 1988; Ablashi et al., 1988), although some studies have not found such an association. Studies to assess active replication of HHV-6 are now underway. At this time, the evidence seems most consistent with the hypothesis that this virus may be secondarily reactivated in this syndrome, as are other viruses; however, a primary role for HHV-6 in the pathogenesis of this illness remains possible.

In this decade of the human retroviruses, it was inevitable that there should be some speculation linking retroviruses to chronic fatigue syndrome. We and others have found no evidence that any of the known human retroviruses are involved with this syndrome. Furthermore, we have found no evidence of reverse transcriptase activity in the supernatants of primary lymphocyte cultures from a number of our sickest patients.

CFS AND PSYCHOLOGICAL ILLNESS

As stated at the outset, most patients seeking medical care for chronic fatigue are probably suffering from a primary affective disorder (depression and/or anxiety). Moreover, most patients seeking medical care for chronic fatigue probably do not have CFS (Kroenke *et al.*, 1988; Manu *et al.*, 1988).

What is the role, if any, of affective disorders in CFS? This is a difficult issue to study, since the affective disorders are defined in part by symptoms that could also reflect a 'physical'illness. In our experience, most patients with CFS perceive themselves as becoming *secondarily* depressed and/or anxious following the (usually sudden) onset of their illness. According to data from a self-administered questionnaire, 80–90% of these same patients deny suffering from depression or anxiety in the years prior to their illness. Yet more intensive interviewing by a trained interviewer, using the Diagnostic Interview Schedule, suggests that affective illness predated the onset of CFS in about 35% of our patients (unpublished data). Kruesi and colleagues, using the same structured interview, found a major depressive disorder in only 7% of CFS patients, in the years *prior to* the onset of their illness (Kruesi *et al.*, 1989), a rate about the same as in the population at large (Robins *et al.*, 1984). (Ironically, Kruesi's report has often been cited as evidence that CFS is a primarily psychological disorder, since many of the patients developed a secondadry, reactive depression.) And the same team, studying largely the same patients, found abnormalities of the hypothalamic–pituitary–adrenal axis that were entirely different from those seen in patients with major affective disorder (Demitrack *et al.*, 1989).

Even if it were true that patients with CFS more frequently have an affective disorder that predates the onset of chronic fatigue, what might that mean? Those who conceive of affective disorders as purely mental phenomena disconnected from the body may conclude that the symptoms in patients with CFS reflect no physical abnormality, just a heightened awareness of and concern about physical sensations, possibly coupled with a desire to attribute their dysfunctional state to a physical illness.

We are more inclined to view affective disorders as biologically determined disorders of neurochemistry, disorders that can affect immune function and that, in turn, can be perturbed by the immune system. According to this model, 'mind' and 'body' are not separate and discrete, but inevitably linked: biological forces that increase the likelihood of affective disorder may also increase vulnerability to disorders of immunity. In patients with CFS, who have a current and/or past affective disorder, and who also have evidence of immune dysfunction and active viral infection, it may never be possible to determine whether the affective disorder, the immune dysfunction or the viral infection came first. Rather, the practical question is what form of therapy will be most effective: psychotherapy, pharmacotherapy of the affective disorder, 'immune modulating' pharmacotherapy, antimicrobial therapy, or some combination of these. There are no good studies of these issues, at this time.

A MODEL FOR THE PATHOGENESIS OF CFS

Knowledge about CFS is limited. The available data permit many models, but provide strong support for none of them. My own current view of this illness is reflected in Figure 1. We currently view CFS as primarily an immunologic disturbance, one that allows reactivation of latent and ineradicable infectious agents, particularly viruses. The reactivation of these viruses may only be an epiphenomenon. However, we feel it is more likely that, once secondarily reactivated, these viruses contribute to the morbidity of CFS—directly, by damaging certain tissues (e.g. the pharyngeal mucosa), and indirectly, by eliciting an ongoing immunologic response. In particular, the elaboration of various cytokines (e.g. interferon-α and interlukin-2) as part of this ongoing immunologic war may produce many of the symptoms of CFS—the fatigue, myalgias, fevers, adenopathy, and even the disorders of mood and cognition. This is suggested by the finding of increased levels of various cytokines in CFS and related conditions (Peter and Wallace, 1988; Wallace and Margolin, 1988; Cheney *et al.*, 1989), and the experience with infusing cytokines made by recombinant DNA techniques for various therapeutic purposes (Muss *et al.*, 1987; Quesada *et al.*, 1986; Erstoff and Kirkwood, 1984; Rosenberg *et al.*, 1987; Belldegrun *et al.*, 1987; Denicoff *et al.*, 1987; Ettinghausen *et al.*, 1988).

Whatever the course, the symptoms of CFS lead to some degree of disability in every patient. As with any illness, the degree of disability must be due, in part, to psychological factors.

What triggers the immune dysfunction in the first place? It is likely that many factors could do so: atopic disorders, exogenous lymphotropic infectious agents, environmental toxins, stress and, as argued earlier, the biology of an underlying affective disorder. This illness seems most likely to have a multifactorial etiology, like most illnesses. While the discovery of a single explanation, such as a novel infectious agent or a specific inherited

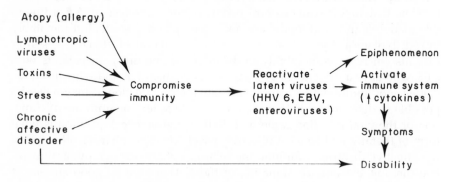

Figure 1 Current favorite model

immunologic defect, might simplify the search for solutions to this illness, such simple explanations are unlikely to be true.

ACKNOWLEDGEMENTS

This work was supported by grants 1RO1A126788 and 1RO1A127314 from the National Institute of Allergy and Infectious Diseases, and grants from the Minann and Rowland Foundations.

REFERENCES

Ablashi, D. V., Salahuddin, S. Z., Josephs, S. F. *et al.* (1987) HBLV (or HHV-6) in human cell lines. *Nature*, **329**, 207.

Ablashi, D. V., Josephs, S. F., Buchbinder, A. *et al.* (1988) Human B-lymphotropic virus (human herpesvirus-6). *Journal of Virological Methods*, **21**, 29–48.

Acheson, E. D. (1959) The clinical syndrome variously called benign myalgic encephalomyelitis, Iceland disease and epidemic neuromyasthenia. *American Journal of Medicine*, **4**, 569–595.

Allan, F. N. (1944) The differential diagnosis of weakness and fatigue. *New England Journal of Medicine*, **231**, 414–418.

Ballow, M., Seeley, J., Purtilo, D. T., St Onge, S., Sakamoto, K. and Rickles, F. R. (1982) Familial chronic mononucleosis. *Annals of Internal Medicine*, **97**, 821–825.

Barsky, A. J. I. (1981) Hidden reasons some patients visit doctors. *Annals of Internal Medicine*, **94**, 492–498.

Belldegrun, A., Webb, D. E., Austin, H. A. I. *et al.* (1987) Effects of interleukin 2 on renal function in patients receiving immunotherapy for advanced cancer. *Annals of Internal Medicine*, **106**, 817–822.

Bengtsson, A., Henriksson, K. G. and Larsson, J. (1986) Reduce high-energy phosphate levels in the painful muscles of patients with primary fibromyalgia. *Arthritis and Rheumatism*, **20**, 817–821.

Benjamin, J. E. and Hoyt, R. C. (1945) Disability following postvaccinal (yellow fever) hepatitis. *Journal of the American Medical Association*, **128**, 319–324.

Bonfede, P., Nelson, D., Clark, S., Goldberg, L. and Bennett, R. (1987) Exercising muscle blood flow in patients with fibrositis. *Arthritis and Rheumatism*, **30**, S14.

Buchwald, D., Saxinger, K. C., Goldenberg, D.L., Gallo, R. C. and Komaroff A. L. (1988) Primary fibromyalgia (fibrositis) and human herpesvirus-6: a serologic association. *Clinical Research*, **36**, 332A.

Caligiuri, M., Murray, C., Buchwald, D. *et al.* (1987) Phenotypic and functional deficiency of natural killer cells in patients with chronic fatigue syndrome. *Journal of Immunology*, **139**, 3306–3313.

Campbell, S. M., Clark, S., Tindall, E. S., Forehand, M. E. and Bennett, R. M. (1983) Clinical characteristics of fibrositis. I. A 'blinded' controlled study of symptoms and tender points. *Arthritis and Rheumatism*, **26**, 132–137.

Caro, X. U., Wolfe, F., Johnston, W. H. and Smith, A. L. (1986) A controlled and blinded study of immunoreactant deposition at the dermal–epidermal junction of patients with primary fibrositis syndrome. *Journal of Rheumatology*, **13**, 1086–1092.

Cathey, M. A., Wolfe, F., Kleinheksel, S. M. and Hawley, D. J. (1986) Socioeconomic impact of fibrositis. *American Journal of Medicine*, **81**, 578–584.

Cheney, P. R., Dorman, S. E. and Bell, D. (1989) Interleukin-2 and the chronic fatigue syndrome. *Annals of Internal Medicine*, **110**, 321.

Cluff, L. L., Trever, R. W., Imboden, J. B. and Canter, A. (1959) Brucellosis II: medical aspects of delayed convalescence. *Archives of Internal Medicine*, **103**, 393–405.

Demitrack, M. A., Dale, J. K., Gold, P. W., Chrousos, G. P. and Straus, S. E. (1989) Neuroendocrine abnormalities in patients with chronic fatigue syndrome. *Clinical Research*, **37**, 532A.

Denicoff, K. D., Rubinow, D. R., Papa, M. X. *et al.* (1987) The neuropsychiatric effects of treatment with interleukin 2 and lymphokine activated killer cells. *Annals of Internal Medicine*, **107**, 293–300.

Dinerman, H., Goldenberg, D. L. and Felson, D. T. (1986) A prospective evaluation of 118 patients with the fibromyalgia syndrome: prevalence of Raynaud's phenomenon, sicca symptoms, ANA, low complement, and Ig deposition at the dermal–epidermal junction. *Journal of Rheumatology*, **13**, 368–373.

DuBois, R. E., Seeley, J. K., Brus, I. *et al.* (1984) Chronic mononucleosis syndrome. *Southern Medical Journal*, **77**, 1376–1382.

Edson, C. M., Cohen, L. K., Henle, W. and Strominger, J. L. (1983) An unusually high-titer human anti-Epstein Barr virus (EBV) serum and its use in the study of EBV-specific proteins synthesized *in vitro* and *in vivo*. *Journal of Immunology*, **130**, 919–924.

Erstoff, M. S. and Kirkwood, J. M. (1984) Changes in the bone marrow of cancer patients treated with recombinant interferon alpha 2. *American Journal of Medicine*, **76**, 593–596.

Ettinghausen, S. E., Puri, R. K. and Rosenberg, S. A. (1988) Increased vascular permeability in organs mediated by the systemic administration of lymphokine activated killer cells and recombinant interleukin 2 in mice. *Journal of the National Cancer Institute*, **80**, 178–188.

Felson, D. T. and Goldenberg, D. L. (1986) The natural history of fibromyalgia. *Arthritis and Rheumatism*, **29**, 1522–1526.

Goldenberg, D. L. (1987) Fibromyalgia syndrome: An emerging but controversial condition. *Journal of the American Medical Association*, **257**, 2782–2787.

Hamblin, T. J., Hussain, J., Akbar, A. N., Tang, Y. C., Smith, J. L. and Jones, D. B. (1983) Immunological reason for chronic ill health after infectious mononucleosis. *British Medical Journal*, **287**, 85–88.

Henderson, D. A. and Shelokov, A. (1959) Epidemic neuromyasthenia—clinical syndrome. *New England Journal of Medicine*, **260**, 757–764.

Hickson, D. D., Gravelyn, T. R. and Wharton, M. (1981) Giant cell arteritis and polymyalgia rheumatica in a conjugal pair. *Arthritis and Rheumatism*, **24**, 1448–1450.

Hoeper, E. W., Nycz, G. R., Cleary, P. D., Regier, D. A. and Goldberg, I. D. (1979) Estimated prevalence of RDC mental disorder in primary medical care. *International Journal of Mental Health*, **8**, 6–15.

Holmes, G. P., Kaplan, J. E., Stewart, J. A., Hunt, B., Pinsky, P. F. and Schonberger, L. B. (1987) A cluster of patients with a chronic mononucleosis-like syndrome: Is Epstein–Barr virus the cause? *Journal of the American Medical Association*, **257**, 2297–2302.

Holmes, G. P., Kaplan, J. E., Gantz, N. M. *et al.* (1988) Chronic fatigue syndrome: A working case definition. *Annals of Internal Medicine*, **108**, 387–389.

Imboden, J. B., Canter, A., Cluff, L. E. and Trever, R. W. (1959) Brucellosis III: psychologic aspects of delayed convalescence. *Archives of Internal Medicine*, **103**, 406–414.

Isaacs, R. (1948) Chronic infectious mononucleosis. *Blood*, **3**, 858–861.

Jones, J. F., Ray, O. G., Minnich, L. L., Hicks, M. J., Kibler, R. and Lucas, D. O. (1975) Evidence for active Epstein–Barr virus infection in patients with persistent unexplained illnesses: Elevated anti-early antigen antibodies. *Annals of Internal Medicine*, **102**, 1–7.

Josephs, S. F., Salahuddin, S. Z., Ablashi, D. V., Schacter, F., Wong-Staal, F. and Gallo, R. C. (1986) Genomic analysis of the human B-lymphotropic virus (HBLV). *Science*, **234**, 601–603.

Kalyan-Raman, U. P., Kalyan-Raman, K., Yunus, M. B. and Masi, A. T. (1984) Muscle pathology in primary fibromyalgia syndrome: a light microscopic, histochemical and ultrastructural study. *Journal of Rheumatology*, **11**, 808–813.

Katerndahl, D. A. (1983) Fatigue of uncertain etiology. *Family Medical Review*, **1**, 26–38.

Kessler, L. G., Cleary, P. D. and Burke, J. D. (1985) Psychiatric disorders in primary care. *Archives of General Psychiatry*, **42**, 583–587.

Kleinman, A. (1982) Neurasthenia and depression: a study of somatization and culture in China. *Culture, Medicine and Psychiatry*, **6**, 117–190.

Komaroff, A. L. (1987) The 'chronic mononucleosis' syndromes. *Hospital Practice*, **22**, 71–75.

Komaroff, A. L. and Geiger, A. (1989) Does the CDC working case definition of chronic fatigue syndrome (CFS) identify a distinct group? *Clinical Research*, **37**, 778A.

Komaroff, A. L., Saxinger, C., Buchwald, D., Geiger, A. and Gallo, R. C. (1983) A chronic 'post-viral' fatigue syndrome with neurologic features: serologic association with human herpesvirus-6. *Clinical Research*, **36**, 743A.

Kroenke, K., Wood, D. R., Mangelsdorff, A. D., Meier, N. J. and Powell, J. B. (1988) Chronic fatigue in primary care. Prevalence, patient characteristics, and outcome. *Journal of the American Medical Association*, **260**, 929–934.

Kruesi, M. J. P., Dale, J. and Straus, S. E. (1989) Psychiatric diagnoses in patients who have chronic fatigue syndrome. *Journal of Clinical Psychiatry*, **50**, 53–56.

Lawton, A. H., Rich, T. A., McLendon, S., Gates, E. H. and Bond, J. O. (1970) Follow-up studies of St. Louis encephalitis in Florida: Reevaluation of the emotional and health status of the survivors five years after acute illness. *Southern Medical Journal*, **63**, 66–71.

Littlejohn, G. O., Weinstein, C. and Helme, R. D. (1987) Increased neurogenic inflammation in fibrositis syndrome. *Journal of Rheumatology*, **14**, 1022–1025.

Lund, N., Bengtsson, A. and Throborg, P. (1986) Muscle tissue oxygen pressure in primary fibromyalgia. *Scandianvian Journal of Rheumatology*, **15**, 165–173.

Manu, P., Lane, T. J. and Matthews, D. A. (1978) The frequency of the chronic fatigue syndrome in patients with symptoms of persistent fatigue. *Annals of Internal Medicine*, **109**, 554–556.

Medical staff of the Royal Free Hospital (1957). An outbreak of encephalomyelitis in the Royal Free Hospital group, London, in 1955. *British Medical Journal*, **2**, 895–904.

Miller, G., Grogan, E. and Rowe, D. (1987) Selective lack of antibody to a component of EB nuclear antigen in patients with chronic Epstein–Barr virus infection. *Journal of Infectious Diseases*, **156**, 26–35.

Moldofsky, H. and Scarisbrick, P. (1976) Induction of neurasthenic musculoskeletal pain syndrome by selective sleep stage deprivation. *Psychosomatic Medicine*, **38**, 35–44.

Moldofsky, H., Scarisbrick, P., England, R. and Smythe, H. (1975) Musculoskeletal symptoms and non-REM sleep disturbance in patients with 'fibrositis syndrome' and healthy subjects. *Psychosomatic Medicine*, **37**, 341–351.

Morrison, J. D. (1980). Fatigue as a presenting complaint in family practice. *Journal of Family Practice*, **10**, 795–801.

Murdoch, J. C. (1983). Cell-mediated immunity in patients with myalgic encephalomyelitis syndrome. *New Zealand Medical Journal*, **101**, 511–512.

Muss, H. B., Costanzi, J. J., Leavitt, R. *et al.* (1987) Recombinant alpha interferon in renal cell carcinoma: a randomized trial of two routes of administration. *Journal of Clinical Oncology*, **5**, 286–291.

Nelson, E., Kirk, J. and McHugo, G. *et al.* (1987) Chief complaint fatigue: a longitudinal study from the patient's perspective. *Family Practice Research Journal*, **6**, 175–188.

Nielsen, A. C. and Williams, T. A. (1980) Depression in ambulatory medical patients. *Archives of General Psychiatry*, **37**, 999–1004.

Olson, G. B., Kanaan, M. N., Gersuk, G. M., Kelley, L. M. and Jones, J. F. (1986a) Correlation between allergy and persistent Epstein–Barr virus infections in chronic-active Epstein–Barr virus-infected patients. *Journal of Allergy and Clinical Immunology*, **78**, 308–314.

Olson, G. B., Kanaan, M. N., Kelley, L. M. and Jones, J. F. (1986b) Specific allergen-induced Epstein–Barr nuclear antigen-positive B cells from patients with chronic-active Epstein–Barr virus infections. *Journal of Allergy and Clinical Immunology*, **78**, 315–320.

Paul, O. (1987) DaCosta's syndrome or neurocirculatory asthenia. *British Heart Journal*, **58**, 306–315.

Peter, J. B. and Wallace, D. J. (1988) Abnormalities of immune regulation in the primary fibromyalgia syndrome. *Arthritis and Rheumatism*, **31**, 24.

Poskanzer, D. C., Henderson, D. A., Kunkle, E. C., Kalter, S. S., Clement, W. B. and Bond, J. O. (1957) Epidemic neuromyasthenia: an outbreak in Punta Gorda, Florida. *New England Journal of Medicine*, **257**, 356–364.

Quesada, J. R., Talpaz, M., Rios, A., Kurzrock, P. and Glutterman, J. U. (1986) Clinical toxicity of interferons in cancer patients. *Journal of Clinical Oncology*, **4**, 234–243.

Reifler, B. V., Okimoto, J. T., Heidrich, F. E. and Inui, T. S. (1979) Recognition of depression in a university-based family medicine residency program. *Journal of Family Practice*, **9**, 623–628.

Robins, L. N., Helzer, J. E., Weissman, M. M. *et al.* (1984) Lifetime prevalence of specific psychiatric disorders in three sites. *Archives of General Psychiatry*, **41**, 949–958.

Rosenberg, S. A., Lotze, M. T., Muul, L. M. *et al.* (1987) A progress report on the treatment of 157 patients with advanced cancer using lymphokine activated killer cells and interleukin 2 or high dose interleukin 2 alone. *New England Journal of Medicine*, **316**, 889–905.

Rosene, K. A., Copass, M. K., Kastner, L. S., Nolan, C. M. and Eschenbach, D. A. (1982) Persistent neuropsychological sequelae of toxic shock syndrome. *Annals of Internal Medicine*, **96**, 865–870.

Russell, I. J., Vipraio, G. A., Tower, Z. *et al.* (1988) Abnormal natural killer cell activity in fibrositis syndrome is responsive *in vitro* to IL-2. *Arthritis and Rheumatism*, **31**, 24.

Salahuddin, S. Z., Ablashi, D. V., Markham, P. D. *et al.* (1986) Isolation of a new virus, HBLV, in patients with lymphoproliferative disorders. *Science*, **324**, 596–601.

Salit, I. E. (1985) Sporadic postinfectious neuromyasthenia. *Canadian Medical Association Journal*, **133**, 659–663.

Schooley, R. T., Carey, R. W., Miller, G. *et al.* (1986) Chronic Epstein–Barr virus infection associated with fever and interstitial pneumonitis. Clinical and serologic features and response to antiviral chemotherapy. *Annals of Internal Medicine*, **104**, 636–643.

Shelokov, A., Habel, K., Verder, E. and Welsh, W. (1957) Epidemic neuromyasthenia: an outbreak of poliomyelitis-like illness in student nurses. *New England Journal of Medicine*, **257**, 345–355.

Sigurdsson, B. and Gudmondsson, K. R. (1956) Clinical findings six years after outbreak of Akureyri disease. *Lancet*, **1**, 766–777.

Sigurdsson, B., Sigurjonsson, J., Sigurdsson, J. H. J., Thorkelsson, J. and Gudmundsson, K. R. (1950) A disease epidemic in Iceland simulating poliomyelitis. *American Journal of Hygiene*, **52**, 222–238.

Stoeckle, J. D., Zola, I. K. and Davidson, G. E. (1964) The quantity and significance of psychological distress in medical patients. *Journal of Chronic Diseases*, **17**, 959–970.

Straus, S. E. (1988) The chronic mononucleosis syndrome. *Journal of Infectious Diseases*, **157**, 405–412.

Straus, S. E., Tosato, G., Armstrong, G. *et al.* (1985) Persisting illness and fatigue in adults with evidence of Epstein–Barr virus infection. *Annals of Internal Medicine*, **102**, 7–16.

Straus, S. E., Dale, J. K., Wright, R. and Metcalfe, D. D. (1988) Allergy and the chronic fatigue syndrome. *Journal of Allergy and Clinical Immunology*, **81**, 791–795.

Tobi, M., Morag, A., Ravid, Z. *et al.* (1982) Prolonged atypical illness associated with serologic evidence of persistent Epstein–Barr virus infection. *Lancet*, **1**, 61–64.

Tosato, G., Straus, S., Henle, W., Pike, S. E. and Blaese, R. M. (1985) Characteristic T cell dysfunction in patients with chronic active Epstein–Barr virus infection (chronic infectious mononucleosis). *Journal of Immunology*, **134**, 3082–3088.

Wallace, D. J. and Margolin, K. (1988) Acute-onset fibromyalgia as a complication of interleukin-2 therapy. *Arthritis and Rheumatism*, **31**, S24.

Wolfe, F. and Cathey, M. A. (1983) Prevalence of primary and secondary fibrositis. *Journal of Rheumatology*, **10**, 965–968.

Wolfe, F., Cathey, M. A. and Kleinheksel, S. M. (1984) Fibrositis (fibromyalgia) in rheumatoid arthritis. *Journal of Rheumatology*, **11**, 814–881.

Wolfe, F., Hawley, D. J., Cathey, M. A., Caro, X. J. and Russell, I. J. (1985) Fibrositis: symptom frequency and criteria for diagnosis. *Journal of Rheumatology*, **10**, 211–222.

Wolfe, F. and Cathey, M. A. (1990) Assessment of functional ability in patients with fibromyalgia. *Archives of Internal Medicine*, **150**, 460.

Yousef, G. E., Bell, E. J., Mann, G. F. *et al.* (1988) Chronic enterovirus infection in patients with postviral fatigue syndrome. *Lancet*, **1**, 146–150.

Yunus, M., Masi, A. T., Calabro, J. J., Miller, K. A. and Feigenbaum, G. L. (1981) Primary fibromyalgia (fibrositis): Clinical study of 50 patients with matched normal controls. *Seminars in Arthritis and Rheumatism*, **11**, 151–171.

3

Enteroviruses and Epstein–Barr Virus in ME

James Mowbray

St Mary's Hospital Medical School, London, UK

INTRODUCTION

The virological basis for some forms of ME arose from several pieces of evidence. The most prominent, and perhaps the most misleading, was that the onset of symptoms was, in a large fraction of patients, preceded by an 'influenzal' illness. The value of this presentation in defining a viral infection is poor, but, worse than that, it does not necessarily imply an infective illness at all. The availability of recombinant interferon has made interferon available for administration to patients in large quantities. It has been used both for chronic viral infections, especially hepatitis B virus (HBV), and for treatment of patients with several kinds of cancer. Administration of a large dose of interferon is rapidly followed by the symptoms of 'flu, although without the superadded bacterial infection with cough and purulent sputum. The lethargy, nasal congestion, myalgia and general illness are quite profound. A number of noninfectious immune reactions can also be associated with similar symptoms, when again the symptoms are produced by liberation of interferon, as part of the immune reaction to a foreign antigen. Immunisation of women with large doses of lymphocytes from another individual produces in some of them a reaction almost identical to 'flu. These symptoms are generally evidence of interferon production as part of the immune response. This is important, but, as the repeated attacks of 'flu-like illness common with ME are often construed as multiple separate infections, rather than fluctuation of interferon production during a single chronic infection, the ME patient may say that they get worse every time they get a virus, or even that they are getting such infections unusually frequently. Instead, they

Post-viral Fatigue Syndrome. Edited by R. Jenkins and J. Mowbray
© 1991 John Wiley & Sons Ltd

have a single chronic infection with fluctuating 'flu-like symptoms related to the interferon response at the time.

It was recognised that a fraction of the patients with ME had some evidence of infection with known viruses, and, as will be shown, there are at least two of these.

The viruses incriminated were predominantly enteroviruses in Britain, and Epstein–Barr virus (EBV) in the USA. The recognition of enteroviruses as a cause largely arose from the serological identification of these viruses from some of the geographical outbreaks of ME (Bell *et al.*, 1988; McCartney *et al.*, 1986). In some of these it was found that there was a widespread epidemic of an enterovirus, when virtually the whole of the population were briefly infected. A few of those infected appear to be unable to eliminate the virus rapidly, and develop the symptom complex called ME. It is not clear in the studies of those outbreaks how many people developed a long-term, asymptomatic infection.

The demonstration of persistent infection with virus does not, of course, prove causality. The findings that the virus is in the muscles or brain fulfil at least one of Koch's postulates for the aetiology of a disease by an infectious agent. Another is the observation that as patients recover from ME those with enteroviruses progressively lose the viral protein detectable in the serum. Additionally, if an agent such as normal human IgG is used to produce remission of symptoms this is also associated with disappearance of detectable IgG from the serum. When the patient relapses after a single dose of the IgG the VP1 antigen of the enteroviruses becomes detectable again in the serum (Figure 1).

STRUCTURE AND REPLICATION OF ENTEROVIRUSES

As most of this chapter is devoted to enteroviral infections producing ME while the virus infection persists, the reader should have some idea of these viruses and the type of infection they cause. There are some contrasts with EBV, which causes a minority of the components of ME syndrome, more commonly being associated with the subacute active infection known as infectious mononucleosis or glandular fever.

The enteroviruses are composed of more than 70 different antigenic types of virus, of which the polio viruses are the most commonly known. Entoviruses are very common in this country and produce epidemics of 'summer colds'. Thus everyone is exposed to about one enterovirus a year, in the summer months. They are highly infectious, but the great majority of the population eliminate the infection in a few days. Only a small minority retain the infection and may go on to develop ME symptoms.

Figure 2 shows the composition of the genome of enteroviruses. They are

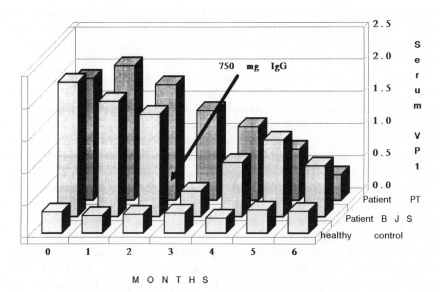

Figure 1 Levels of VP1 protein in serum of patients with ME. The back row shows an untreated patient with declining levels of VP1 as she improved over the months. The middle row shows a patient who was given a single dose of human IgG (750 mg) with marked amelioration of symptoms for about four weeks. The VP1 disappeared from the serum during the period of remission but reappeared as symptoms recurred. IgG injection given as arrow

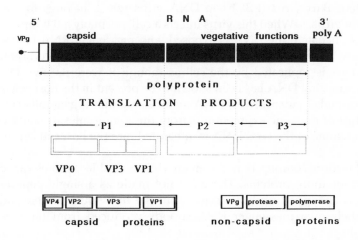

Figure 2 The genome of enteroviruses. The viral RNA encodes a single polyprotein which is subject to proteolytic digestion in the cell after its production into the individual viral proteins. These are the capsid proteins VP1–4 and two virus-coded enzymes. RNA polymerase and a protease

small, simple RNA viruses. Their genes code for two enzyme proteins which are not a structural part of the virus, and the structural proteins, VP1, VP2, VP3 and VP4. There is a nonstructural protein which is essential for replication of the virus, the RNA polymerase.

Whereas in mammalian cells messenger RNA is made from a DNA template, in the enteroviruses RNA polymerase, an enzyme found in picornaviruses, of which the enteroviruses from a part, is used to make new messenger RNA directly from an RNA template. The messenger RNA within the virus is used inside the infected cell to make a single long peptide, the polyprotein. This is cleaved by proteolytic enzymes, some of which are coded for in the RNA, into separate proteins. The newly synthesised RNA is combined with the viral structural proteins and assembled in the cell to become a complete infectious viral particle. This is only released from the cell by death and disruption of the host cell. The released particle then attaches to another cell surface, and penetrates the cell membrane. This is rapidly associated with removal of the protein coat from the virus, revealing the viral RNA, when the replication process starts again. Each cell cycle produces hundreds of particles in each infected cell which are released when the cytopathic effect of the virus replication results in cell death and disruption. Incomplete virus, unable to complete assembly of infectious virus within the cell, is not usually associated with cell death, but fragments of the virus may persist for a while within the cell. As will be seen this appears to be the state of virus infecting muscle cells in ME. Elsewhere in the body, cells are disrupting having made complete, infectious viral particles.

Epstein–Barr virus (EBV) is a DNA virus which belongs to the herpes group of viruses. When this virus infects a cell, normally a B lymphocyte, the virus is uncoated, the DNA is exposed, and messenger RNA is made from the DNA. This RNA is used by the cell to make the viral-coded proteins. The viral DNA is replicated by the cell as though it were its own DNA. The majority of viral DNA has been shown to be present in the host cell nuclei as the episomal circular form of DNA molecules, and it is generally considered that most of the gene expression is from these molecules. It is not yet clear whether some of the viral DNA is integrated into the host cell chromosomal DNA.

EBV is more complex than the enteroviruses, and its genome carries information for more proteins. These are not made as a single peptide strand which is choopped up by enzymes, but the individual proteins are made from their own messenger RNA strands produced from the viral DNA template.

Although EBV as a DNA virus has a mechanism for remaining dormant in the cell, enteroviruses cannot do this, and there is no mechanism for them to be dormant, or for their genome to survive in the cell without virus replication. There is another difference in EBV compared with enteroviruses, and that is that the host cell can survive, producing virus particles, which are extruded through the cell membrane. At this time they gain the outer viral coat wrapping, the surface protein having been previously inserted in the cell membrane. Cell death is not therefore a necessity for virus release, and a cell may survive for prolonged periods as a virus factory, continuing to release very large numbers of infectious virus particles.

IMMUNE RESPONSES TO ENTEROVIRUSES AND EPSTEIN–BARR VIRUS

A cell, infected by either virus, has viral proteins inserted in the cell membrane. This means that the infected cell can be identified by these as infected, and is susceptible to attack by specifically immune lymphocytes, cytotoxic T lymphocytes (CTL), which can kill the infected cells, but not uninfected cells which do not have viral proteins on the outside of the cell membrane. Antibody-binding cells may also be able to kill the infected cells and anti-viral antibodies with complement may result in their phagocytosis and destruction. The most important role of antibodies is, however, their ability to neutralise the virus. Here, antibodies bound to surface proteins of the virus may prevent the virus attachment to cells, and hence neutralise their infectivity.

There are some specific differences in human immune responses to viruses and other infections, but for the most part similar mechanisms are involved. Our ability to recover from acute virus infections is somewhat different from the processes which may occur when there is a long-term virus infection, without elimination of the virus.

Viruses elicit immune responses against any of the immunogenic parts of the virus, but the protective responses are involved in cellular and humoral responses to the external protein components. Antibodies directed against these components may neutralise infectivity of the virus. Any class of immunoglobulin can neutralise viruses, but IgG is most potent. The IgA antibodies are important as the neutralising antibodies present on mucosal surfaces, preventing initial infection of a cell by the virus. This represents a very important part of resistance to a new infection in an immune individual.

The actual process of virus infection goes in stages. The first is the initial infection of a few cells, with replication of the virus in those cells. Depending on the virus, the infection spreads to other cells either by death of the cell releasing a large number of formed, infectious intracellular virus particles, or by the virus budding from the cell surface of a cell which survives as a virus factory. When a virus enters a cell, and the protein coat is removed inside it, the virus nucleic acid can switch off the host genes. The cell reads the virus genes in preference to its own genes, and will have its own genes suppressed to varying degrees. It may function fairly normally, or may lose quite a lot of its specialised functions as a differentiated cell.

When viruses infect cells they may make the cell produce α or β-interferon. In addition, when lymphocytes recognise the viral antigens and start to respond to them, they produce a number of cytokines, one of which is δ-interferon. Thus interferons may come from a number of sources, and can be picked up by normal cells. The interferon makes the cells more resistant to viral infection, acting in more than one way on the cell. The uncoating of the virus after entry into the cell may be prevented, and the replication process may be blocked at several points. This is a first part of the treatment of the infection, resulting in diminished spread of virus. This is aided by the liberation of neutralising antibody from lymphocytes, which can neutralise the virus before it is able to infect another cell.

CTL cells appear coincident with the appearance of IgG antibody. These are the most specific method by which the infection is overcome, as they result in death of the virus-infected cells, whereas the uninfected cells of the same type are not affected. If the factories budding infectious virus are killed, this represents a very considerable reduction in the new cells which are going to be infected and produce more virus. This is more important than the neutralising antibody in reducing the number of infected cells in the course of an infection. Obviously cure is the point when there are no virus-infected cells left. As was made clear in World War II, a more effective way of destroying an air force, better than shooting down planes, was to bomb the factories that produced them. Antiviral immunity appears to know that this is the most effective mechanism.

The viruses which most commonly produce ME are enteroviruses, and these viruses are cytopathic. Although the viruses do not bud from the surface, there is apparently some expression of virus antigens on the surface. There is thus still a mechanism for attack on the infected cells, but one must assume that neutralising antibody may represent a more important mechanism of control of infection with this virus. Herpes viruses, which include EBV, are budding viruses, and the infected cells are readily susceptible to the action of specifically immune cytotoxic T lymphocytes. When we come to consider the reasons why a patient may become chronically infected by these two kinds of virus, we will see different aspects of immunity at work.

Before discussing the tissue sites of virus infection in ME, or indeed the related chronic viral illnesses, one should look at the changes that can be produced by immunity itself. As already stated, there are cytokines produced by the infected cells, and γ-interferon from lymphocytes. In the early stage of the immune response there is the production of interleukin-1 (IL-1), another cytokine, from macrophages which have ingested viral antigens. This has several important actions in initiating the immune response, but IL-1 has one very important feature, and that is the production of fever. Fever is a presenting feature of many infections, but there is a great difference in the persistence of fever in ME due to enteroviruses, and that during the course of glandular fever. In the latter there may be several recurrences of fever, before final resolution of the disease, but with the enteroviruses in ME, although patients may complain that they feel feverish from time to time, measured pyrexia is found only in the initial phases. This might be interpreted as showing that the ME patients stop being immunised by the virus soon after onset, and this could be important in understanding why that patient had a chronic infection with the enterovirus, which the rest of the population will have eliminated in a few days.

DEMONSTRATION OF PERSISTENT ENTEROVIRAL INFECTION IN ME

As already stated, the United States was the place where it was assumed that the set of fatigue syndromes encompassed in the term CFS, or chronic fatigue syndrome, was due to EBV. It was largely the failure to substantiate this view that led them to use the term CFS, which excluded viruses from the definition, although there were several fatigue syndromes within the umbrella of CFS, and not just the syndrome which we recognise as ME. Nevertheless, even when the ME group was studied by Crawford and Smith, evidence for reactivation of EBV as a cause was only found in about 20% (Hotchin *et al.*, 1989). Their studies showed that this 20% had elevated levels of IgG antibody to the early antigen (EA) of EBV-infected lymphocytes, generally associated with antibody to the viral capsid antigen (VCA) as well. These are both found when there is reactivation of an old EBV infection, although in particular circumstance of ME it would seem more appropriate to call it persistent activation, rather than reactivation. It is of great interest that patients who had evidence of persistent enterovirus infection by the detection of VP1 in the blood, or IgM anti-enteroviral antibody, did not overlap with the EA IgG positive patients, so that ME may be associated with either virus. It remains to be seen if there are clinical differences in ME caused by the two types of virus, although my clinical experience is that muscle fatigue on exercise is a feature of the enteroviral patients, more than the EBV group. Certainly, some of the latter group appear to have central problems more than specific excessive muscle fatigue on exercise. They tend to show lethargy and inanition and do not wish to exercise, in contrast with the very poor exercise tolerance seen normally in the enteroviral group.

ARE THERE OTHER VIRUSES WHICH MIGHT BE INVOLVED?

When large-scale screening of ME patients for the VP1 antigen of enteroviruses was started, about 65% of all samples examined were positive. Continuing to screen the members of the ME Association over the next two years, during which time its membership increased about 20-fold, the fraction positive stayed about the same for one year, but then declined to about 30% of the total examined. At the same time Crawford and Smith found that about 20% of samples from ME patients were positive for the IgG antibody to the EA of EBV, and that these patients did not overlap the enteroviral ones (Hotchin *et al.*, 1989). This left about 15% not in either virus camp. The more recent drop in enteroviral fraction probably represents a fall in the fraction of membership of the ME Association seeking tests who have ME. Probably there is a considerable dilution with patients having other related syndromes, many of which will not be even of viral aetiology.

Is there evidence for another virus or viruses producing the muscle fatigue syndrome of ME? As we have considered with non-viral infections, 'fatigue states' exist with many infections, probably as a result of interferon production. Some of the 15% of ME patients might be in this category, or have another virus capable of producing the same muscle and brain changes. There is little, very poor, clinical evidence for *Varicella zoster*, and although many other viruses have been invoked, the evidence for them is zero. There was a preliminary report of a high incidence of herpes virus-6 in CFS in the United States, but when appropriate normal controls were examined, it was found that antibody, indicating exposure, was present in about 40% of both groups.

NON-VIRAL FATIGUE SYNDROMES

Before one can set out to see how many ME patients are infected with a particular virus, it is necessary to identify the subset of fatigue syndromes which constitute ME as accurately as possible. As I have already stated, some 'fatigue' occurs with the administration of interferon, and it is important to realise that some of the syndromes are common in association with organic disease (Figure 2).

Among the noninfectious diseases which produce fatigue is cancer, and especially during chemotherapy or radiotherapy courses. Of infectious disease caused by agents other than virus, the most well-known is probably tuberculosis. In parts of the world where giardiasis is common it is recognised that this is a subacute cause of a sometimes severe fatigue syndrome. One of the questions that needs addressing is what are the mediators of these infectious fatigue syndromes. In some cases, for example tuberculosis, the fatigue is of long duration, and cured when the infection is overcome. The long-term production of cytokines may explain some or all of the features. By study of interferon production by stimulated lymphocytes in these conditions as well as ME associated with virus infections, it may be possible to show that there is an additional muscle fatigue problem, not produced by cytokines.

TISSUE INFECTION WITH VIRUSES

After we had been able to culture different strains of enterovirus from at least a fraction of patients with ME, we showed that the same strain of enterovirus could be isolated a year later (Yousef *et al.*, 1988). This was good evidence for the persistence of the same infection, rather than infection repeatedly with different viruses. To do this we took samples of faeces, removed neutralising antibody from the virus with acid, and then separated the two. We were then able to culture viruses which previously would not grow because of the neutralising antibody on them. It was next necessary to look for the virus in the affected tissues, and the blood as a route for transmission from gastrointestinal (GI) tract to muscle and brain, if it were present in the latter tissues. To look at the muscle biopsies was comparatively simple, but to examine the virus in CNS tissues required the availability of autopsy material. Some of this has been available as a result of accident and suicide, but it is still too early to say how many ME patients have detectable virus in the brain. There are undoubtedly some patients with virus detectable in the brain tissue, but we cannot yet say how common this is.

In muscle, two techniques have been used to look for virus. From previous studies it was known that culture of the tissue did not reveal infectious virus. Using the monoclonal antibody against VP1 we were unable to demonstrate the synthesis of viral protein in the tissue, but both Len Archard and ourselves were able to show that viral RNA was present in the tissue. Archard used a gene probe to look for enteroviral gene sequences in RNA extracted from the tissue (Archard *et al.*, 1988). This only allowed him to say that the RNA was present in about a quarter of the samples studied, but its localisation could not be determined this way. We used the technique of *in vitro* hybridisation, in which the labelled gene probe is applied to sections of the tissue. The sites of binding were determined by the use of a streptavidin–peroxidase complex, which has a very high affinity for the biotin label of the gene probe. The peroxidase was then used to produce staining of the sites where the gene probe had bound to the viral RNA (Yousef, 1989). Using this technique we were able to see that a few muscle cells, about 1% of the total, contained viral RNA and were infected (Figure 3). The remainder did not show evidence of infection, thus leading me to the conclusion that it must be these few infected cells that were the cause of symptoms. An important corollary is that one would not expect to find changes in composition or metabolism of whole muscle as a result of infection of so few cells. The reduction in protein turnover, and the decrease in ribosomal-associated RNA, so elegantly studied in ME biopsies by Peters (T. Peters, personal communication) probably represents to a large extent disuse atrophy. The absence of general metabolic changes or histological changes led Smith, who provided the patients for his study, to conclude that there was no change in muscles other than disuse atrophy.

The few infected cells shown by *in vitro* hybridisation to be infected may have deranged metabolic processes, as a result of the virus infection, and may have their own genes suppressed *vide supra*. These cells may then

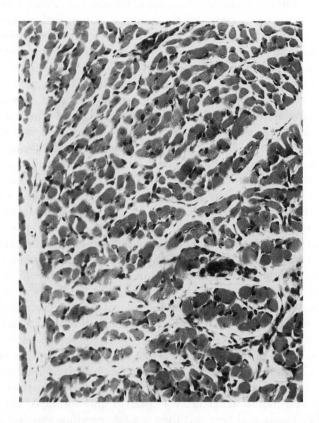

Figure 3 *In situ* hybridisation of enteroviral RNA in a muscle biopsy of a patient with ME. Only a very few myocytes are infected. Infected cells hybridise a cDNA probe for enteroviruses which has been labelled with biotin. Subsequent addition of peroxidase-labelled streptavadin localises the place where the viral RNA has bound the probe to the section

produce pain signals on limited muscle exercise, which is interpreted as fatigue. Protracted muscular effort is normally limited by the development of severe pain on exercise. This is usually interpreted as 'fatigue'. It is now necessary to see if the infected cells do indeed elaborate chemical signals which may be interpreted as premature pain on exertion. ME patients do not, even with extended exercise, usually develop true weakness on prolonged effort, only pain too severe for them to continue. A few ME patients with very long histories appear to develop some progressive and true weakness of muscle, even at rest, but the normal situation in ME is of a muscle which starts to exercise normally, but fatigues rapidly. The fatigue pain would be seen in a normal when running or walking a long distance. The middle- or long-distance runner knows that it is pain that limits exertion, not weakness. In ME, therefore, it may be that a few infected cells may produce pain which limits exercise, but the bulk of the muscle, uninfected, still produces forceful contraction. This is an important contrast with the muscle weakness on exercise of disease such as motor neurone disease, or the painless weakness on exercise which occurs in *myasthenia gravis*.

Archard and his colleagues have used probes for EBV DNA to see if this could be detected in some of the muscle biopsies (Archard and Bowles, 1988). They did find that a small number of specimens, negative for enteroviral RNA, did have EBV DNA present. It is possible that this may have come from a few lymphocytes in the biopsies, as in reactivation of EBV there are large numbers of copies of the viral DNA in infected B lymphocytes. Whether there are in fact some muscle cells infected would seem unlikely, as there is no receptor for EBV on muscle cells, unlike the B lymphocytes which are the usual cells infected by EBV.

It should be appreciated that the cells which are infected in muscle do not apparently have new virus being synthesised within them. Enterovirus RNA will not survive long in the cell, and hence the RNA detected must have been from recent infection. This would require some other site of persistence of infectious virus which can act as a source of infection of the muscle cells. We were able to show that infectious virus was present in the GI tract, and that could be the site of persistence. The presence of quite large amounts of VP1 in the blood suggests that there is likely to be active infection in cells which are in close approximation to or within the circulation. Circulating white cells, endothelium and Kuppfer cells are sites worthy of further study. In these sites, where infectious virus is assumed to be assembled, the sites could be detected by using the monoclonal against VP1, as well as with the gene probe. The former is a tool much easier to use in hunting for virus-infected cells. Cells producing infectious complete virus particles must produce VP1 and, if they are the source of the VP1 in blood, must produce it in quite large quantities.

POSSIBLE MECHANISMS AND SITES OF PERSISTENCE

As has already been discussed, there is a possibility that persistence of a virus in ME might be in a different site from the muscle and brain. It is virtually certain that the site, wherever it is, allows the production of complete infectious virus. Indeed our studies have shown that the muscle appears to be infected with a virus incapable of causing production of infectious virus or even viral proteins in the infected cell. It is very unlikely that such an infection can persist long in the cell, as the uncoated viral RNA will be degraded rapidly. Infection of cells from another site would be required. As I have already considered, the infectious virus we have detected in the faeces probably does not represent the main source of virus for systemic spread. What then would be the appropriate scenario for a source of infection?

The site should be in a tissue with rapid turnover of the cells to provide a continuing source of uninfected cells which can be infected by the particles released by the cells which die of the cytopathic effect of virus replication in the cell. Thus when enteroviruses are infecting intestinal cells, the mucosa is turning over rapidly, and there is a continuous shedding of mucosal cells into the lumen. It is quite easy then for a cytopathic virus to be established, continuously infecting new cohorts of cells arising in the basal layers and moving towards the lumen. It matters not that cells die in order to release virus particles, as there are always new ones on the way. An interesting theoretical possibility arises in this circumstance. If viral replication can be held for only a few days, all the infected cells will be shed into the lumen of the gut, and the infection may be lost. Equally the infection can only survive as long as the cell population is dividing. Prevention of cell division for a time, with temporary severe depletion of cell numbers, may result in a substantial decrease in the number of infected cells after recovery. Not entirely in jest, I have suggested that a short, sharp attack of staphylococcal enterocolitis with shedding of most of the mucosa might be a good way of treating a chronic intestinal enteroviral infection.

The continuously dividing cell populations which might be a reservoir of infection would include gut epithelium, skin, and bone marrow derived, circulating cells. This last population would include macrophage/ monocytes, granulocytes and precursors, and lymphocytes. If the infection were sited in the marrow, infected cells might be liberated to circulate, and possibly carry the virus to other tissues.

When we had isolated virus from the GI tract of ME patients we were able, in co-operation with Eleanor Bell in Glasgow, to show that the serum of each patient contained neutralising antibodies against their own virus serotype. If blood were to be the route for transmission of the infection to muscle (and probably brain as well), the neutralising antibody would not permit the virus to reach the target issue in an infectious form. If, however, it were transmitted in circulating cells, the virus would not be exposed to antibody until release, presumably by lysis of the carrier cell. It is clearly urgent to hunt for the sites of infection, other than the GI tract, where a chronic infection results in continuing from muscle, or brain, when 'exhausted' to the sites of persistence. This would increase the production of virus, since relapses caused by exhaustion of either tissue are both associated with a rise in VP1. The relapse affects both tissues, albeit sometimes rather unequally, but it does not matter from which tissue the signal came. It is realistic to assume that either can produce a signal which increases virus production, and the latter affects both tissue in consequence.

The nature of such a putative signal remains to be determined, if indeed it is present, but knowledge of the mechanisms involved in either afferent signals or efferent exacerbation of symptoms would be useful. With that information we might be close to manipulating the situation to the patient's benefit.

THE FUTURE OF STUDIES OF PERSISTENT ENTEROVIRAL INFECTION AND ME

A better understanding of the sites and mechanism of persistence, and the signals which may control viral replication in those sites must be important in attempting rational management of the condition of ME. To see how much of any central CNS effects are mediated by cytokines such as interferon would also be needed for a complete view of the symptom complex. It may be some time before antiviral agents that could truncate the infection, and hence the disease, are available. Understanding of the control of virus production would help in other approaches to amelioration of the condition while the virus is still present. These might be somewhat more effective than the exhortations which we all give to patients: 'do *not* get exhausted'—easy to say, difficult to take to heart, when so much time has been lost with illness before improvement begins!

REFERENCES

Archard, L. A. and Bowles, N. (1988) Detection of EBV-DNA in muscle biopsies of patients with postviral fatigue syndrome. *Proceedings 3rd International Symposium on EBV and Associated Malignancies, Rome 1988*, p. 132.

Archard, L., Bowles, N. E., Behan, P. O., Bell, E. J. and Doyle, D. J. (1988) Postviral fatigue syndrome: persistence of enterovirus RNA in muscle and elevated creatine kinase. *Journal of the Royal Society of Medicine*, **81**, 326–329.

Bell, E. J., McCartney, R. A. and Riding, M. H. (1988) Coxsackie B viruses and myalgic encephalomyolitis. *Journal of the Royal Society of Medicine*, **81**, 329–331.

Hotchin, N. A., Read, R., Smith, D. G. and Crawford, D. H. (1989) Active Epstein–Barr virus infection in post viral fatigue syndrome. *Journal of Infection*, **18**, 143–150.

McCartney, R. A., Banatvala, J. E. and Bell, E. J. (1986) Routine use of M-capture ELISA for the serological diagnosis of coxsackie B virus. *Journal of Medical Virology*, **19**, 205–212.

Yousef, G. E. (1989) Entovirus infection and muscle disease. *PhD Thesis*, University of London.

Yousef, G. E., Mann, C. F., Smith, D. G., Bell, E. J., Murugesan, V., McCartney, R. A. and Mowbray, J. F. (1988) Chronic enterovirus infection in patients with post viral fatigue syndrome. *Lancet* **i**, 146–150.

4

Chronic Viral Infections of the Brain

Peter Portegies and Jaap Goudsmit

University of Amsterdam, Amsterdam, The Netherlands

INTRODUCTION

Chronic viral infections of the brain are characterized by a long incubation period, ranging from several months to many years, followed by a slowly progressive course, ending in severe disease or death. The term slow infections is often used for this group of viral infections. This term has been introduced by Sigurdsson, an Icelandic pathologist who worked with chronic sheep diseases (Sigurdsson, 1954). Scrapie (or rida) and visna (Sigurdsson *et al.*, 1957) are the prototypes of these slow infections of sheep. Since its introduction the term has been used for several viral infections of the nervous system, not precisely fulfilling the original criteria.

Chronic or persistent infection means that there is continuous virus production, although this might be at very low levels. In contrast, in latent infection the viral genome is present in the host cell, even sometimes as messenger RNA, but no virus is produced. The definitions of persistence and latency are not used very properly, and sometimes persistence is equated with chronic or dynamic latency. In some infections described in this chapter a latent stage is followed by a persistent stage and a stage of viral replication at a higher level.

The mechanisms of viral latency and persistence are complex, and depend on a number of viral and host factors (Wolinsky and Johnson, 1980). Chronic viral infections of the brain are of two general types: (1) those due to conventional viruses—subacute sclerosing panencephalitis, progressive rubella panencephalitis, progressive multifocal leucoencephalopathy, and HIV-1 encephalopathy; and (2) those due to unconventional agents or

Post-viral Fatigue Syndrome. Edited by R. Jenkins and J. Mowbray

prions—kuru, Creutzfeldt–Jakob disease and Gerstmann–Sträussler syndrome.

Although the causative agents (a paramyxovirus (measles), a togavirus (rubella), a papovavirus (PML), a retrovirus (HIV-1) and prions) differ markedly, the diseases caused by them share many characteristics. The retrovirus HTLV-1 is associated with a chronic myelopathy.

This chapter reviews the above-mentioned chronic viral infections of the brain, emphasizing clinical aspects and recent progress in virology and pathophysiology. Prions will be discussed in some detail separately.

SUBACUTE SCLEROSING PANENCEPHALITIS

Subacute sclerosing panencephalitis (SSPE) is a rare, usually fatal neurological disease seen in children and young adults, due to persistent infection with measles virus following primary and usually uncomplicated measles several years earlier.

Patients present with personality and behavioural changes and gradual loss of intellectual function. The disease progresses to convulsions, myoclonic movements, increasing spasticity of the limbs and dementia (Jabbour et al., 1969). Eventually neurological deterioration leads to coma and death (Metz et al., 1964). The course is usually steadily progressive, death occurring within one to three years. Atypical presentations, with myoclonus or headache, vomiting and papilloedema, have been described. Claims of successful therapy with isoprinosine for patients with SSPE evoke great controversy (Mattson, 1974).

The majority of affected children have high titres of measles antibody in the serum, and both IgM and IgG measles-specific antibodies in the cerebrospinal fluid (CSF) (Connolly et al., 1967). The CSF of such a symptomatic child generally contains few or no cells.

In this disorder the electroencephalograms (EEG) show recurrent slow-wave complexes, sometimes with associated transient sharp waves. The complexes usually last for up to three seconds, but their form and interval may show considerable variation. When myoclonic jerking is a clinical feature of the patient's illness, the jerks are usually time-related to the periodic complexes.

Early in the course of the disease the computed tomography (CT) of the brain can be normal or show some brain swelling, but later atrophy and hypodense areas in the white matter appear.

Pathologically SSPE is characterized by eosinophilic intranuclear inclusion bodies, which are seen in all cell types, but which are most common in oligodendrocytes (Dawson, 1934). Viral antigen can be detected in neurons and glial cells. Abnormalities are present in both grey and white matter. Demyelination, gliosis and microglial reaction are found (Silva et al., 1981).

The virus has been recovered from the brain tissue only with difficulty. The pathogenesis of SSPE is unknown. It is not known why a small proportion of children infected by the measles virus develops a progressive fatal disease years later. Patients have no generalized immune deficiency. They tend to be unvaccinated, male children who had natural measles before age 2 (Detels *et al.*, 1973). There might be a delay in the development of the immune response during the initial infection, leading to persistence and multiplication of the virus in an abnormal form, eventually causing disease. Another hypothesis is that in SSPE the matrix (M) protein of the measles virus is not synthesized in brain cells, leading to a block in virus replication (Hall and Choppin, 1979). The absence of M protein has been attributed to a decrease in translation of the corresponding mRNA (Haase *et al.*, 1985). Probably the low level of viral antigen enables the infected cell to evade detection and destruction by the immune system (Hall *et al.*, 1979). Recently viral RNA sequences have been detected in peripheral blood lymphocytes of SSPE patients (Fournier *et al.*, 1985). It is not known whether these infected lymphocytes carry the virus to the brain.

RUBELLA

In children with the congenital rubella syndrome a progressive neurological deterioration has been observed after a prolonged latent period (Weil *et al.*, 1975). The syndrome, which is extremely rare, has been called progressive rubella panencephalitis. It has also been described in previously normal children (Lebon and Lyon, 1974). Clinically the syndrome is comparable with subacute sclerosing panencephalitis: progressive impairment of mental functions, seizures, spasticity, dysarthria and ataxia. However, the course can last as long as 10 years. Besides a mild lymphocytic pleocytosis, the CSF shows a moderate elevation of protein, with oligoclonal bands demonstrated in the gammaglobulin region (Wolinsky *et al.*, 1976). The CSF and serum rubella antibody titres are elevated. EEG abnormalities are less specific. Periodic EEG complexes have not been described, and detailed EEG studies of this syndrome have not been published.

Pathological examination of the brain showed a panencephalitis, without inclusion-bearing cells, and mainly affecting the white matter (Townsend *et al.*, 1976).

PROGRESSIVE MULTIFOCAL LEUCOENCEPHALOPATHY

Progressive multifocal leucoencephalopathy (PML) is a subacute demyelinating disease resulting from infection of oligodendrocytes by a

papovavirus, called the JC virus. It occurs almost exclusively in immunocompromised patients and can be considered as an opportunistic viral
infection. The condition was first recognized in 1958 (Astrom *et al.*, 1958).

The most common associated conditions are Hodgkin's disease, chronic
leukaemia and other lymphoproliferative diseases, sarcoidosis and AIDS
(Richardson, 1961; Berger *et al.*, 1987). The onset of the disease is usually
insidious, with symptoms and signs suggesting multifocal disease. Hemi-
paresis, visual field defects, cortical blindness, aphasia, ataxia, and dementia
may occur (Richardson, 1961). Headaches and seizures are rare and there
are no signs of raised intracranial pressure. The disease evolves relentlessly,
until the patient dies, usually within four to six months. However, stabiliza-
tion or spontaneous remissions have been described.

The CSF is generally normal. EEG shows only nonspecific changes. CT of
the brain shows hypodense non-enhancing white matter lesions. With magnetic resonance imaging (MRI) high-intensity signal lesions are found in the
white matter on T2-weighted spin-echo images (Guilleux and Steiner, 1986).
MRI is more sensitive than CT in detecting lesions; MRI shows more extensive or a greater number of lesions, or both, than CT scan.

Treatment of PML has been unsuccessful, despite occasional reports of a
positive response to cytarabine (Bauer *et al.*, 1973).

Pathologically there are multifocal areas of demyelination, which are most
prominent in the subcortical white matter, but cerebellum, brain stem and
basal ganglia may also be affected. Many of these lesions join, forming
multilobulated lesions. Histologically, loss of myelin is obvious, with relative sparing of axons. Within the lesions oligodendrocytes are absent, while
at the margin oligodendrocytes are greatly enlarged and may contain large
intranuclear inclusion bodies. Astrocytes are enlarged too (giant astrocytes)
with distorted nuclei. Usually there is no inflammatory response (Walker,
1985).

In nearly all cases, PML is the result of infection of the brain by the JC
virus (Zu Rhein and Chou, 1965; Silverman and Rubinstein, 1965; Padgett *et
al.*, 1971). JC virus is one of the papovaviruses of which the best known is
simian virus 40 (SV 40), which infects monkeys but is not pathogenic for
humans. The JC virus is almost ubiquitous among adults all over the world.
Seroconversion occurs during childhood, usually without producing
disease.

The pathogenesis of PML has remained obscure, but important progress
has been published recently. Houff and colleagues demonstrated with *in situ*
DNA hybridization and immunocytochemical studies that, in PML, JC virus
DNA and capsid antigen are present in B lymphocytes in the bone marrow
and spleen (Houff *et al.*, 1988). The presence of virion capsid antigen suggests ongoing replication in these cells. Further studies on replication of the
JC virus and on host cell factors have been stimulated by these findings.

HIV-1 ENCEPHALOPATHY

One of the most common neurological syndromes in patients with the acquired immune deficiency syndrome (AIDS) is the human immunodeficiency virus type 1 (HIV-1) encephalopathy or AIDS dementia complex, which is
directly related to infection of the brain with HIV-1 (Price *et al.*, 1988).

The epidemiology of the AIDS dementia complex has not yet been precisely defined, but without treatment at least a third of all patients with
AIDS eventually develop a mild or severe form of the AIDS dementia
complex.

Clinically AIDS dementia complex is characterized by abnormalities in
cognition, motor performance, and behaviour (Navia *et al.*, 1986a). Usually
the onset of the syndrome is insidious. Early cognitive symptoms include
poor concentration, forgetfulness, and slowness of thought. Concomitantly
patients appear apathetic, lose spontaneity and withdraw socially. Patients
complain of poor balance, clumsiness and leg weakness. Neurological examination reveals impaired rapid movements, slight paraparesis with gait ataxia, hyperreflexia, snout response, tremor and impaired smooth eye
movements. Although the course is highly variable, in time progression to
moderate or severe global dementia occurs in all patients. In end stages
patients are nearly or absolutely mute, paraplegic and incontinent. A staging
scheme for quantifying clinical abnormalities has been devised by Price
(Price and Brew, 1988).

Diagnosis of AIDS dementia complex is established on clinical grounds.
Neuropsychological testing reveals abnormalities conforming to a 'subcortical dementia', with slowing of both mental and motor functions. CT scan or
MRI of the brain and CSF analysis are useful for excluding opportunistic
infections and tumours of the central nervous system. CT and MRI show
widened cortical sulci and enlarged ventricles. MRI shows white matter
abnormalities. CSF abnormalities reported in patients with AIDS dementia
complex include elevated protein, pleocytosis, HIV-1 isolation, HIV-1 p24
antigen detection, increased levels of neopterin, and beta-2-microglobulin.
HIV-1 p24 antigen and beta-2-microglobulin correlate best with clinical neurological status (Portegies *et al.*, 1989a; Sönnerborg *et al.*, 1989).

Some beneficial effects of zidovudine treatment in patients with the AIDS
dementia complex have been described (Yarchoan *et al.*, 1987; Pizzo *et al.*,
1988; Schmitt *et al.*, 1988) and since the introduction of zidovudine the incidence of AIDS dementia complex has declined (Portegies *et al.*, 1989b). These
results suggest that, with antiviral treatment, it might be possible to inhibit
viral replication of HIV-1 in the brain, and in doing so to prevent or improve
neurological dysfunction. The characteristic pathological abnormalities are
most prominent in the central white matter, deep grey structures (basal ganglia, thalamus), brain stem and spinal cord (Navia *et al.*, 1986b). There is relative

sparing of the cortex. Histopathologically, characteristics include diffuse pallor of the white matter, multinucleated cell encephalitis (with some reactive infiltrates consisting of foamy macrophages, microglia, lymphocytes and multinucleated cells), and a vacuolar myelopathy. In children, in which the syndrome has been called progressive encephalopathy, the pathology is similar except that it also includes a calcific vasculopathy.

Substantial evidence for a direct aetiological role of HIV-1 came from Southern blot analysis, *in situ* hybridization and immunohistochemical studies (Shaw *et al.*, 1985; Koenig *et al.*, 1986; Wiley *et al.*, 1986). HIV-1 has been cultured from the brain and CSF in affected patients and HIV-1 virions have been detected by electron microscopy. There is emerging evidence now that macrophages and multinucleated cells derived from macrophages are the major target cells in the brain (Ho *et al.*, 1987). The mechanism underlying the neurological dysfunction is poorly understood. There is no productive infection or lysis of neurones, oligodendrocytes or astrocytes. So instead of tissue destruction, indirect mechanisms predominate in pathogenesis. Persistence of unintegrated viral DNA (Pang *et al.*, 1990), or interference of viral proteins or cytokines with neurotransmission, may play an important role (Gendelman *et al.*, 1989).

HTLV-1 INFECTIONS

The human T cell leukaemia virus type 1 (HTLV-1), a retrovirus, is an aetiological agent of adult T cell leukaemia. Recently, the virus was found to be associated with a chronic myelopathy, known by several names: tropical spastic paraparesis (TSP), HTLV-1-associated myelopathy (HAM) and chronic progressive myelopathy (CPM) (Roman, 1987; Johnson and McArthur, 1987; Brew and Price, 1988). Clinically the main manifestations are a slowly spastic paraparesis with hyperreflexia of the legs (and often of the arms), with mild sensory and bladder disturbances, leading to chronic disability rather than death.

Intrathecal synthesis of antibodies against HTLV-1, isolation of the virus from peripheral blood and CSF mononuclear cells, and identification of HTLV-1 nucleic acid sequences in blood and CSF cells (Bhagavati *et al.*, 1988), strengthen the proposition that HTLV-1 is involved in the pathogenesis of this chronic myelopathy. Although increased replication of HTLV-1 in lymphocytes in patients with HTLV-1 myelopathy has been described (Yoshida *et al.*, 1989), the agent has not been demonstrated in the spinal cord, and the underlying pathogenetic mechanisms remain to be elucidated.

Favourable responses to glucocorticoids have been reported (Osame *et al.*, 1987).

SPONGIFORM ENCEPHALOPATHIES

Scrapie in sheep and kuru, Creutzfeldt–Jakob disease and Gerstmann–Sträussler syndrome in man are transmissible degenerative diseases of the central nervous system grouped as spongiform encephalopathies, as spongiform neuronal degeneration is one of the characteristic histological features. Their aetiological agents are probably small proteins, designated prions (proteinaceous infectious particles) by Prusiner and co-workers.

Scrapie

Scrapie is a progressive neurological disease, affecting both sheep and goats in many countries of the world. After a long incubation period, from two to five years, affected sheep suffer from excitability, behavioural changes, incoordination, ataxia, tremor and continuous scratching or rubbing due to sensory neurological disturbance. The progressive ataxia leads to death in six weeks to six months (Johnson and Johnson, 1969).

Pathological changes, which are most prominent in cerebellar cortex and brain stem, consist of neuronal degeneration with cytoplasmic vacuolization and astrocytic proliferation (Beck *et al.*, 1964).

The disease is transmitted by contact in flocks of sheep, but the incubation time and the susceptibility to scrapie can be influenced by the genetic background of the host (Dickinson and Fraser, 1977).

Since scrapie has been experimentally transmitted to laboratory rodents by intracerebral or subcutaneous inoculation using the brains of infected sheep (Chandler, 1961), the transmissible scrapie agent has been studied extensively. The unconventional agent does not evoke cytopathic effects in cell cultures or non-neural tissues, does not evoke an immune response, has not been seen by electron microscopy, is highly resistant to ultraviolet irradiation, formaldehyde and heat, and appears not to have a nucleic acid genome (Prusiner, 1982). Scrapie and the human spongiform encephalopathies are caused by proteins (Prusiner, 1987). The characteristics of these proteins will be discussed at the end of this chapter.

Kuru

Kuru is a degenerative disease of the brain found only among the Foré-speaking people in New Guinea (Gajdusek and Zigas, 1957). Kuru is a native word meaning shivering or trembling. The disease was common in the Foré-speaking people in the late 1950s, but the incidence declined rapidly and kuru is dying out now.

The disease has a very characteristic pattern (Hornabrook, 1968), that starts with unsteadiness in walking, truncal ataxia and postural instability.

With time, ataxia increases and voluntary movements are poorly controlled, leading to movements resembling chorea or myoclonus. Speech becomes slurred, but no nystagmus occurs. Late in the disease patients cannot walk without support because of muscle weakness and wasting. In the terminal stages patients become progressively paralysed and dementia is common. The course is always progressive; remissions have never been documented. Death occurs within three to 24 months. During the course of the disease patients remain afebrile. The CSF shows no abnormalities. Pathological examination reveals cerebellar atrophy and microscopic neuronal degeneration with neuronal vacuolization, astrocytosis, and gliosis, without inflammatory infiltrates. There is no demyelination, and some patients have plaques of amyloid-like material, so-called kuru plaques (Lampert *et al.*, 1972). Pathological changes are not limited to the cerebellum; brain stem and cortex are involved too.

The disease was most common in adult females, less common in children and uncommon in adult males, who did not usually take part in cannibalistic feasts, while women and children ate viscera and brains of relatives, including those who died of kuru. Therefore this ritual cannibalism has been held responsible for transmission of the disease (Gajdusek, 1977). Cannibalism was generally stopped around 1957 and afterwards the incidence of kuru declined.

Transmission of kuru to a chimpanzee, reported by Gajdusek in 1966, was the first demonstration of a slow infection of man (Gajdusek *et al.*, 1966). The kuru agent passes filters of 100-nm pore diameter, is present in infected brain tissue and in spleen, liver and kidney of infected animals, and can be transmitted peripherally as well as intracerebrally; no antibody to the agent has been detected. Kuru is therefore one of the so-called human 'prion' diseases.

Creutzfeldt–Jakob disease

Creutzfeldt described a progressive dementia illness in a 22-year-old woman in 1920 (Creutzfeldt, 1920). Jakob described five older patients with a comparable clinical presentation in 1921 (Jakob, 1921). The following year Spielmeyer, for the first time, used the term Creutzfeld–Jakob disease. Subsequently at least 20 synonyms have been used, but Creutzfeldt–Jakob disease is still generally accepted in the English literature.

Creutzfeld–Jakob disease (CJD) is a rare disease (incidence less than 1/million) with a peak incidence in the fifth to seventh decades (Matthews and Will, 1982).

In the prodromal stage patients may complain of tiredness, apathy, change in mood, insomnia, anorexia and weight loss. Then, sometimes very abruptly, overt neurological symptoms and signs appear. The patient develops ataxia, dysarthria, dysphasia, focal limb weakness with progressive spasticity, and visual hallucinations. Intellectual impairment becomes evident. With time the disease progresses steadily to a severe dementia with mutism and involuntary movements such as myoclonic jerks or choreo-athetoid movements (Jones and Nevin, 1954; Nevin *et al.*, 1960). Most patients die within 12 months of onset.

The CSF is usually normal, although some patients have a mild elevation of protein.

The EEG is characterized by periodic complexes occurring on a diffusely abnormal, slowed background. The complexes consist of brief waves of rather variable, often triphasic, form and sharpened outline that recur about once every second and may show a temporal relationship to the myoclonic jerking. Sometimes serial recordings are necessary to register this periodic activity.

CT scan can be normal in subacute cases, but usually it shows some degree of atrophy.

Pathologically, CJD is characterized by neuronal loss, astrocytosis, and cytoplasmic vacuolization of neurones and astrocytes, causing status spongiosus (Brownell and Oppenheimer, 1965; Masters and Richardson, 1978). These abnormalities are localized in the grey matter of the cerebral cortex, cerebellum, basal ganglia and brain stem. In a minority of patients amyloid plaques can be found.

Antiviral agents have been ineffective.

The disease is reproduced in chimpanzees and other monkeys after intracerebral inoculation of brain tissue from cases of the disease (Gibbs *et al.*, 1968). Peripheral routes (combined intravenous, intraperitoneal and intramuscular routes) are also effective. The incubation period is from 11 to 14 months.

Although the natural route of infection is unknown, the disease has been accidentally transmitted by corneal transplantation, by neurosurgery, via electrodes used for electroencephalography and by injections of human growth hormone (Gibbs *et al.*, 1985). Transmission to laboratory workers has never been described.

Prusiner and colleagues have proposed that CJD, like scrapie and kuru, is caused by prions (Prusiner, 1987).

Gerstmann–Sträussler disease

Gerstmann–Sträussler disease, which was first observed in an Austrian family by Gerstmann in 1936 (Gerstmann *et al.*, 1936), and which has been known as Sträussler's disease, Gerstmann–Sträussler–Scheinker disease, and spinocerebellar ataxia with dementia and plaque-like deposits, can be considered to be the third of the spongiform encephalopathies. There is still much controversy about whether this is a familial (autosomal dominant) variant of CJD, or an entity which can be distinguished from CJD and kuru.

Clinically, patients present with a slowly progressive dysarthria and cerebellar ataxia, followed by bradykinesia, pyramidal signs, with in some cases areflexia in the lower limbs, and a form of dementia (Farlow *et al.*, 1989). The mean duration of the disease is four to five years. Pathological examination reveals abundant amyloid plaques (so-called kuru bodies), mainly in the cerebellar cortex, degeneration of fibre systems and grey matter and slight spongy change in the cerebral cortex and caudate nuclei (Kuzuhara *et al.*, 1983; Azzarelli *et al.*, 1985; Ghetti *et al.*, 1989). Some of the anterior horn cells show chromatolysis. The syndrome possibly represents the genetic form of 'prion' disease (Prusiner, 1987).

'PRIONS' OR TRANSMISSIBLE PROTEINS: VIRUSES?

Prions are novel, transmissible pathogens causing degenerative diseases in humans and animals. Stanley B. Prusiner and his colleagues at the University of California, San Francisco, have contributed, following the era of Gajdusek, Gibbs, Dickinson, Kimberlin and others, most significantly to the characterization of these novel 'unconventional' agents, and a large amount of the experimental data available about these infectious proteins has been generated in his laboratory (Prusiner, 1989). Prions have been defined as 'small proteinaceous infectious particles that resist inactivation by procedures which modify nucleic acids' (Prusiner, 1982).

Although both prions and viruses multiply, their properties, structures, and modes of replication seem to be fundamentally different. Viruses contain nucleic acid genomes, that encode for viral proteins, while prions contain no nucleic acids, and the prion protein is encoded by a cellular gene (Oesch *et al.*, 1985). Viruses usually evoke an immune response during infection, while prions appear not to do so. Furthermore, prions do not evoke cytopathic effects in cell cultures or non-neural tissues, are highly resistant to disinfection, and have not been visualized by electron microscopy.

Prions are composed largely, if not entirely, of an abnormal form of the prion protein (PrP), a glycoprotein of molecular weight 27000–30000. Molecular genetic studies have revealed that PrP molecules are encoded by the host, by a gene located on human chromosome 20 (Westaway *et al.*, 1989) and they may play a role in the regulation of neurochemical receptor production in the central nervous system. Why and how normal, probably necessary, proteins (derived from cell membranes) are converted into malignant, lethal molecules is unknown. It is possible that infectious, environmental and genetically programmed events may signal this conversion.

In animals 'prions' are the cause of scrapie of sheep and goats, of transmissible mink encephalopathy, of chronic wasting disease of mule deer and elk and of bovine spongiform encephalopathy. In humans prions cause kuru, CJD and Gerstmann–Sträussler syndrome (GSS). Of all these 'prion' diseases scrapie has been studied most extensively (Prusiner *et al.*, 1984; Carp *et al.*, 1985; Prusiner, 1989).

All these 'prion' diseases are degenerative neurological disorders, which can be transmitted by inoculation, and which progress to death in the absence of a detectable immune response. The human prion diseases kuru, CJD and GSS illustrate three manifestations of a central nervous system degenerative disorder: a slow infection (kuru), a sporadic disease (CJD) and a genetic disorder (GSS).

The pathological features of 'prion' diseases include neuronal vacuolation, astrocytic gliosis, deposition of amyloid plaques, and a lack of any inflammatory response. Usually the grey matter is most affected. The vacuoles in neurones may coalesce into larger ones, leading to what has been called spongiform degeneration (Beck and Daniel, 1979). However, these changes are rare in scrapie and in some cases of CJD. 'Prion' proteins or the human prion–gene complex are not likely to be involved in the pathogenesis of the more common central nervous system degenerative diseases, such as Alzheimer's disease, Parkinson's disease, and amyotrophic lateral sclerosis. Still, CJD and Alzheimer's disease share many clinical and pathological features, suggesting a common pathogenetic pathway. And, although Alzheimer's disease has not been transmitted to laboratory animals (Goudsmit *et al.*, 1980), the resemblance of the aggregated scrapie-associated fibrils to the amyloid observed in brains of patients with Alzheimer's disease is remarkable (Prusiner *et al.*, 1984).

Despite considerable progress in research on prion proteins and prion diseases, the pathological mechanisms leading to central nervous system dysfunction (possibly by interference of prion proteins with receptor production and neurotransmission) in prion diseases remain to be elucidated.

CONCLUDING REMARKS

Chronic viral infections of the central nervous system are rare diseases, caused by conventional viruses and unconventional agents or 'prions'. Clinically, a progressive course, lasting between several months and many years, leads to severe disability or death. Some of these disorders are limited to certain age groups (SSPE, rubella) or certain risk groups (PML, HIV-1 encephalopathy) (Table 1), which can give important clues in differential diagnosis. The results of treatment in most of these infections have been disappointing. However, in HIV-1 encephalopathy promising benefits of antiviral treatment have been described recently and this retroviral infection of the brain is closest to being resolved.

Table 1

Disease	Age-group	Risk factor/ underlying disease	Course and prognosis	Treatment
SSPE	4–20 years	Early age measles?	Progression to death in 1–2 years	Isoprinosine?
Rubella	8–19 years	Congenital rubella syndrome	Slow progression over 8–10 years	None
PML	6th decade AIDS (20–40 years)	Immuno-suppression, e.g. AIDS, chronic leukaemia	Progression to death in 2 months to 2 years	Cytarabine?
HIV-1 encephalopathy	0–12 years 20–40 years	Homosexual men, i.v. drug abusers, haemophiliacs, children of infected mothers, blood products recipients	Without treatment progression to death in 3 months to 1 year	Zidovudine
Kuru	4 years–all ages	Cannibalism (children, and their mothers) in New Guinea	Progression to death in 3 months to 2 years	None
CJD	5th–7th decade sometimes 15–25 years	Not known	Progression to death in 12 months	None
GSS	3rd–6th decade	Possible familial (autosomal dominant)	Progression to death in 6 months to 2 years	None
TSP	3rd–6th decade	Geographically determined (Japan, the Caribbean)	Slow progression to moderate or severe disability	Corticosteroids?

SSPE, subacute sclerosing panencephalitis; PML, progressive multifocal leucoencephalopathy; HIV-1, human immunodeficiency virus type 1; CJD, Creutzfeldt–Jakob disease; GSS, Gerstmann–Sträussler syndrome; TSP, tropical spastic paraparesis.

In the last decade, the rapid development of molecular biology has enabled important developments in the understanding of chronic viral infections of the brain. It is to be expected that further progress will be made in the near future.

REFERENCES

Astrom, K. E., Mancall, E. L. and Richardson, E. P. Jr (1958) Progressive multifocal leucoencephalopathy: a hitherto unrecognized complication of chronic lymphatic leukaemia and Hodgkin's disease. *Brain*, **81**, 93–111.

Azzarelli, B., Muller, J., Ghetti, B., Dyken, M. and Conneally, P. M. (1985) Cerebellar plaques in familial Alzheimer's disease (Gerstmann–Sträussler–Scheinker variant?). *Acta Neuropathologica (Berlin)*, **65**, 235–246.

Bauer, W. R., Turel, A. P. and Johnson, K. P. (1973) Progressive multifocal leucoencephalopathy and cytarabine. Remission with treatment. *Journal of the American Medical Association*, **226**, 174–175.

Beck, E. and Daniel, P. M. (1979) Kuru and Creutzfeldt–Jakob disease; neuropathological lesions and their significance. In S. B. Prusiner and W. J. Hadlow (eds) *Slow Transmissible Diseases of the Nervous System*, Vol. 1, pp. 253–270. Academic Press, New York.

Beck, E., Daniel, P. M. and Parry, H. B. (1964) Degeneration of the cerebellar and hypothalamo-neurohypophysial systems in sheep with scrapie, and its relation to human system degeneration. *Brain*, **87**, 153–176.

Berger, J. R., Kaszovitz, B., Donovan Post, M. J. and Dickinson, G. (1987) Progressive multifocal leucoencephalopathy associated with human immunodeficiency virus: a review of the literature with a report of sixteen cases. *Annals of Internal Medicine*, **107**, 78–87.

Bhagavati, S., Ehrlich, G., Kula, R. W., Kwok, S., Sninsky, J., Udani, V. and Poiesz, B. J. (1988) Detection of human T-cell lymphoma/leukemia virus type I DNA and antigen in spinal fluid and blood of patients with chronic and progressive myelopathy. *New England Journal of Medicine*, **318**, 1141–1147.

Brew, B. and Price, R. W. (1988) Another retroviral disease of the nervous system; Chronic progressive myelopathy due to HTLV-I. *New England Journal of Medicine*, **318**, 1195–1197.

Brownell, B. and Oppenheimer, D. R. (1965) An ataxic form of subacute presenile polioencephalopathy (Creutzfeldt–Jakob disease). *Journal of Neurology, Neurosurgery and Psychiatry*, **28**, 350–361.

Carp, R. I., Merz, P. A., Kascsak, R., Merz, G. S. and Wisniewski, H. M. (1985) Nature of the scrapie agent: current status of facts and hypothesis. *Journal of General Virology*, **66**, 357–1368.

Chandler, R. L. (1961) Encephalopathy in mice produced by inoculation with scrapie brain material. *Lancet*, **1**, 1378–1379.

Connolly, J. H., Allen, I. V., Hurwitz, L. J. and Millar, J. H. D. (1967) Measles-virus antibody and antigen in subacute sclerosing panencephalitis. *Lancet*, **i**, 542–544.

Creutzfeldt, H. G. (1920) Uber eine eigenartige herdformige Erkrankung des Zentralnervensystems. *Zeitschrift fur die gesamte Neurologie und Psychiatrie*, **57**, 1–18.

Dawson, J. R. Jr (1934) Cellular inclusions in cerebral lesions of epidemic encephalitis. *Archives of Neurology and Psychiatry*, **31**, 685–700.

Detels, R., Brody, J. A., McNew, J. and Edgar, A. H. (1973) Further epidemiological studies of subacute sclerosing panencephalitis. *Lancet*, **ii**, 11–14.

Dickinson, A. G. and Fraser, H. (1977) Scrapie: Pathogenesis in inbred mice: An assessment of host control and response involving many strains of agent. In V. ter Meulen and M. Katz (eds) *Slow Virus Infections of the Central Nervous System*, pp. 3–14. Springer-Verlag, New York.

Farlow, M. R., Yee, R. D., Dlouhy, S. R., Conneally, P. M., Azarelli, B. and Ghetti, B. (1989) Gerstmann–Sträussler–Scheinker disease. I. Extending the clinical spectrum. *Neurology*, **39**, 1446–1452.

Fournier, J. G., Tardieu, M., Lebon, P. *et al.* (1985) Detection of measles virus RNA in lymphocytes from peripheral-blood and brain perivascular infiltrates of patients with subacute sclerosing panencephalitis. *New England Journal of Medicine*, **313**, 910–915.

Gajdusek, D. C. (1977) Unconventional viruses and the origin and disappearance of kuru. *Science*, **197**, 943–960.

Gajdusek, D. C. and Zigas, V. (1957) Degenerative disease of the central nervous system in New Guinea: The endemic occurrence of 'kuru' in the native population. *New England Journal of Medicine*, **257**, 974–978.

Gajdusek, D. C., Gibbs, C. J. Jr and Alpers, M. (1966) Experimental transmission of a kuru-like syndrome to chimpanzees. *Nature*, **209**, 794–796.

Gendelman, H. E., Orenstein, J. M., Baca, L. M., Weiser, B., Burger, H., Kalter, D. C. and Meltzer, M. S. (1989) The macrophage in the persistence and pathogenesis of HIV infection. *AIDS*, **3**, 475–495.

Gerstmann, J., Sträussler, E. and Scheinker, I. (1936) Uber eine iegenartige hereditär-familiäre Erkrankung des Zentralnervensystems. Zugleich ein Beitrag zur Frage des vorzeitigen lokalen Alterns. *Zeitschrift für die gesamte Neurologie und Psychiatrie*, **154**, 736–762.

Ghetti, B., Tagliavini, F., Masters, C. L., Beyreuther, K., Giaccone, G., Verga, L., Farlow, M. R., Conneally, P. M., Dlouhy, S. R., Azzarelli, B. and Bugiani, O. (1989) Gerstmann–Sträussler–Scheinker disease. II. Neurofibrillary tangles and plaques with PrP-amyloid coexist in an affected family. *Neurology*, **39**, 1453–1461.

Gibbs, C. J., Gajdusek, D. C., Asher, D. M., Alpers, M. P., Beck, E., Daniel, P. M. and Matthews, W. B. (1968) Creutzfeldt–Jakob disease (spongiform encephalopathy): transmission to the chimpanzee. *Science*, **161**, 388–389.

Gibbs, C. J., Joy, A., Heffner, R., Franks, M., Miyazaki, M., Asher, D. M. *et al.* (1985) Clinical and pathological features and laboratory confirmation of Creutzfeldt–Jakob disease in a recipient of pituitary-derived growth hormone. *New England Journal of Medicine*, **313**, 734–738.

Goudsmit, J., Marrow, C. H., Asher, D. M., Yanagihara, R. T., Masters, C. L., Gibbs, C. J. Jr and Gajdusek, D. C. (1980) Evidence for and against the transmissibility of Alzheimer disease. *Neurology (Minneapolis)*, **30**, 945–950.

Guilleux, M. H. and Steiner, R. E. (1986) MR imaging in progressive multifocal leucoencephalopathy. *American Journal of Neuroradiology*, **7**, 1033–1035.

Haase, A. T., Gantz, D., Eble, B. *et al.* (1985) Natural history of restricted synthesis and expression of measles virus genes in subacute sclerosing panencephalitis. *Proceedings of the National Academy of Sciences of the USA*, **82**, 3020–3024.

Hall, W. W. and Choppin, P. W. (1979) Evidence for lack of synthesis of the M polypeptide of measles virus in brain cells in subacute sclerosing panencephalitis. *Virology*, **99**, 443–447.

Hall, W. W., Lamb, R. A. and Choppin, P. W. (1979) Measles and subacute sclerosing panencephalitis virus proteins: Lack of antibodies to the M protein in patients with subacute sclerosing panencephalitis. *Proceedings of the National Academy of Sciences of the USA*, **76**, 2047–2051.

Ho, D. D., Pomerantz, R. J. and Kaplan, J. C. (1987) Pathogenesis of infection with human immunodeficiency virus. *New England Journal of Medicine*, **317**, 278–286.

Hornabrook, R. W. (1968) Kuru—a subacute cerebellar degeneration. *Brain*, **91**, 53–74.

Houff, S. A., Major, E. O., Katz, D. A., Kufta, C. V., Sever, J. L. Pittaluga, S., Roberts, J. R., Gitt, J., Saini, N. and Lux, W. (1988). Involvement of JC virus-infected mononuclear cells from the bone marrow and spleen in the pathogenesis of progressive multifocal leucoencephalopathy. *New England Journal of Medicine*, **318**, 301–305.

Jabbour, J. T., Garcia, J. H., Lemmi, H., Rayland, J., Duenas, D. A. and Sever, J. L. (1969) Subacute sclerosing panencephalitis. A multidisciplinary study of eight cases. *Journal of the American Medical Association*, **207**, 2248–2254.

Jakob, A. (1921) Uber eine der multiplen Sklerose klinisch nahestehende Erkrankung des Zentralnervensystems (spastische Pseudosklerose) mit bemerkswerten anatomischen Befunde. *Medizinische Klinik*, **13**, 372–376.

Johnson, R. T. and Johnson, K. P. (1969) Slow and chronic infections of the nervous system. In F. Plum (ed.) *Recent Advances in Neurology*, pp. 33–78. F. A. Davis, Philadelphia.

Johnson, R. T. and McArthur, J. C. (1987) Myelopathies and retroviral infections. *Annals of Neurology*, **21**, 113–116.

Jones, D. P. and Nevin, S. (1954) Rapidly progressive cerebral degeneration (subacute vascular encephalopathy) with mental disorder, focal disturbances and myoclonic epilepsy. *Journal of Neurology, Neurosurgery and Psychiatry*, **17**, 148–159.

Koenig, S., Gendelman, E., Orenstein, J. M., Dal Canto, M. C., Pezeshkpour, G. H., Yungbluth, M., Janotta, F., Aksamit, A., Martin, M. A. and Fauci, A. S. (1986) Detection of AIDS virus in macrophages in brain tissue from AIDS patients with encephalopathy. *Science*, **233**, 1089–1093.

Kuzuhara, S., Kanazawa, I., Sasaki, H., Nakanishi, T. and Shimamura, K. (1983) Gerstmann–Sträussler–Scheinker's Disease. *Annals of Neurology*, **14**, 216–225.

Lampert, P. W., Gajdusek, D. C. and Gibbs, C. J. Jr (1972) Subacute spongiform virus encephalopathies. *American Journal of Pathology*, **68**, 626–652.

Lebon, P. and Lyon, G. (1974) Non-congenital rubella encephalitis. *Lancet*, **ii**, 468.

Masters, C. L. and Richardson, E. P. (1978) Subacute spongiform encephalopathy (Creutzfeldt–Jakob disease). *Brain*, **101**, 333–344.

Matthews, W. B. and Will, R. G. (1982) Epidemiology of Creutzfeldt–Jakob disease in Britain. *Neurology (NY)*, **32**, A186.

Mattson, R. H. (1974) Subacute sclerosing panencephalitis: recovery associated with isoprinosine therapy. *Neurology (Minneapolis)*, **24**, 383.

Metz, H., Gregoriou, M. and Sandifer, P. (1964) Subacute sclerosing panencephalitis: A review of 17 cases with special reference to clinical diagnostic criteria. *Archives of Disease in Childhood*, **39**, 554.

Navia, B. A., Jordan, B. D. and Price, R. W. (1986a) The AIDS dementia complex: I. Clinical features. *Annals of Neurology*, **19**, 517–524.

Navia, B. A., Cho, E. S., Petito, C. K. and Price, R. W. (1986b) The AIDS dementia complex II. Neuropathology. *Annals of Neurology*, **19**, 525–535.

Nevin, S., McMenemey, W. H. Behrman, S. and Jones, D. P. (1960) Subacute spongiform encephalopathy—a subacute form of encephalopathy attributable to vascular dysfunction (spongiform cerebral atrophy). *Brain*, **83**, 519–564.

Oesch, B., Westaway, D., Walchli, M., McKinley, M. P., Kent, S. B. H. *et al.* (1985) A cellular gene encodes scrapie PrP 27–30 protein. *Cell*, **40**, 735–746.

Osame, M., Matsumoto, M., Usuku, K. *et al.* (1987) Chronic progressive myelopathy associated with elevated antibodies to human T-lymphotropic virus type I and adult T-cell leukemia-like cell. *Annals of Neurology*, **21**, 117–122.

Padgett, B. L., Walker, D. L., ZuRhein, G. M. and Eckroade, R. J. (1971) Cultivation of papova-like virus from human brain with progressive multifocal leucoencephalopathy. *Lancet*, **i**, 1257–1260.

Pang, S., Koyanagi, Y., Miles, S., Wiley, C., Vinters, H. and Chen, I. S. Y. (1990) High levels of unintegrated HIV-1 DNA in brain tissue of AIDS dementia patients. *Science*, **343**, 85–89.

Pizzo, P. A., Eddy, J., Falloon, J., Balis, F. M., Murphy, R. F., Moss, H., Wolters, P., Brouwers, P., Jarosinski, P., Rubin, M., Broder, S., Yarchoan, R., Brunetti, A., Maha, M., Nusinoff-Lehrman, S. and Poplack, D. G. (1988) Effect of continuous intravenous infusion of zidovudine (AZT) in children with symptomatic HIV infection. *New England Journal of Medicine*, **319**, 889–896.

Portegies, P., Epstein, L. G., Tjong, A. Hung, S., De Gans, J. and Goudsmit, J. (1989a) Human immunodeficiency virus type 1 antigen in cerebrospinal fluid. Correlation with clinical neurologic status. *Archives of Neurology*, **46**, 261–264.

Portegies, P., De Gans, J., Lange, J. M. A., Derix, M. M. A., Speelman, H., Bakker, M., Danner, S. A. and Goudsmit, J. (1989b) Declining incidence of AIDS dementia complex after introduction of zidovudine treatment. *British Medical Journal*, **299**, 819–821.

Price, R. W., Brew, B., Sidtis, J., Rosenblum, M., Scheck, A. C. and Cleary, P. (1988) The brain in AIDS: central nervous system HIV-1 infection and AIDS dementia complex. *Science*, **239**, 586–592.

Price, R. W. and Brew, B. (1988) AIDS commentary: The AIDS dementia complex. *Journal of Infectious Diseases*, **158**, 1079–1083.

Prusiner, S. B. (1982) Novel proteinaceous infectious particles cause scrapie. *Science*, **216**, 136–144.

Prusiner, S. B. (1987) Prions and neurodegenerative diseases. *New England Journal of Medicine*, **317**, 1571–1581.

Prusiner, S. B. (1989) Scrapie prions. *Annual Review of Microbiology*, **43**, 345–374.

Prusiner, S. B., Groth, D. F., Bolton, D. C., Kent, S. B. and Hood, L. E. (1984) Purification and structural studies of a major scrapie prion protein. *Cell*, **38**, 127–134.

Richardson, E. P. Jr (1961) Progressive multifocal leucoencephalopathy. *New England Journal of Medicine*, **265**, 815–823.

Roman, G. C. (1987) Neurological review: Retrovirus-associated myelopathies. *Archives of Neurology*, **44**, 659–663.

Schmitt, F. A., Bigley, J. W., McKinnis, R., Logue, P. E., Evans, R. W., Drucker, J. L. and the AZT Collaborative Working Group (1988) Neuropsychological outcome of zidovudine (AZT) treatment of patients with AIDS and AIDS related complex. *New England Journal of Medicine*, **319**, 1573–1578.

Shaw, G. M., Harper, M. E., Hahn, B. H., Epstein, L. G., Gajdusek, D. C., Price, R. W., Navia, B. A., Petito, C. K., O'Hara, C. J., Groopman, J. E., Cho, E.–S., Oleske, J. M., Wong-Staal, F. and Gallo, R. C. (1985) HTLV-III infection in brains of children and adults with AIDS encephalopathy. *Science*, **227**, 177–181.

Sigurdsson, B. (1954) Rida; a chronic encephalitis of sheep. With general remarks on infections which develop slowly and some of their special characteristics. *British Veterinary Journal*, **110**, 341–354.

Sigurdsson, B., Palsson, P. A. and Grimsson, H. (1957) Visna, a demyelinating transmissible disease of sheep. *Journal of Neuropathology and Experimental Neurology*, **15**, 389–403.

Silva, C. A., Paula-Barbosa, M. M. and Pereira, S. (1981) Two cases of rapidly progressive subacute sclerosing panencephalitis: Neuropathological findings. *Archives of Neurology*, **38**, 109–113.

Silverman, L. and Rubinstein, L. J. (1965) Electron microscopic observations on a case of progressive multifocal leucoencephalopathy. *Acta Neuropathologica (Berlin)*, **5**, 215–224.

Sönnerborg, A. B., Von Stedingk, L.–V., Hansson, L. O. and Strannegard, O. O., (1989). Elevated neopterin and beta-2-microglobulin levels in blood and cerebrospinal fluid occur early in HIV-1 infection. *AIDS*, **3**, 277–283.

Townsend, J. J., Wolinsky, J. S. and Baringer, J. R. (1976) The neuropathology of progressive rubella panencephalitis of late onset. *Brain*, **99**, 81–90.

Walker, D. L. (1985) Progressive multifocal leucoencephalopathy. In P. J. Vinken, G. W. Bruyn and H. L. Klawans (eds) *Handbook of Clinical Neurology*, Vol. 47, P. J. Vinken, G. W Bruyn, H. L. Klawans and J. C. Koetsier (eds) *Demyelinating Diseases*, pp. 503–524. Elsevier Press, Amsterdam.

Weil, M. L., Itabashi, H. H., Cremer, N. E., Oshiro, L. S., Lennett, E. H. and Carnay, L. (1975) Chronic progressive panencephalitis due to rubella virus simulating subacute sclerosing panencephalitis. *New England Journal of Medicine*, **292**, 994–998.

Westaway, D., Carlson, G. A. and Prusiner, S. B. (1989) Unraveling prion diseases through molecular genetics. *Trends in Neurological Sciences*, **12**, 221–227.

Wiley, C. A., Schrier, R. D., Nelson, J. A., Lampert, P. W. and Oldstone, M. B. A. (1986) Cellular localization of human immunodeficiency virus infection within the brains of acquired immune deficiency syndrome patients. *Proceedings of the National Academy of Sciences of the USA*, **83**, 7089–7093.

Wolinsky, J. S. and Johnson, R. T. (1980) Role of viruses in chronic neurological diseases. In H. Fraenkel-Conrat and R. R. Wagner (eds) *Comprehensive Virology 16*, pp. 257–296. Plenum, New York.

Wolinsky, J. S., Berg, B. O. and Maitland, C. J. (1976) Progressive rubella panencephalitis. *Archives of Neurology*, **33**, 722–723.

Yarchoan, R., Brouwers, P., Spitzer, A. R., Grafman, J., Safai, B., Perno, C. F., Larson, S. M., Berg, G., Fischl, M. A., Wichman, A., Thomas, R. V., Brunetti, A., Schmidt, P. J., Meyers, Ch. E. and Broder, S. (1987) Response of human-immunodeficiency-virus-associated neurological disease to 3′-azido-3′-deoxythymidine. *Lancet*, **i**, 132–135.

Yoshida, M., Osame, M., Kawai, H., Toita, M., Kuwasaki, N., Nishida, Y., Hiraki, Y., Takahashi, K., Nomura, K., Sonoda, S., Eiraku, N., Ijichi, S. and Usuku, K. (1989) Increased replication of HTLV-I in HTLV-I-associated myelopathy. *Annals of Neurology*, **26**, 331–335.

Zu Rhein, G. M. and Chou, S. M. (1965) Particles resembling papova viruses in human cerebral demyelinating disease. *Science*, **148**, 1477–1479.

5

Interpreting the Role of Depression in Chronic Fatigue Syndrome

Colette Ray

Brunel University, Uxbridge, UK

Chronic fatigue syndrome, post-viral fatigue syndrome, and myalgic en-cephalomyelitis each refer to a cluster of symptoms of which the key feature is persistent, excessive and debilitating fatigue. The syndrome does not sit comfortably with conventional medical concepts, and the clinical presenta-tion is complex with patients describing a variety of muscular, neuro-psychological and autonomic symptoms in addition to fatigue. It is an intriguing disorder, and one that has attracted much controversy. Indeed, it is not even clear whether we are dealing with a single syndrome, or with a heterogeneous group of disorders which share some common characteris-tics. For example, Ramsay (1988) has argued that post-viral fatigue syn-drome and myalgic encephalomyelitis are distinct conditions, the latter being marked by its tendency to become chronic, by an almost unique form of muscular fatigability, and by the fluctuating nature of the symptoms. It may, perhaps, be premature to differentiate at this stage, and chronic fatigue syndrome (CFS) will be used throughout this chapter as an umbrella term. It has the advantage of referring directly to a major symptom, while making no assumptions about aetiology (Holmes *et al.* 1988; Lloyd *et al.*, 1988).

Sporadic cases of the disorder have been linked in the literature with epidemics of a similar illness, which are similarly unexplained, and one of which occurred at the Royal Free Hospital, London, in 1955 (Ramsay, 1988). Though it was suspected that an infectious agent might be involved in the Royal Free outbreak, an organic cause was not established, and this invited speculation that the victims had succumbed to mass hysteria. Some years later, two psychiatrists presented a defence of this hypothesis, basing their argument on a *post hoc* analysis of the case notes of affected nurses

Post-viral Fatigue Syndrome. Edited by R. Jenkins and J. Mowbray

(McEvedy and Beard, 1970), and on a finding of higher neuroticism scores for affected nurses compared with controls (McEvedy and Beard, 1973). The mass hysteria hypothesis has been widely challenged (Hyde and Bergmann, 1988; Kendell, 1967; Ramsay, 1988), but the debate continues (Dawson, 1987). There is an analogous debate about the aetiology of sporadic cases of CFS. There is a growing body of evidence, reviewed elsewhere in this volume, that CFS is related to viral infection and immunological abnormalities. However, this evidence is not unambiguous and there are, in parallel, findings which suggest that psychological factors are implicated in the illness.

Some of these studies have employed standard interviews designed to elicit psychiatric symptoms, such as the Diagnostic Interview Schedule (Robins et al., 1981) or the Schedule for Affective Disorders and Schizophrenia (Endicott and Spitzer, 1978). The absence or presence of psychiatric disorder is then determined, together with the diagnosis of type of disorder, on the basis of classification systems such as DSM-III (American Psychiatric Association, 1980) or the Research Diagnostic Criteria (Spitzer et al., 1978). Another approach has been to employ self-rating scales which provide a score on the psychological dimension of interest. The scores obtained for fatigued patients are then compared with those of a control group, or with normative scores. An example of such a scale is the Beck Depression Inventory (Beck, 1978). The relevant studies, with the samples and assessment procedures they employed, are summarised in Table 1.

From Table 1 it can be seen that, in studies which attempted a psychiatric diagnosis, a significant percentage of patients with fatigue appeared to have a psychiatric disorder, with major depression being the most common diagnosis. Where rating scales were employed, patients with chronic fatigue had higher scores than controls, or higher than would be expected on a normative basis, in a direction indicating affective or other disturbance. These studies adopted different criteria for defining their samples, but the findings are relatively consistent. Might it then be that depression can provide us with an explanation of CFS? Alternatively, should we exclude from the diagnosis those who meet the criteria for psychiatric disorder (Holmes et al., 1988)? Manu et al. (1988) (see Table 1) found that the majority of patients in their sample had either a medical or psychiatric diagnosis, or failed to meet minor criteria for CFS. They concluded that, if CFS is discounted in these cases, then CFS is rare indeed.

The section that follows puts the arguments in favour of attributing CFS to depression. There are, however, alternative ways of interpreting the data and subsequent sections will consider each of these in turn. First, there are complex issues involved in assessing psychological disorder in the context of medical illness, and these call into question the appropriateness of using standard procedures for determining depression. Second, a depressive syndrome may form part of the symptomatology of an organic illness. Third,

Table 1 Psychological status of patients with chronic fatigue

Authors	Samples	Assessments	Outcomes
Kroenke *et al.* (1988)	(1) 102 patients who identified fatigue as a major problem, lasting more than 30 days; not under the care of a psychiatrist, or with major medical disease. Mean duration of illness = 3.3 years (2) 26 non-fatigued controls, demographically matched with 26 of the fatigued patients	(a) Beck Depression Inventory (b) Modified Somatic Perceptions Questionnaire (c) Millon Health Behavioral Inventory	(a) 56% of the fatigued group had scores suggestive of depression (>10), and none of the controls (b) 57% of the fatigued group had high scores for somatic anxiety (>7), compared with 12% of the controls (c) The fatigued group had higher scores on all six psychogenic scales of the Millon Health Behavioral Inventory, especially for premorbid pessimism and somatic anxiety. On the coping attitude scales, the fatigued patients were more inhibited, less sociable and more sensitive
Kruesi *et al.* (1989)	28 patients who met Centers for Disease Control case definition criteria for CFS. Patients were required to have been ill for at least one year, and to be EBV-seropositive and to have antibodies to the diffuse or restricted components of EBV early antigen at titres of at least 1:40 or to lack antibodies to EBV nuclear antigens. Mean duration of illness = 6.8 years	Diagnostic Interview Schedule, with DSM–III criteria, but symptoms typically characterising CFS were not included	Lifetime prevalence of psychiatric diagnosis was 75%. Major depressive episode: $N = 13$ Simple phobia: $N = 8$ Dysthymia: $N = 7$ Alcohol abuse/dependence: $N = 3$ Somatisation disorder: $N = 2$ Antisocial personality: $N = 1$ Panic/agoraphobia: $N = 1$

(continued)

Table 1 (contd.)

Authors	Samples	Assessments	Outcomes
Manu et al. (1988)	135 patients with six months or more of debilitating fatigue	Diagnostic Interview Schedule	91 patients had one or more psychiatric disorders that were clinically active. Major depression: 50% Somatisation disorder: 14% Panic disorder: 8% Dysthymia: 6% Social phobia: 2% Bipolar disorder: 1%
Millon et al. (1989)	24 patients with both serological profiles and clinical symptomatology indicative of CEBV/CFS infection	(a) Millon Clinical Multiaxial Inventory (b) Profile of Mood States (c) Hamilton Rating Scale of Depression	(a) Compared with normative data, patients had high scores on some personality scales, and on the clinical syndrome scales of anxiety, somatoform disorder and dysthymia (b) Compared with normative data for college students, patients had elevated scores for fatigue and depression, and diminished vigour (c) 19 patients had scores indicative of at least moderate depression, with retardation/depression, anxiety/somatisation and diurnal variation featuring in particular

Table 1 (contd.)

Authors	Samples	Assessments	Outcomes
Taerk *et al.* (1987)	(1) 24 neuromyasthenic patients with subjective weakness or exhaustion, absence of significant physical findings, duration of symptoms for at least three months, onset after an apparent acute infective episode. Mean duration of illness = 18.1 months	(a) Diagnostic Interview Schedule, with DSM-III criteria	(a) There was a significant difference in the lifetime prevalence of major depression (patients 67%; controls 29%). There were no significant differences between the groups for anxiety disorders or substance use disorders
	(2) 24 non-clinical volunteers	(b) Beck Depression Inventory	(b) On the Beck Depression Inventory, 67% patients and 17% controls reported mild to severe depression
Wessely and Powell (1989)	(1) 47 CFS patients with a primary complaint of fatigue, lasting six months or more, and an absence of abnormalities on conventional investigation. Mean duration of illness = 67 months	(a) Schedule for Affective Disorder and Schizophrenia, with Research Diagnostic Criteria, but excluding fatigue as a criterion	(a) 72% of the CFS patients were cases of psychiatric disorder, compared with 36% of the neuromuscular controls. Major depression: 47% Somatisation disorder: 15%
	(2) 33 patients with peripheral neuromuscular fatiguing illnesses. Mean duration of illness = 75 months	(b) General Hospital Questionnaire	
	(3) 21 patients with major depression, diagnosed by Research Diagnostic Criteria. Mean duration of illness = 37 months	(c) Hospital Anxiety and Depression Scale	(b,c) The CFS group had higher scores than the neuromuscular controls, but lower scores than the patients with a primary diagnosis of major depression

chronic illness produces a psychological challenge, and patients who are depressed may be so as a reaction to their illness. Finally, psychological states may interact with organic factors in producing illness, thus playing a contributory role but without being causally sufficient. Though the discussion that follows centres on depression, many of the issues are pertinent also to other categories of psychological disturbance referred to in Table 1.

THE FORCE OF DEPRESSION AS AN EXPLANATION

If we look at the symptoms commonly cited for CFS, they show a considerable overlap with those of depression. Symptoms such as fatigue, headache, chest pain, dyspnoea, dizziness, dysuria and gastrointestinal disturbance may be present in both (David *et al.*, 1988). Somatic symptoms are a common feature of depressive disorder. Weckowicz *et al.* (1967) factor analysed the scores of hospitalised depressed patients for separate items of the Beck Depression Inventory, and found three factors: affective or guilty depression, retarded depression, and somatic disturbance. Items contributing to the latter included weight loss, loss of appetite and sleep disturbance, while the retardation factor included fatigue and somatic preoccupation. Wilson *et al.* (1983) noted that 51% of depressed patients in a family practice had somatoform complaints, in particular, sleep disorder, fatigue, dizziness, and diet-related and gastrointestinal complaints. The most commonly identified somatic complaints in another study of depressed patients were autonomic symptoms, wakefulness, a dry mouth and fatigue (Wittenborn and Buhler, 1979). These findings strongly suggest that affective disorder can play a role in the development and the continuation of somatic problems (Brenner, 1979; Cadoret *et al.*, 1980; Wilson *et al.*, 1983; Wittenborn and Buhler, 1979). Studies in the general population are also compatible with the existence of a relationship between somatic symptoms and depression. In a national sample of adults, fatigue was found to be related to depression, anxiety and stress, when these were rated as either present or absent in the past month (Chen, 1986). Similarly, in a study of undergraduates, fatigue was correlated with depression as measured by the Beck Depression Inventory, and also with cognitive anxiety or worry (Montgomery, 1983).

Fatigue and somatic complaints in general are thus commonly implicated in depression and other emotional disturbance, though they are not universal and the nature and severity of the complaints varies from patient to patient (Wittenborn and Buhler, 1979). At least in the context of clinical depression, such complaints are commonly attributed to the affective disorder. But what if, as is the case in CFS, patients feel that their disorder is physical, and claim that they are not depressed or that depression is not the key to their problem? This, too, can be encompassed within the framework of depression, on the assumption that people may be psychologically distressed but express this in physical terms, either being unaware of their psychological distress or declining to attribute physical symptoms to this. Several, interrelated conceptual frameworks are relevant to this view: somatisation, masked depression and abnormal illness behaviour.

Somatisation disorder, as described by DSM-III, is a specific diagnostic category, referring to a history of physical symptoms of several years' duration and beginning before the age of 30. The criteria specify at least 14 symptoms for women and 12 for men. These may include pseudoneurological, gastrointestinal, female reproductive, psychosexual and cardiopulmonary symptoms, and pain. In studies of patients with chronic fatigue, a few patients have attracted diagnoses of somatisation disorder (see Table 1). However, *somatisation* as a process, rather than as a specific disorder, might have a more widespread relevance in CFS. It occurs in the context of disorders such as major depression, where it has been defined as 'the selective perception and focus on the somatic manifestations of depression with denial or minimization of the affective and cognitive changes' (Katon *et al.*, 1982, p. 127). A similar concept is that of *masked depression* (Lesse, 1968; Lesse and Mathers, 1968), and this refers to depression which manifests as hypochondriacal or psychosomatic complaints, rather than as affective disturbance. In such cases there may or may not be a medical condition underlying the somatic complaints but, if there is such a condition, its symptoms are exaggerated or amplified. Goldberg and Bridges (1988) have argued that somatisation is a phenomenon which occurs within the general, non-psychiatric population, with some people choosing to express their distress in physical terms while others choose to psychologise theirs. Factors which might affect the somatisation of distress include cultural norms and family influences, sanctions against the expression of emotional states, and lay models of causation which govern the interpretation of bodily change (Katon *et al.*, 1982). Goldberg and Bridges (1988) highlight the blame-avoiding function of somatisation:

. . . it is a great way for not seeing oneself as mentally ill, and not seeing oneself as responsible for the life predicament that one happens to be in . . . It is this blame-avoiding function of somatization that seems to us to be its key feature, and perhaps explains why patients do not report such great levels of depression. (p. 142)

Illness behaviour is the term employed to describe the ways in which people monitor their bodies, define and interpret symptoms, take remedial action, and utilise sources of help; broadly, it refers to how they view bodily indications and the conditions under which they come to see these as abnormal (Mechanic, 1986). Abnormal illness behaviour implies a biased and distorted view, and the term is used to indicate

The persistence of a maladaptive mode of experiencing, perceiving, evaluating and responding to one's own health status, despite the fact that a doctor has provided a lucid and accurate appraisal of the situation and management to be followed (if any), with opportunities for discussion, negotiation and clarification, based on adequate assessment of all relevant biological, psychological, social and cultural factors. (Pilowsky, 1986, p. 76)

(It is admitted that this definition raises issues about the accuracy of the medical opinion!) Analysis of an Illness Behavior Questionnaire, administered to patients with intractable pain, yielded seven factors (Pilowsky and Spence, 1975). These included disease conviction, that is, a firm belief that a somatic disorder is present and a reluctance to accept reassurance, and somatic focusing, indicating the tendency to reject the possibility of a psychological dimension to the condition and to focus on somatic problems (Pilowsky and Spence, 1975). It is suggested that abnormal illness behaviour should perhaps be best regarded neither as a physical disorder nor as an affective disorder, but as the achievement of a form of psychological equilibrium through adopting a particular sick role.

What then is the difficulty in attributing CFS to psychological distress? A ready and well-established diagnosis of major depression is available for those patients who meet the criteria for this disorder, while patients who report little affective disturbance may be regarded as somatising their distress and presenting this in the form of abnormal illness behaviour. Nevertheless, in order to prove a hypothesis, it is not sufficient to demonstrate its plausibility. Recognised physical conditions such as cancer and tuberculosis have in the past been construed in terms of psychological causation, with such models being abandoned with the advance of medical knowledge (Angell, 1985; Sontag, 1977). There are a number of alternative explanations for the consistently observed association between CFS and psychological disorder, and these need to be considered alongside the hypothesis that psychological factors play a role in the aetiology and maintenance of CFS.

THE SPURIOUS DIAGNOSIS OF DEPRESSION IN MEDICAL ILLNESS

We have already noted the overlap between the somatic symptoms of CFS and depression. However, if we assume that CFS is essentially a medical disorder primarily caused by viral or immunological factors, then it can be argued that the somatic symptoms are a direct outcome of this illness process rather than of depression. Kathol and Delahunt (1986) have pointed to the cross-over of symptoms between hyperthyroidism, depression and anxiety. When major depressive disorder was defined according to DSM-III, but excluding the requirement that the symptoms should not be due to organic disease, 10 of 32 hyperthyroid patients were identified as depressed. When somatic symptoms associated with their condition were de-emphasised, and significant social incapacity was included in their place, only three patients could be described as depressed. The researchers concluded that the incidence of depression varies significantly, depending upon the criteria that are employed; they warned that systems such as DSM-III are intended for the evaluation of patients without medical illness, and that their use in patients with physical conditions can lead to false positive psychiatric diagnoses. Somewhat different findings have been obtained in the context of diabetes mellitus. Lustman *et al.* (1986a) noted a high rate of psychiatric disorder in these patients, most commonly major depression and anxiety, even when symptoms which physicians had consistently attributed to the physical illness were excluded as criteria (for depression, these were weight loss, feeling tired out, hypersomnia, feeling slowed down and loss of sexual interest). Then, subsequently, the symptoms which had been excluded were re-included (Lustman *et al.*, 1986b). This procedure resulted in only a marginal increase in the diagnoses of depression. It was concluded that the Diagnostic Interview Schedule is appropriate for the detection of psychiatric illness in diabetes, though the researchers cautioned that a generalisation of this conclusion to other disorders would be injudicious.

The issue at stake here is that the diagnosis of depression is determined in part by the presence of somatic symptoms, when such symptoms may be produced by a medical condition in the absence of affective disorder. It is thus possible for patients to be assigned to a category of major depression largely on the basis of symptoms produced by their physical illness (Popkin *et al.*, 1987; Snaith, 1987). For a diagnosis of a major depressive episode, the Research Diagnostic Criteria require five out of eight symptoms in addition to dysphoric mood. These include changes in appetite or weight, sleep difficulties, fatigability, psychomotor retardation and diminished ability to think or concentrate (Spitzer *et al.*, 1978). The criteria for DSM-III-R similarly include symptoms which are not specific to depression. There are parallel difficulties when rating scales are used for the assessment of depression or other dimensions of psychological distress. The Hamilton Depression Scale includes six items which relate to somatic disturbance, and these account for 31% of the possible variance (Snaith, 1987), while seven of the 21 items of the Beck Depression Inventory refer to somatic function. One study compared psychiatric with medical patients on individual items of the Beck Depression Inventory (Cavanaugh *et al.*, 1983). It was found that somatic items such as fatigue, weight loss and worry about health did not discriminate between the two groups, and that the groups were more clearly differentiated by cognitive and affective items. Furthermore, cognitive and affective symptoms increased both in frequency and intensity with the overall severity of depression, while somatic symptoms increased in intensity but only minimally in frequency. The authors concluded that somatic symptoms are a poor indicator of depression in the medically ill.

ASSESSING DEPRESSION IN CFS

Are, then, standard measures of depression appropriate in the context of CFS? Some of the somatic symptoms commonly reported by patients, including the key feature of fatigue itself, overlap with symptoms of depression. If we were to assume that this is not a physical illness, then it would certainly be appropriate to include such symptoms as criteria for depression. If, on the other hand, we admit the possibility that this is a medical condition with somatic features in common with depression, then such symptoms should perhaps not be included. The situation is complex, given the currently ambiguous nature of the disorder. It is complex even in the case of an illness such as cancer (Endicott, 1984) which is, relatively speaking, well understood. Two studies have addressed the issue with regard to CFS. Wessely and Powell (1989) excluded just fatigue as a criterion for depression in their study of patients with CFS; they nevertheless found higher rates of depressive disorder in the CFS than in the neuromuscular control group. Another study followed Lustman et al.'s procedure described earlier, omitting as criteria symptoms which typically characterise CFS; a high rate of psychiatric disorder was still obtained and this was not significantly changed by rescoring the excluded symptoms as psychiatrically relevant (Kruesi et al., 1989). The latter finding suggests that, in terms of psychiatric assessment, CFS might be like diabetes mellitus for which standard procedures may be appropriate (Lustman et al., 1986b), rather than like thyroid disorder for which highly variable rates of disorder are obtained depending upon whether standard or adjusted criteria are applied (Kathol and Delahunt, 1986). Given the range and variability of symptoms associated with CFS, it may be difficult to decide which symptoms should and should not be included as legitimate criteria for depression, and this issue needs to be considered further. The report of the study described above (Kruesi et al., 1989) did not specify the symptoms excluded.

If rating scales are used, then these should, arguably, be appropriate to the setting of medical illness. One study has noted that CFS patients showed high scores particularly on those affective scales with a large somatic component (Millon et al., 1989). The Beck Depression Inventory is one of the most widely used self-report measures, but in the context of physical illness cognitive and affective items should be scored separately from somatic items. Items which provide an index of severity of depression in the medically as well as psychiatrically ill are suicidal ideation, sense of failure, sense of punishment, loss of social interest, indecision and dissatisfaction (Clark *et al.*, 1983). The Hospital Anxiety and Depression Scale (Zigmund and Snaith, 1983) was designed with the problem of confounding between symptoms of medical illness and affective disturbance in mind. Items for depression on this scale are based largely upon the anhedonic state. Even more appropriate are measures which provide a multifactorial assessment of psychological status. The Profile of Mood States (McNair *et al.*, 1981) yields separate assessments for depression, fatigue, vigour, confusion, tension and anger; several of these dimensions are relevant in the context of CFS, and the measure was used by Millon *et al.* (1989) (see Table 1). Unfortunately, since it focuses on mood states, there is no assessment of specific somatic concerns. Another broad measure of psychological distress is the SCL-90R (Derogatis *et al.*, 1976; Derogatis, 1977). As well as producing an overall score for distress, it comprises a number of factorially distinct subscales, one of which assesses depression primarily as an affective state, while cognitive and somatic symptoms are represented on separate subscales (these factors are labelled, respectively, obsessive-compulsive and somatisation).

DEPRESSION AS A SYMPTOM OF MEDICAL ILLNESS

A somewhat different issue is that a medical condition can produce a full-blown depressive syndrome, irrespective of any overlap in somatic features. Patients with neurological, endocrinal, metabolic and nutritional disorders may show symptoms of such a syndrome (Derogatis and Wise, 1989), and viral illness is also associated with mood changes. Sachar (1975) notes a study by Sachar and Juter, in which it was found that 25% of a sample of influenza victims reported depressed mood, pessimism, self-deprecation, diminished libido, anorexia, sleep disturbance and decreased ambition three weeks after the illness had subsided. Long-term psychological effects have been noted following infectious mononucleosis. In one study, patients filled in the Middlesex Hospital Questionnaire a year after their illness; the women in the sample had higher scores than a normative sample on anxiety, depression and somatic symptoms, though there were no differences for male subjects (Cadie *et al.*, 1976). It has been suggested that this illness can have persistent neurological and psychiatric consequences in a minority of cases, and that depression here may be organically caused and secondary to nervous system involvement (Hendler and Leahy, 1978; Hendler, 1987).

Where depression arises as a direct result of a medical condition, it is possible that there may be processes at work which are common to primary affective disorder. The depression of viral and post-viral illness could reflect a neurochemical change induced by the virus (Sachar, 1975). One might speculate that CFS involves a shift in the activity of biogenic amines, producing changes similar to those of depressive illness. Their decreased activity or availability has long been cited as a basis for depression, though the status of findings relating to these various amine hypotheses remains unsettled (Baldessarini, 1983) and the overall pattern of neurotransmitter activity, rather than any one factor considered in isolation, may be important in understanding the varied phenomenology (Whybrow *et al.*, 1984).

Depressive illness has also been associated with abnormalities of function in the hypothalamo–pituitary–adrenal axis (Charlton and Ferrier, 1989), characterised by raised basal cortisol but normal levels of basal ACTH. A significant proportion of patients show a resistance to cortisol suppression by oral dexamethasone (Carroll *et al.*, 1981). Taerk *et al.* (1987) (see Table 1) administered the Dexamethasone Suppression Test to 16 of the fatigued patients in their sample, but found normal responses in 15 of these. However, not all patients diagnosed with major depression show a positive response, and the test may be sensitive only in the most severe cases (Christie *et al.*, 1986). A recent study has investigated neuroendocrine abnormality in CFS (Demitrack *et al.*, 1989), with challenging results. Compared with healthy controls, the fatigued patients had low basal cortisol levels and high basal ACTH, a pattern which contrasts with that observed in depression. Such comparisons offer the prospect of clarifying our understanding of both CFS and depression, though it will be important to consider the complexity and variability of biochemical features in the latter when designing and interpreting studies.

DEPRESSION AS A REACTION TO CHRONIC ILLNESS

If a person is physically ill and depressed, their emotional state could reflect a dispositional tendency to depression or it could represent a symptom of the illness. There is also a third possibility, which is that their depression is a reaction to the distressing situation in which they find themselves. In one study of patients covering the spectrum of medical illness, irritability, anxiety and depression were noted in 78%, 75% and 50% of the sample respectively, though such symptoms were not as severe as in psychiatric patients (Schwab *et al.*, 1966). The physically ill patient has to cope with the frustration of malaise and debility and, where the illness is chronic, may be forced to re-evaluate long-term expectations and life plans. Psychological well-being depends upon a positive self-evaluation, the perception of control or mastery, and an optimism about the future (Taylor and Brown, 1988). All of these will be challenged, and the patient may have difficulty in achieving the goals and maintaining incentives which previously gave meaning to life.

Whatever the role of psychological factors in contributing to CFS, the syndrome would thus be likely to give rise to a depressive *reaction* to the impairment that is involved. Kroenke *et al.* (1988), in their study of patients who identified fatigue as a major problem, found elevated scores on as many as 10 of the 12 subscales of the Sickness Impact Profile, which is a measure of functional impairment. It would be surprising if patients did not become demoralised as they find their activity curtailed and sources of reward lost to them. According to one model of depression (Klinger, 1975, 1977), the first response when incentives become difficult to maintain is one of invigoration; there will be a focus on overcoming obstacles, and anger and aggression may increase. As the expectation of success declines, so there will be a feeling of loss and hopelessness, and invigoration will give way to disengagement and depression. This model suggests a progression from invigoration to depression, but the patient with CFS might equally well shift between these different responses, at times despairing and at times striving for a resolution. This shifting perspective could contribute to what has been described as the fraught interplay between patients and their doctors (David *et al.*, 1988). Social and family relationships may also suffer as a result of chronic illness. The plight of the cancer patient has been vividly described, and elements of this may apply similarly to CFS:

So, most . . . patients find themselves in an uncomfortable situation, a 'catch-22': either they can express their feelings and be themselves, thereby incurring others' avoidance and rejection, or they can enact a charade, pretending that everything is fine, and obtain at least some support from others. Because neither of these alternatives is satisfactory, the patient may vacillate between them, sometimes putting on a good face, and sometimes confronting others with their pain and anxiety. This vacillation, of course, pollutes the social environment still further . . . (Wortman and Dunkel-Schetter, 1979, pp. 142–143)

INTERACTIONS BETWEEN PSYCHOLOGICAL AND ORGANIC FACTORS

The intention in this chapter is to present possible interpretations of the role of depression in CFS, rather than to argue for any one of these. If there is an argument, it is that we should remain for the time being open-minded, hastening neither to discount psychological influences nor to seize upon these as an explanation for the disorder. Four positions have been considered:

(a) The symptoms of CFS can be regarded as a manifestation of psychological distress, given the high rate of depressive and other disorder in these patients. However, not all patients meet psychiatric criteria, and there is recent evidence of differences between CFS and primary affective disorder when specific features of the depressive syndrome are considered.

Biological and functional symptoms, together with mood change, are the predominant features in the former, and depressed CFS patients are less likely to report guilt and low self-esteem than affective patients (Powell *et al.*, 1990). This suggests that we are dealing at least with a particular subtype of depression, though it is unclear whether this should be taken to indicate a different biological basis or merely the patient's avoidance of self-blame by attributing symptoms to a physical rather than a psychological illness. Can, however, psychological disorder fully explain the physical and immunological aberrations found in CFS (Kruesi *et al.*, 1989; Straus, 1988)?

(b) Estimates of the rate of depression and other psychological disorder in CFS may be inflated by the fact that somatic symptoms which characterise this, and other medical illness, are also criteria for depression. It is unlikely that this in itself could account for the findings, but it is a methodological problem that needs to be addressed in future studies. Assessment procedures that are valid in the absence of medical illness may not be so in CFS, but this will be a difficult issue to resolve given our poor understanding of the structure not only of CFS but also of depression (Kendell, 1976).

(c) The depressive syndrome observed in CFS may result from pathological processes whose aetiology is distinct from that of major affective disorder. Different causes can produce the same phenomenon, and commonalities between symptoms do not indicate that they have the same cause. Within the terms of DSM-III, a diagnosis of organic affective syndrome rather than major depression is appropriate where affective disturbance is thought to be a direct pathophysiological function of a medical condition, and the manual specifically notes that viral illness may cause a depressive syndrome.

(d) To some extent at least, the depression observed in patients with CFS will be a reaction to the malaise and chronicity of the illness, and its impact on functioning. DSM-III recommends that, where major depression is a psychological reaction to the impairment caused by physical illness, then this should be the diagnosis recorded, with the physical disorder being noted on a separate axis. It is, however, difficult in these circumstances to determine whether depression is indeed a response to impairment, or whether the patient's disposition is such that they would be depressed irrespective of the illness. A preceding history of mood disorder would suggest that a depressed state is more than just a reaction to circumstances. In the absence of such a history, we should beware of what has been termed the 'fundamental attribution error' (Heider, 1958; Ross, 1977). It seems that when we make judgements about others, but not when judging ourselves, we have a bias towards attributing behaviour to enduring personal characteristics and fail to give due explanatory weight to situational pressures.

It is in principle possible to interpret the affective disorder of CFS as a symptom of the medical condition or reaction to the impairment produced by this. However, there is evidence that psychological problems precede the onset of fatigue in some patients, and this suggests that they may indeed play a contributory role. Taerk *et al.* (1987) found that 50% of patients in their sample had had a major depressive episode prior to the development of neuromyasthenia, and Wessely and Powell (1989) observed that patients in their CFS group were more likely to have a psychiatric history than were the neuromuscular controls. It was concluded by Kruesi *et al.* (1989) that psychiatric problems are more likely to precede the syndrome than to follow the syndrome; in 10 patients, the problem antedated the onset of chronic fatigue though, in the majority of these cases, the diagnosis was one of anxiety rather than depression. These observations are retrospective and should be treated with caution but, even if taken at face value, they do not in themselves imply that CFS is no more than a psychological disorder. The latter may interact with an organic condition, reinforcing its effects. There are several ways in which such an interaction might occur, adding to the list of possibilities summarised above.

ENHANCING OR PROLONGING SYMPTOMS

Psychological factors could interact with an organic illness through their influence on illness behaviour. First, they might exacerbate the symptoms of an ongoing disorder. A patient's general emotional status may determine the distress produced by symptoms (Zigmund and Snaith, 1983), and the adaptiveness of their response. Second, the symptoms of an infective illness might be prolonged in the absence of continuing organic involvement. Thus, in the context of chronic brucellosis, it has been argued that depression causes the normally transient symptoms of lassitude and fatigability to be perpetuated, as these merge with depressive lassitude and fatigue (Imboden *et al.*, 1959). Similarly, in neurasthenia, it has been suggested that 'while the precipitant to the illness is an acute (usually viral) illness, the development of chronicity could be related to a particular response to the illness and its associated debilitation, which triggers a depressive syndrome' (Taerk *et al.*, 1987, p. 54). Wessely and colleagues (Wessely *et al.*, 1989; Chapter 2) describe in detail cognitive and behavioural factors which may foster such chronicity. Avoidance of activity and mood disorder could sustain symptoms, and create a vicious circle including expectations of failure, a belief in the continuation of the original illness, decreased physiological and psychological tolerance, and feelings of helplessness and loss of control.

INCREASED PHYSICAL VULNERABILITY

Psychological factors can affect susceptibility to viral illness (Laudenslager, 1987). Cluff et al. (1966) assessed psychological vulnerability in a group of employees and found that this was related to subsequent illness in an influenza epidemic. In this study, as in many others in this area, it may have been illness behaviour that was affected rather than illness per se, with vulnerable patients being more likely to respond to symptoms and to seek help. However, a long-term prospective study of military cadets found that psychosocial risk factors predicted both those who developed clinical infectious mononucleosis and seroconverters who developed high antibody titres without apparent disease (Kasl et al., 1979). Psychological factors can enhance the severity and duration of illness, as well as susceptibility. In one study (Canter, 1972), subjects were assessed before being experimentally exposed to tularaemia; those who were psychologically vulnerable on the basis of this prior assessment experienced higher levels of symptoms and had more hours of fever. Greenfield et al. (1959) studied a sample of undergraduates who had suffered from infectious mononucleosis. Though the psychological tests were administered after their recovery, the duration of their illness was determined by objective haematological criteria; a relationship was found between the latter and the psychological dimension of ego strength. In line with this finding, psychosocial risk factors were found to predict length of hospitalisation among cadets who developed clinical infectious mononucleosis (Kasl et al., 1979).

The expanding field of psychoneuroimmunology is concerned with the interconnections between emotions and behaviour, the central nervous system, and the immune system (Ader, 1981; Solomon, 1985). There is evidence that short- and long-term stressors, ranging from sitting an examination to caring for a relative with Alzheimer's disease, produce changes in immune function (Kennedy et al., 1988). Some studies have found altered cell-mediated immunity in patients with major depressive disorder, though it seems that this is restricted to certain subgroups (Schleifer et al., 1989). It is not yet clear whether such changes are clinically significant (Hall, 1987; King and Cooper, 1989), but it has been suggested that links between psychological factors and the immune system could be relevant to the understanding of CFS (David et al., 1988; Straus, 1988). These pathways of influence might be bidirectional. There is reason to believe that immune function can influence affect, cognition and behaviour (Adams et al., 1984), and Straus (1988) has suggested that an initiating virus could lead to sustained immunological activation in CFS, this in itself perpetuating fatigue, malaise and depression. This raises the possibility of there being a vicious circle at a biological level, as well as at the level of illness behaviour, with emotion influencing immunity and immune factors further compromising psychological status.

Three sets of factors are commonly cited in the explanation of CFS: viral, immunological and psychological. It would be misleading to assume that these are rival hypotheses. The syndrome may prove to have multiple causes (Straus, 1988; Swartz, 1988), though one set of factors could be more important than another in the individual case. Furthermore, the syndrome may result from a reciprocal interplay of causes, with psychological status potentially having an impact on both physical vulnerability and the response to the illness, and being in turn affected by the illness process. The significance of a psychological influence is still a matter for debate, since the findings are open to multiple interpretations. However, to accept such an influence is not to deny the involvement of other factors. All illness may be multifactorial (Lipowski, 1986; Plaut and Friedman, 1981), and the distinction between psychosomatic and organic categories has become increasingly difficult to sustain: 'There are no psychosomatic illnesses because all illness (and health, along a continuum) is psychosomatic. To speak of psychosomatic illness is to court error by suggesting that there are nonpsychosomatic illnesses' (Oken, 1987, p. 110).

REFERENCES

Adams, F., Quesada, J. R. and Guiterman, J. V. (1984) Neuropsychiatric manifestations of human leucocyte interferon therapy in patients with cancer. *Journal of the American Medical Association*, **252**, 938–941.

Ader, R. (ed.) (1981) *Psychoneuroimmunology*. Academic Press, New York.

American Psychiatric Association (1980) *Diagnostic and Statistical Manual of Mental Disorders (DSM-III)*, 3rd edn, revised 1987. American Psychiatric Association, Washington, DC.

Angell, M. (1985) Disease as a reflection of the psyche. *New England Journal of Medicine*, **312**, 1570–1572.

Baldessarini, R. (1983) *Biomedical Aspects of Depression and its Treatment*. American Psychiatric Press, Washington, DC.

Beck, A. T. (1978) *Depression Inventory*. Center for Cognitive Therapy, Philadelphia.

Brenner, B. (1979) Depressed affect and somatic problems. *Psychological Medicine*, **9**, 737–746.

Cadie, M., Nye, F. J. and Storey, P. (1976) Anxiety and depression after infectious mononucleosis. *British Journal of Psychiatry*, **128**, 559–564.

Cadoret, R. J., Widmer, R. B. and Troughton, E. P. (1980) Somatic complaints: Harbinger of depression in primary care. *Journal of Affective Disorders*, **2**, 61–70.

Canter, A. (1972) Changes in mood during incubation of acute febrile disease and effects of pre-exposure psychologic status. *Psychosomatic Medicine*, **34**, 424–430.

Carroll, B. J., Feinberg, M., Greden, J. F., Tarika, J., Albala, A. A., Haskett, R. F., James, N. M., Kronfol, Z., Lohr, N., Steiner, M., de Vigne, J. P. and Young, E. (1981) A specific laboratory test for the diagnosis of melancholia. *Archives of General Psychiatry*, **38**, 15–22.

Cavanaugh, S., Clark, D. and Gibbons, R. (1983) Diagnosing depression in the hospitalised medically ill using the Beck Depression Inventory. *Psychosomatics*, **24**, 809–815.

Charlton, B. G. and Ferrier, I. N. (1989) Hypothalamo–pituitary–adrenal axis abnormalities in depression: A review and a model. *Psychological Medicine*, **19**, 331–336.

Chen, M. K. (1986) The epidemiology of self perceived fatigue among adults. *Preventive Medicine*, **15**, 74–81.

Christie, J. E., Whalley, L. J., Dick, H., Blackwood, D. H. R., Blackburn, I. M. and Fink, G. (1986) Raised plasma cortisol concentrations are a feature of drug-free psychotics and are not specific to depression. *British Journal of Psychiatry*, **148**, 58–67.

Clark, D. C., Cavanaugh, S. and Gibbons, R. D. (1983) The core symptoms of depression in medical and psychiatric patients. *Journal of Nervous and Mental Disease*, **171**, 705–713.

Cluff, L. E., Canter, A. and Imboden, J. B. (1966) Asian influenza: Infection, disease and psychological factors. *Archives of Internal Medicine*, **117**, 159–163.

David, A. S., Wessely, S. and Pelosi, A. J. (1988) Postviral fatigue syndrome: Time for a new approach. *British Medical Journal*, **296**, 696–699.

Dawson, J. (1987) Royal Free disease: Perplexity continues. *British Medical Journal*, **294**, 327–328.

Demitrack, M., Dale, J. K., Gold, P. W., Chrousos, G. and Straus, S. E. (1989) Neuroendocrine abnormalities in patients with chronic fatigue syndrome. *Clinical Research*, **37**, 532A.

Derogatis, L. R. (1977) *The SCL-90 Manual I: Scoring, Administration and Procedures for the SCL-90.* Clinical Psychometric Research, Baltimore.

Derogatis, L. R. and Wise, T. N. (1989) *Anxiety and Depressive Disorders in the Medical Patient.* American Psychiatric Press, Washington, DC.

Derogatis, L. R., Rickels, K. and Rock, A. F. (1976) The SCL-90 and the MMPI: A step in the validation of a new self report scale. *British Journal of Psychiatry*, **128**, 280–289.

Endicott, J. (1984) Measurement of depression in patients with cancer. *Cancer*, **53**, 2243–2248.

Endicott, J. and Spitzer, R. L. (1978) A diagnostic interview: The schedule for affective disorders and schizophrenia. *Archives of General Psychiatry*, **35**, 835–844.

Goldberg, D. and Bridges, K. (1988) Somatic presentations of psychiatric illness in primary care setting. *Journal of Psychosomatic Research*, **32**, 137–144.

Greenfield, N. S., Roessler, R. and Crosley, A. P. (1959) Ego strength and length of recovery from infectious mononucleosis. *Journal of Nervous and Mental Disease*, **128**, 125–128.

Hall, J. G. (1987) Depression, stress and immunity. *Lancet*, **ii**, 221.

Heider, F. (1958) *The Psychology of Interpersonal Relations.* Wiley, New York.

Hendler, N. (1987) Infectious mononucleosis and psychiatric disorders. In E. Kurstak, Z. J. Lipowski and P. V. Morozov (eds) *Viruses, Immunity and Mental Disorders*, pp. 81–94. Plenum, New York.

Hendler, N. and Leahy, W. (1978) Psychiatric and neurologic sequelae of infectious mononucleosis. *American Journal of Psychiatry*, **135**, 842–844.

Holmes, G. P., Kaplan, J. E., Gantz, N. M., Komaroff, A. L., Schonberger, L. B., Straus, S. E., Jones, J. F., Dubois, R. E., Cunningham-Rundles, C., Pahwa, J., Tosato, G., Zegans, L. S., Purtilo, D. T., Brown, N., Schooley, R. T. and Brus, I. (1988) Chronic fatigue syndrome: A working case definition. *Annals of Internal Medicine*, **108**, 387–389.

Hyde, B. and Bergmann, S. (1988) Akureyri disease (myalgic encephalomyelitis), forty years later. *Lancet*, **ii**, 1191–1192.

Imboden, J. B., Canter, A., Cluff, L. E. and Trever, R. W. (1959) Brucellosis III. Psychologic aspects of delayed convalescence. *Archives of Internal Medicine,* **103,** 406–414.

Kasl, S. V., Evans, A. S. and Niederman, J. C. (1979) Psychosocial risk factors in the development of infectious mononucleosis. *Psychosomatic Medicine,* **41,** 445–466.

Kathol, R. G. and Delahunt, J. W. (1986) The relationship of anxiety and depression to symptoms of hyperthyroidism using operational criteria. *General Hospital Psychiatry,* **8,** 23–28.

Katon, W., Kleinman, A. and Rosen, G. (1982) Depression and somatization: A review. *American Journal of Medicine,* **72,** 127–135.

Kendell, R. E. (1967) The psychiatric sequelae of benign myalgic encephalomyelitis. *British Journal of Psychiatry,* **113,** 837–846.

Kendell, R. E. (1976) The classification of depression: A review of the contemporary confusion. *British Journal of Psychiatry,* **129,** 15–28.

Kennedy, S., Kiecolt-Glaser, J. K. and Glaser, R. (1988) Immunological consequences of acute and chronic stressors: Mediating role of interpersonal relationships. *British Journal of Medical Psychology,* **61,** 77–85.

King, D. J. and Cooper, S. J. (1989) Viruses, immunity and mental disorder. *British Journal of Psychiatry,* **154,** 1–7.

Klinger, E. (1975) Consequences of commitment to and disengagement from incentives. *Psychological Review,* **82,** 1–24.

Klinger, E. (1977) *Meaning and Void.* University of Minnesota Press, Minneapolis.

Kroenke, K., Wood, D. R., Mangelsdorff, A. D., Meier, N. J. and Powell, J. B. (1988) Chronic fatigue in primary care. *Journal of the American Medical Association,* **260,** 929–934.

Kruesi, M. J. P., Dale, J. and Straus, S. E. (1989) Psychiatric diagnoses in patients who have chronic fatigue syndrome. *Journal of Clinical Psychiatry,* **50,** 53–56.

Laudenslager, M. L. (1987) Psychosocial stress and susceptibility to infectious disease. In *Viruses, Immunity and Mental Disorders* E. Kurstak, Z. J. Lipowski and P. V. Morozov (eds) *Viruses, Immunity and Mental Disorders,* pp. 391–402. Plenum, New York.

Lesse, S. (1968) The multivariate masks of depression. *American Journal of Psychiatry,* **124,** 35–40.

Lesse, S. and Mathers, J. (1968) Depression sine depression. *New York Journal of Medicine,* **68,** 535–543.

Lipowski, Z. J. (1986) What does the word 'psychosomatic' really mean? A historical and semantic inquiry. In M. J. Christie and P. G. Mellett (eds) *The Psychosomatic Approach: Contemporary Practice of Whole-person Care,* pp. 17–38. Wiley, London.

Lloyd, A., Wakefield, D., Boughton, C. and Dwyer, J. (1988) What is myalgic encephalomyelitis? *Lancet,* **i,** 1286–1287.

Lustman, P. J., Griffith, L. S., Clouse, R. E. and Cryer, P. E. (1986a) Psychiatric illness in diabetes mellitus: Relationship to symptoms and glucose control. *Journal of Nervous and Mental Disease,* **174,** 736–742.

Lustman, P. J., Harper, G. W., Griffith, L. S. and Clouse, R. E. (1986b) Use of the Diagnostic Interview Schedule in patients with diabetes mellitus. *Journal of Nervous and Mental Disease,* **174,** 743–746.

Manu, P., Lane, T. and Matthews, D. (1988) The frequency of Chronic Fatigue Syndrome in patients with symptoms of persistent fatigue. *Annals of Internal Medicine,* **109,** 554–556.

McEvedy, C. P. and Beard, A. W. (1970) Royal Free epidemic of 1955: A reconsideration. *British Medical Journal,* **1,** 7–11.

McEvedy, C. P. and Beard, A. W. (1973) A controlled follow-up of cases involved in an epidemic of 'benign myalgic encephalomyelitis'. *British Journal of Psychiatry*, **122**, 141–150.

McNair, D. M., Lorr, M. and Droppleman, L. F. (1981) *Profile of Mood States*. Educational and Industrial Testing Service, San Diego.

Mechanic, D. (1986) The concept of illness behaviour: Culture, situation and personal predisposition. *Psychological Medicine*, **16**, 1–17.

Millon, C., Salvato, F., Blaney, N., Morgan, R., Mantero-Atienza, E., Klimas, N. and Fletcher, M. A. (1989) A psychological assessment of Chronic Fatigue Syndrome/Chronic Epstein–Barr Virus patients. *Psychology and Health*, **3**, 131–141.

Montgomery, G. (1983) Uncommon tiredness among undergraduates. *Journal of Consulting and Clinical Psychology*, **51**, 517–525.

Oken, D. (1987) Coping and psychosomatic illness. In. A. Baum and J. E. Singer (eds) *Handbook of Psychology and Health*, Vol. 5, *Stress*, pp. 109–135. Lawrence Erlbaum, Hillsdale, New Jersey.

Pilowsky, I. (1986) Abnormal illness behavior (dysnosognia). *Psychotherapy and Psychosomatics*, **46**, 76–84.

Pilowsky, I. and Spence, N. D. (1975) Patterns of illness behaviour in patients with intractable pain. *Journal of Psychosomatic Research*, **19**, 279–287.

Plaut, S. M. and Friedman, S. B. (1981) Psychosocial factors in infectious disease. In R. Ader (ed.) *Psychoneuroimmunology*, pp. 3–30. Academic Press, New York.

Popkin, M. K., Callies, A. L. and Colon, E. A. (1987) A framework for the study of medical depression. *Psychosomatics*, **28**, 27–33.

Powell, R., Dolan, R. and Wessely, S. (1990) Attributions and self esteem in depression and chronic fatigue syndromes. *Journal of Psychosomatic Research*, **34**, 665–673.

Ramsay, A. M. (1988) *Myalgic Encephalomyelitis and Postviral Fatigue States: The Saga of Royal Free Disease*. Gower Medical Publications, London.

Robins, L. N., Helzer, J. E., Croughan, J. and Ratcliff, K. S. (1981) National Institute of Mental Health Diagnostic Interview Schedule: Its history, characteristics and validity. *Archives of General Psychiatry*, **38**, 381–389.

Ross, L. (1977) The intuitive psychologist and his shortcomings: Distortions in the attribution process. In L. Berkowitz (ed.) *Advances in Experimental Social Psychology*, Vol. 10, pp. 173–220. Academic Press, New York.

Sachar, E. J. (1975) Evaluating depression in the medical patient. In J. J. Strain and S. Grossman (eds) *The Psychological Care of the Medically Ill: A Primer in Liaison Psychiatry*, pp. 64–75. Appleton Century Crofts, New York.

Schleifer, S. J., Keller, S. E., Bond, R. N., Cohen, J. and Stein, M. (1989) Major depressive disorder and immunity: Role of age, sex, severity and hospitalisation. *Archives of General Psychiatry*, **46**, 81–87.

Schwab, J. J., Bialow, M. R., Clemmons, R. S. and Holzer, C. E. (1966) The affective symptomatology of depression in medical inpatients. *Psychosomatics*, **7**, 214–217.

Snaith, R. (1987) The concept of mild depression. *British Journal of Psychiatry*, **150**, 387–393.

Solomon, G. F. (1985) The emerging field of psychoneuroimmunology with a special note on AIDS. *Advances*, **2**, 6–19.

Sontag, S. (1977) *Illness as Metaphor*. Allen Lane, London.

Spitzer, R. L., Endicott, J. and Robins, E. (1978) Research Diagnostic Criteria: Rationale and reliability. *Archives of General Psychiatry*, **35**, 773–782.

Straus, S. E. (1988) The chronic mononucleosis syndrome. *Journal of Infectious Diseases*, **157**, 405–412.

Swartz, M. N. (1988) The chronic fatigue syndrome—one entity or many? *New England Journal of Medicine*, **319**, 1726–1728.

Taerk, G. S., Toner, B. B., Salit, I. E., Garfinkel, P. E. and Ozersky, S. (1987) Depression in patients with neuromyasthenia (benign myalgic encephalomyelitis). *International Journal of Psychiatry in Medicine*, **17**, 49–56.

Taylor, S. E. and Brown, J. D. (1988) Illusion and well-being: A social psychological perspective on mental health. *Psychological Bulletin*, **103**, 193–210.

Weckowicz, T. E., Muir, W. and Cropley, A. J. (1967) A factor analysis of the Beck Inventory for Depression. *Journal of Consulting Psychology*, **31**, 23–28.

Wessely, S. and Powell, R. (1989) Fatigue syndrome: A comparison of 'postviral' fatigue with neuromuscular and affective disorder. *Journal of Neurology, Neurosurgery and Psychiatry*, **52**, 940–948.

Wessely, S., David, A., Butler, S. and Chalder, T. (1989) Management of chronic (postviral) fatigue syndrome. *Journal of the Royal College of General Practitioners*, **39**, 26–29.

Whybrow, P. C., Akiskal, H. S. and McKinney, W. T. (1984) *Mood Disorders: Towards a New Psychobiology*. Plenum, New York.

Wilson, D., Widmer, R., Cadoret, R. and Judiesch, K. (1983) Somatic symptoms: A major feature of depression in a family practice. *Journal of Affective Disorder*, **5**, 199–207.

Wittenborn, J. and Buhler, R. (1979) Somatic discomforts among depressed women. *Archives of General Psychiatry*, **36**, 465–471.

Wortman, C. B. and Dunkel-Schetter, C. (1979) Interpersonal relationships and cancer: A theoretical analysis. *Journal of Social Issues*, **35**, 120–155.

Zigmund, A. S. and Snaith, R. P. (1983) The Hospital Anxiety and Depression Scale. *Acta Psychiatrica Scandinavica*, **67**, 361–370.

Part II

The Host Response

6

Laboratory Abnormalities in Chronic Fatigue Syndrome

Dedra Buchwald

University of Washington and Chronic Fatigue Clinic, Seattle, Washington, USA

The heterogeneity of patients with chronic fatigue syndrome (CFS) is rivaled only by the diversity of laboratory abnormalities, particularly those involving the immune system, associated with this syndrome. This chapter will review the function and measurement of selected components of the immune system and specific laboratory findings in CFS. First, however, the following words of caution are appropriate:

(a) Studies on chronic fatigue may describe different clinical syndromes with fatigue as the common denominator. Entry criteria are not consistent and until recently a good case definition was lacking.
(b) Indications for obtaining tests vary between both patients and studies and are often unclear. Specific tests are often performed only in highly selected patients and therefore may not be representative.
(c) Tests are obtained at various, usually unspecified, points in the clinical course. This is important if abnormalities are transient or fluctuate over time.
(d) Abnormalities often fail to correlate with the severity of complaints or the clinical course, making interpretation difficult.
(e) Multiple laboratories perform these tests with no standardization between them.
(f) Results are often reported with inappropriate or no control data.

OVERVIEW OF THE IMMUNE RESPONSE

The immune system responds to invading organisms by a series of reactions designed to eradicate infection while not responding adversely to 'self'. This

Post-viral Fatigue Syndrome. Edited by R. Jenkins and J. Mowbray
© 1991 John Wiley & Sons Ltd

involves the activities of a natural defense system that can be summarized in six words: encounter, recognition, activation, deployment, discrimination and regulation (Nossal, 1987). The immune response is carried out by immunologically specific T and B lymphocytes whose functions are mediated by a large number of nonspecific components such as natural killer cells and the complement system. Antigen is first encountered by phagocytic cells such as macrophages, processed in a complex fashion, and then re-expressed on cell surfaces. In conjunction with major histocompatibility complex (MHC) molecules, antigen recognition by helper or cytotoxic T cells takes place. This specific encounter leads to cell activation and the production of a wide variety of growth and differentiation factors by both the antigen-presenting cells and T cells. These factors, known as cytokines, lymphokines or interleukins, participate in the expansion, differentiation and deployment of T and B cells and also collaborate with nonspecific components of the immune system such as phagocytes. These complex interactions result not only in an appropriate immune response but also in the ability to discriminate between 'self' and 'non-self'. Finally, regulation involves the balance and control of factors that amplify or attenuate the immune response.

Immunoglobulins and immune complexes

Immunoglobulins are folded polypeptide chains produced by B cells. A single antibody molecule consists of two heavy and two light chains arranged in the shape of a 'Y'. Both heavy and light chains make up the arms of the 'Y' while only heavy chains are found in the stem. The antigen-combining sites, or variable regions, are located at the ends of the arms and confer immunologic specificity. The stem, or constant region, also has biological activity such as the ability to activate the complement system and to combine with cell surface receptors on certain leukocytes.

There are five major classes and several subclasses of immunoglobulins that are heterogeneous with respect to structure and function. IgG is the most prevalent antibody. It has antiviral and antibacterial action, is a potent opsonin and toxin neutralizer and fixes complement by the classical pathway. IgA is the principal secretory antibody in the respiratory, genitourinary and gastrointestinal tracts. Secretory IgA is composed of two IgA molecules and a peptide called the secretory component. IgM molecules are predominantly macroglobulins formed by five individual IgM molecules linked by joining chains. IgM is present on the surface of B cells early in their maturation and is the first antibody produced by activated B cells in response to an antigen. IgM can also activate the classical complement pathway. IgD is found on B cell surfaces and in low concentrations in serum. Little is known about its biological function. Although IgE is the least abundant antibody in serum, its affinity for mast cells and basophils makes it one of the most important. When receptors on these cells bind IgE, the cells degranulate, releasing mediators of immediate hypersensitivity and anaphylaxis.

Individual immunoglobulins can be identified and quantified by a variety of methods, most commonly immunoelectrophoresis. This method combines electrophoretic separation with an immune precipitation reaction.

Immune complexes are antigen–antibody complexes that are generated in a wide variety of diseases, particularly infections. They may be circulating or deposited in various tissues. Because immune complexes are immunoglobulins from different classes combined with a wide variety of antigens, there is no single method of quantification which is adequate for all types of complexes. In general, the measurement of immune complexes has a relative lack of diagnostic or prognostic specificity.

Complement

Complement is a system of serum proteins that mediates antigen–antibody reactions. Its functions include opsonizing the targets of phagocytic cells to facilitate ingestion, inducing inflammation and directly damaging target cells or tissues. Complement can be activated by two pathways—the classical or alternative pathway. The classical pathway is usually activated when antigen is bound by IgM or by a subclass of IgG. Although the alternative pathway is more efficient in the presence of antibody, it can be activated by the presence of a target surface alone. After complement activation, there is a single common effector pathway mediated by proteins called 'components'. Because components behave like acute phase reactants, their turnover is rapid, and the range of normal is wide, component levels are a poor index of complement activation and, in general, are not helpful in the diagnosis and prognosis of disease. Nonetheless, there are a large number of functional and immunochemical tests for individual components and total complement activity.

Interferon

Interferon is a protein produced by cells in response to viral infections that exerts a protective effect against attack by other viruses. It also possesses immunomodulating and antineoplastic activity. Interferon may regulate the immune response by increasing the expression of MHC cell surface antigens, surface receptors for cytokines or the stem portion of immunoglobulins. Interferon may also induce or be induced by other cytokines. There are three main types of interferon—alpha, beta and gamma. Interferon-alpha and -beta possess antiviral and antitumor activity and are commonly stimulated by viruses, bacteria and double-stranded RNA.

Interferon-alpha may also exert a negative influence on antibody and hypersensitivity responses. Interferon-alpha is produced by leukocytes and interferon-beta by fibroblasts and epithelial cells. Interferon-gamma, reflecting its more central immunomodulatory role, is produced by activated lymphocytes and induced by mitogens and antigens. It has been shown to activate macrophages, cytotoxic T cells and natural killer cells. It also stimulates T cell and natural killer cell growth and B cell differentiation. Notably, interferons induce the production of 2',5'-oligosynthetase, an enzyme that inhibits protein translation used as a marker of viral infection.

Interleukins

Interleukins are small molecules lacking specificity that have important roles in the regulation of antigen-specific humoral and cellular immune responses. They are produced by lymphocytes, primarily T cells, and a wide variety of other cell types. Interleukins have widespread effects and may mediate several different effects in a single target cell population.

These are at least seven distinct interleukins of which the best known are interleukin-1 and -2. Interleukin-1 is produced by endothelial, epithelial and hematopoietic cells, particularly macrophages. It has a role both as a mediator of the inflammatory response and as an inducer or enhancer of the immune system. The functional properties of interleukin-1 include stimulation of helper T cell and B cell proliferation and hemapoietic cell growth and differentiation. It can also induce the production of prostaglandins and other cytokines, including interleukin-2. Interleukin-2 is secreted by activated T cells. In addition to its function as a growth factor for mature T cells and thymocytes, interleukin-2 induces T cell cytotoxicity, stimulates natural killer cell activity and may cause B cells to differentiate into antibody-secreting cells.

T lymphocytes

Thymus-derived lymphocytes, or T cells, are components of the immune system partially responsible for immunologic specificity and memory. In contrast to B cells, T cells rarely display immunoglobulins on their surface. Instead, they have a distinctive receptor which is similar, but not identical, to an immunoglobulin molecule. This difference accounts for the fact that, unlike B cells, T cells only recognize antigen in conjunction with MHC antigens. T cells also have a variety of other surface molecules that play important roles in T cell differentiation and function.

T cell activation

Specific activation occurs when antigen is presented to a T cell with the appropriate receptor and MHC. The resulting complex, in conjunction with interleukin-1 elaborated by the presenting cell, leads to T cell activation, clonal expansion and production of interleukin-2.

Cell expansion can be quantified by uptake of radioisotopes (e.g. [³H]thymidine) by proliferating cells after stimulation with specific antigens. This assay can also be used to assess T cell response to nonspecific stimulation by mitogens. Mitogens such as phytohemagglutinin stimulate the nonclonal expansion of T cells, providing another estimate of T cell function.

T cell subsets

T cells mediate two general types of functions: effector and regulatory. Effector functions depend on the ability of the T cells to secrete lymphokines and kill cells. Regulatory functions require the synthesis of lymphokines. These different functions are often associated with specific T cell subsets defined by cell surface markers that can be detected by monoclonal antibodies.

The major functions of effector T cells are cytotoxicity and delayed-type hypersensitivity. Cytotoxic T cells, recognized by OKT8 monoclonal antibodies, play an important role in the host defense against viruses. If primed with antigen and specific MHC molecules they can lyse target cells. For example, individuals immune to rubella will have cytotoxic T cells capable of lysing rubella-infected cells only in the context of these MHC molecules. Delayed-type hypersensitivity T cells react with OKT4 monoclonal antibodies and combine with other MHC components to carry out their functions, mainly through production of lymphokines. Delayed hypersensitivity is important in the defense against viruses, fungi, mycobacteria and other organisms that replicate intracellularly. The reaction is 'delayed' because of the time required for lymphokine synthesis and action to take place.

Regulator T cells control the development of effector T and B cells by mediating T and B cell interactions. There are two types of regulator T cells, helper and suppressor cells. Helper, or T_4^+, cells react with OKT4 monoclonal antibodies and recognize antigen in conjunction with specific MHC components. They produce interleukin-2 when activated and 'help' B cells to make antibodies. Suppressor, or T_8^+, cells suppress the proliferative response of other T cells and inhibit B cell immunoglobulin production and secretion.

B lymphocytes

B cell maturation

B lymphocyte maturation can be defined both by cell surface markers and functional capabilities. Precursor B cells, generated in fetal liver and then in bone marrow, lack immunoglobulin on their surface. As B cell development proceeds, IgM, then IgD, is displayed on the surface membrane. Resting, mature B cells use surface IgM as an antigen receptor but the function of the more predominant IgD is unclear.

B cell activation

Resting B cells can be stimulated to enlarge, proliferate, mature and secrete antibody via a complex process which can be specific, or nonspecific and polyclonal. Specific activation is T cell dependent and involves an antigen complementary to the cells' surface immunoglobulin. After stimulation, B cells differentiate into plasma cells that secrete large amounts of immunoglobulin or they divide and return to a resting state as memory B cells. Memory B cells can rapidly differentiate following a second exposure to the same antigen—the anamnestic response. Efficient antibody production by plasma cells requires a specific antigen and the secretion of lymphokines by activated helper T cells. This process involves a switch in the class of immunoglobulin produced from IgM early in the primary response to IgG, IgA or occasionally IgE in the late primary or an amnestic response.

Nonspecific, or T-independent, activation can occur in the presence of B cell mitogens such as the polysaccharide polymer, dextran. Without T cell help, the B cell response is usually weak, induces mainly IgM and results in little immunologic memory.

Quantification of T and B cells can be accomplished by tests performed with peripheral blood mononuclear cells isolated by centrifugation on Ficoll-Hypaque solutions or on whole blood with the use of laser flow cytometry. Up to 70% of mononuclear cells are lymphocytes. Of these, approximately 80% are T cells based on their ability to form rosettes with sheep erythrocytes or bind T-cell-specific monoclonal antibodies. Ten per cent to 15% are B cells and the remainder are null cells, which include the population of natural killer cells. B cells are identified by cell surface immunoglobulins detected with fluorescein-labelled antiserum or by specific surface antigens.

Using monoclonal antibodies directed against unique cell surface antigens and flow cytometry, two distinct populations of T cells have been identified. One subset, bearing T_3 and T_4 determinants, constitutes approximately 60%

of T cells and has helper-inducer functions. Another subset with T_3 and T_8 markers makes up 20–30% of peripheral T cells and has cytotoxic-suppressor functions.

The simplest way to examine T cell function is intradermal skin testing. Normal individuals will respond with at least 5 mm of induration in 24–48 hours in response to ubiquitous antigens (e.g. mumps, candida). Unreactive individuals are called anergic.

Natural killer cells

Natural killer cells are a population of large granular lymphocytes that can functionally be defined by their ability to lyse target cells without prior sensitization or MHC restriction. There is evidence suggesting that natural killer cell activity is important in the defense against malignancy, rejection of bone marrow transplants and graft-versus-host disease. It acts to regulate cellular development, and as a major producer of interferon and an effector of its action. Natural killer cells also appear to play a significant role in host defense against microbial, particularly viral, infections and to participate in antibody-dependent cell-mediated cytotoxicity against antibody-coated target cells. All natural killer cells express the NKH1 surface antigen; over 75% of these lack the T_3 antigen.

Natural killer cells can be enumerated by specific monoclonal antibodies that detect a variety of receptors and antigens such as NKH1 and T_3. Functional testing is assessed by the ability of these cells to kill target cells such as the erythroleukemia cell line K562. In this assay, cytotoxicity is quantified by measuring the amount of chromium-51 released by the lysed target cells.

LABORATORY FINDINGS IN CFS

I have reviewed 57 articles and abstracts and will present data from these, as well as from studies done by myself and others. Only studies describing patients who *seem* to fit the Centers for Disease Control case definition of CFS are included. More specifically, studies describing children, patients with astronomical Epstein–Barr virus (EBV) titers or familial or acquired immune deficiencies have been excluded. For each individual test, the data from all studies have been combined and a 'pooled average' and range calculated.

As shown in Table 1, on standard hematologic testing, leukocytosis is seen in 18% of patients (Aoki *et al.*, 1987; Kaslow *et al.*, 1989; Komaroff, unpublished; Komaroff and Buchwald, unpublished) and leukopenia in a similar number (Aoki *et al.*, 1987; Kaslow *et al.*, 1989; Komaroff, unpublished; Komaroff and Buchwald, unpublished; Lloyd *et al.*, 1989). A relative lymphocytosis has been found in 22% ranging from 0% to 71% (Behan *et al.*,

1985; Borysiewicz *et al.*, 1986; DuBois *et al.*, 1984; Kaslow *et al.*, 1989; Komaroff, unpublished; Salit, 1985; Tobi *et al.*, 1982) and one study found lymphopenia in 28% of patients (Lloyd *et al.*, 1989). Atypical lymphocytes have been reported in 0–30% of patients (Behan *et al.*, 1985; Borysiewicz *et al.*, 1986; Hamblin *et al.*, 1983; Jones *et al.*, 1985; Kaslow *et al.*, 1989; Gold *et al.*, 1990; Komaroff, unpublished; Komaroff and Buchwald, unpublished; Salit, 1985; Straus *et al.*, 1985). In contrast to a smaller study (Kaslow *et al.*, 1989), 48% of our patients have a monocytosis (Komaroff, unpublished). An elevated erythrocyte sedimentation rate (ESR) is seen in 18% of these otherwise healthy patients (Behan *et al.*, 1985; DuBois *et al.*, 1984; Kaslow *et al.*, 1989; Komaroff, unpublished; Komaroff and Buchwald, unpublished; Kroenke *et al.*, 1988; Salit, 1985; Straus *et al.*, 1985). Perhaps more interestingly, an average of 40% have a low ESR (Kaslow *et al.*, 1989; Komaroff, unpublished; Komaroff and Buchwald, unpublished). With the exception of sickle cell disease, there are few conditions associated with sedimentation rates that are consistently 0, 1 or 2 mm/hr. Lastly, an average of 15% of patients have a positive heterophile or monospot test (Borysiewicz *et al.*, 1986; DuBois *et al.*, 1984; Jones *et al.*,1985; Komaroff, unpublished; Kroenke *et al.*, 1988; Straus *et al.*, 1985; Tobi *et al.*, 1988).

Other standard laboratory tests have revealed that 20% of patients have modestly elevated transaminases (DuBois *et al.*, 1984; Komaroff, unpublished; Komaroff and Buchwald, unpublished; Roubalová *et al.*, 1988; Straus *et al.*, 1985; Tobi *et al.*, 1982). About 7% of patients have evidence of hypothyroidism usually manifested by a modest elevation in the thyroid stimulating hormone (Borysiewicz *et al.*, 1986; Kaslow *et al.*, 1989; Komaroff, unpublished; Komaroff and Buchwald, unpublished; Kroenke *et al.*, 1988; Lane *et al.*, 1988; Prieto *et al.*, 1989).

Table 1   Hematologic abnormalities

| | No. of studies | Patients with abnormalities (%) | |
		Pooled average	Range
Leukocytosis	4	18	0–21
Leukopenia	5	20	0–26
Lymphocytosis	7	22	0–71
Lymphopenia	1	28	—
Atypical lymphocytes	10	11	0–30
Monocytosis	2	45	0–48
Elevated ESR*	8	18	0–32
Decreased ESR	3	40	0–42
Positive heterophile	7	15	0–50

* Erythrocyte sedimentation rate

The serologic profiles are generally unremarkable (Table 2). Antinuclear antibodies (Jones *et al.*, 1985; Gold *et al.*, 1990; Komaroff, unpublished; Komaroff and Buchwald, unpublished; Prieto *et al.*, 1989; Salit, 1985; Straus *et al.*, 1985; Tobi *et al.*, 1982) and rheumatoid factor (Jones *et al.*, 1985; Kaslow *et al.*, 1989; Komaroff, unpublished; Komaroff and Buchwald, unpublished; Prieto *et al.*, 1989; Salit, 1985; Straus *et al.*, 1985; Tobi *et al.*, 1982) are occasionally present, typically in low concentrations without other evidence for lupus or rheumatoid arthritis. In four studies antithyroid antibodies were found in an average of 29% of selected patients (Behan *et al.*, 1985; Komaroff, unpublished; Tobi *et al.*, 1982; Weinstein, 1987) and in another study anti-smooth muscle antibodies were found in 36% (Behan *et al.*, 1985). Anti-gastric parietal cell, anti-insulin and insulin receptor antibodies, elevated cryoglobulins, cold agglutinins and false positive VDRL (Venereal Disease Research Laboratory of the Public Health Service) tests have all been looked for and found in 0–8% of patients (Behan *et al.*, 1985; Straus *et al.*, 1985).

Table 3 illustrates the unusual and often conflicting findings noted in a large number of immunologic studies. In nine studies, an average of 31% of patients were noted to have decreased immunoglobulins of the IgA, IgD, IgG or IgM class (DuBois *et al.*, 1984; Komaroff, unpublished; Komaroff and Buchwald, unpublished; Lloyd *et al.*, 1989; Read *et al.*, 1988; Roubalová *et al.*, 1988; Salit, 1985; Straus *et al.*, 1985; Tosato *et al.*, 1985). IgG subclass deficiencies, usually IgG_1, or IgG_3, have been reported in 45% of patients studied (Komaroff *et al.*, 1988a; Linde *et al.*, 1988; Lloyd *et al.*, 1989; Read *et al.*, 1988). In contrast, we found increased immunoglobulin levels in 29% (Komaroff, unpublished; Komaroff and Buchwald, unpublished) and normal levels were found in two other studies (Behan *et al.*, 1985; Borysiewicz *et al.*, 1986). Spontaneous (Hamblin *et al.*, 1983) and mitogen-induced diminutions in immunoglobulin synthesis *in vitro* have also been reported in 10% of CFS patients (Borysiewicz *et al.*, 1986; Hamblin *et al.*, 1983; Tosato *et al.*, 1985). An average of 53% of patients have low levels of circulating immune complexes (Behan *et al.*, 1985; Borysiewicz *et al.*, 1986; Komaroff, unpublished; Straus *et*

Table 2 Serologic abnormalities

	No. of studies	Patients with abnormalities (%)	
		Pooled average	Range
Antinuclear antibodies	8	7	0–32
Rheumatoid factor	8	4	0–10
Antithyroid antibodies	4	29	15–100
Anti-smooth muscle antibodies	1	36	—

Table 3 Abnormalities in humoral immunology

	No. of studies	Patients with abnormalities (%)	
		Pooled average	Range
Decreased immunoglobulins	9	31	4–100
Increased immunoglobulins	2	29	11–40
IgG subclass deficiency	4	45	17–100
Decreased mitogen-induced Ig synthesis	3	10	0–66
Immune complexes	4	53	0–73
Depressed complement	4	13	0–25

al., 1985); however, only 0–25% of patients have depressed complement as measured by different assays (Behan *et al.*, 1985; Borysiewicz *et al.*, 1986; DuBois *et al.*, 1984; Salit, 1985).

Several groups have noted abnormalities in lymphokine and interleukin responses (Table 4). The activity of the interferon-induced enzyme, 2',5'-oligoadenylate synthetase, was almost always elevated in the leukocytes from a small number of CFS patients (Morag *et al.*, 1982; Straus *et al.*, 1985). The pooled data from six studies suggest circulating interferon is present in 3% of patients (Aoki *et al.*, 1987; Borysiewicz *et al.*, 1986; Ho-Yen *et al.*, 1988; Jones *et al.*, 1985; Lloyd *et al.*, 1988a; Straus *et al.*, 1985). Of three studies

Table 4 Lymphokine and interleukin abnormalities

	No. of studies	Patients with abnormalities (%)	
		Pooled average	Range
Increased 2',5'-oligodenylate synthetase	2	100	—
Increased circulating interferon	6	3	0–20
Increased interferon synthesis by mitogen-stimulated lymphocytes	1	—	—
Decreased interferon synthesis by mitogen-stimulated lymphocytes	1	—	—
Increased circulating interleukin-2	1	—	—
Decreased interleukin-2 synthesis by mitogen-stimulated lymphocytes	2	—	—

reporting results on *in vitro* gamma-interferon synthesis by mitogen-stimulated lymphocytes, one reported increased (Altman *et al.*, 1988), one decreased (Kibler *et al.*, 1985) and one normal production (Morte *et al.*, 1988). In addition, elevated levels of circulating interleukin-2 (Cheney *et al.*, 1989) and decreased interleukin-2 synthesis *in vitro* have been found (Gold *et al.*, 1990; Kibler *et al.*, 1985).

Paradoxical cellular immune abnormalities have also been noted (Table 5). Normal numbers of T_4^+ and T_8^+ cells (Behan *et al.*, 1985; Borysiewicz *et al.*, 1986; Jones *et al.*, 1985; Straus *et al.*, 1985; Tosato *et al.*, 1985) are common; however, increases and decreases in T_4^+ and T_8^+ cells have been reported (Behan *et al.*, 1985; Komaroff, unpublished; Linde *et al.*, 1988). We and others (DuBois *et al.*, 1984) have found a higher than normal T_4/T_8 ratio; among patients we studied from the Lake Tahoe area, this generally reflects a diminution in suppressor cells rather than an absolute increase in helper cells (Komaroff and Buchwald, unpublished). This is in contrast to a large number of other studies which demonstrated a decreased T_4/T_8 ratio in 2–100% of patients (Aoki *et al.*, 1987; DuBois *et al.*, 1984; Hamblin *et al.*, 1983; Jones *et al.*, 1985; Komaroff, unpublished; Komaroff and Buchwald, unpublished; Linde *et al.*, 1988). As with T cells, both increased and decreased numbers of B cells have been reported (Borysiewicz *et al.*, 1986; Komaroff, unpublished; Komaroff and Buchwald, unpublished; Linde *et al.*, 1988). In our studies, a small number of patients have dramatically increased raw numbers and percentages of B cells (Komaroff and Buchwald, unpublished).

Evidence of deranged lymphocyte function has also been demonstrated in a number of studies (Table 6). A small percentage of patients are anergic (Borysiewicz *et al.*, 1986; DuBois *et al.*, 1984; Lloyd *et al.*, 1989; Murdoch, 1988; Straus *et al.*, 1985); however, a larger percentage have decreased responsiveness *in vitro* to standard mitogen stimulation assays (Aoki *et al.*,

Table 5 Lymphocyte number

		Patients with abnormalities (%)	
	No. of studies	Pooled average	Range
Increased T_4^+ cells	1	50	—
Decreased T_4^+ cells	2	51	12–86
Increased T_8^+ cells	2	14	14–100
Decreased T_8^+ cells	1	11	—
Increased T_4/T_8 ratio	2	31	30–40
Decreased T_4/T_8 ratio	7	17	2–100
Increased B cells	4	10	0–50
Decreased B cells	1	7	—

1987; Behan *et al.*, 1985; Borysiewicz *et al.*, 1986; Jones *et al.*, 1985; Komaroff and Buchwald, unpublished; Tobi *et al.*, 1982). Additional evidence of T cell dysfunction is manifested by increased spontaneous suppressor activity (Hamblin *et al.*, 1983) and T cell suppression of *in vitro* immunoglobulin synthesis by normal allogeneic B cells (Tosato *et al.*, 1985). Others have reported decreased EBV-specific cytotoxic T cell activity (Borysiewicz *et al.*, 1986) and antibody-dependent cell-mediated cytotoxicity (DuBois, 1986; Straus *et al.*, 1985). A recent controlled study found a significant reduction in the display of the CD_3 (T_3) cell surface marker on T cells in patients with CFS (Subirá *et al.*, 1989). Since CD_3 appears to play an important role in T cell activation, this finding suggests a mechanism for the observed T cell dysfunction in CFS. Several investigators have reported difficulty in establishing spontaneous outgrowth of EBV-transformed B cell lines (Komaroff and Buchwald, unpublished; Straus *et al.*, 1985; Tosato *et al.*, 1985).

Natural killer cell deficiencies have been confirmed in a number of independent laboratories (Table 7). A diminution in natural killer cell number or percentage has been seen in 0–73% of patients (Aoki *et al.*, 1987; Behan *et al.*, 1985; Caligiuri *et al.*, 1987). We have found that 73% of CFS patients have a decreased number of natural killer cells and the normally dominant subset, the NKH1 positive, T_3 negative subset, is reduced by 50% in patients compared to age- and sex-matched controls (Caligiuri *et al.*, 1987).

Natural killer cell function has been found to be increased (Gold *et al.*, 1990), decreased (Aoki *et al.*, 1987; Caligiuri *et al.*, 1987; Kibler *et al.*, 1985) and normal (Borysiewicz *et al.*, 1986) as measured by cytolytic activity against a number of different target cell lines. We have found that stimulation with

Table 6 Lymphocyte function

	No. of studies	Patients with abnormalities (%)	
		Pooled average	Range
T cells			
Anergy	5	32	0–54
Decreased response to mitogens	6	30	0–70
T cell suppression of Ig synthesis	1	100(?)	—
Decreased EBV-specific cytotoxic T cell activity	1	100	—
B cells			
Spontaneous outgrowth of transformed B cells in EBV-seropositive patients	3	0	—

Table 7 Natural killer cell phenotype and function

	No. of studies	Patients with abnormalities (%)	
		Pooled average	Range
Decreased cell number	3	32	0–73
Decreased cell function	3	77	0–100
Increased cell function	1	—	—

interleukin-2 resulted in no improvement in cytolytic activity in many patients. This dysfunction in cytolytic activity was greatest with the EBV-infected LAZ 388 target cell line (Caligiuri *et al.*, 1987). These abnormalities of natural killer cell phenotype and function are interesting, given the central role played by natural killer cells in containing viral infections, particularly infections with the herpes virus family.

Klimas has recently reported multiple abnormalities of cellular immunity in 30 CFS patients, including decreases in natural killer cell cytotoxicity, the suppressor inducer subset of T_4 cells, gamma interferon production and lymphoproliferation after mitogen stimulation. In contrast, increases were noted in the percentages of T_8 cells, particularly those with activation markers, the suppressor–cytotoxic T_8 subset, and numbers of B cells.

Although early studies linked EBV and CFS (DuBois *et al.*, 1984; Jones *et al.*, 1985; Straus *et al.*, 1985), further investigations of CFS patients and evidence from two seroepidemiologic surveys have made this hypothesis less attractive (Hellinger *et al.*, 1988; Horwitz *et al.*, 1985; Lamy *et al.*, 1982). These studies suggest that the serologic differences between patient and controls probably reflect statistical rather than etiologic differences. As Table 8 illustrates, elevated viral capsid antigen IgG (VCA-IgG) and early antigen (EA) are not universally found (Borysiewicz *et al.*, 1986; Buchwald *et al.*, 1987; Holmes *et al.*, 1987; Hotchin *et al.*, 1989; Jones *et al.*, 1985; Kaslow *et al.*, 1989; Komaroff, unpublished; Komaroff and Buchwald, unpublished; Kroenke *et al.*, 1988; Prieto *et al.*, 1989; Tobi *et al.*, 1982; Tosato *et al.*, 1985; Waters-Peacock *et al.*, 1988) and VCA-IgM is unusual (Borysiewicz *et al.*, 1986; Buchwald *et al.*, 1987; Holmes *et al.*, 1987; Jones *et al.*, 1985; Komaroff, unpublished; Komaroff and Buchwald, unpublished; Kroenke *et al.*, 1988; Lloyd *et al.*, 1989; Prieto *et al.*, 1989; Roubalová *et al.*, 1988; Straus *et al.*, 1985; Tobi *et al.*, 1982; Tosato *et al.*, 1985; Waters-Peacock *et al.*, 1988). Although most studies have found higher geometric mean antibody titers in patients, there is extensive overlap between patients and healthy control subjects. A low or absent Epstein–Barr nuclear antigen (EBNA) has been found in 0–75% of CFS patients (Borysiewicz *et al.*, 1986; Jones *et al.*, 1985; Gold *et al.*,

Table 8   EBV serology

	No. of studies	Patients with abnormalities (%)	
		Pooled average	Range
Elevated VCA-IgG	13	47	7–100
Elevated VCA-IgM	14	10	0–100
Elevated EA	13	44	6–100
Low or absent EBNA	10	22	0–75
Decreased EBNA1/EBNA2 ratio	1	—	—
Antibody to K antigen absent	2	11	10–12
Anti-DNase or DNA polymerase	1	5	—
EBV VCA-specific IgG$_3$	1	98	—

1990; Komaroff, unpublished; Komaroff and Buchwald, unpublished; Kroenke *et al.*, 1988; Roubalová *et al.*, 1988; Straus *et al.*, 1985; Tobi *et al.*, 1982; Tosato *et al.*, 1985).

Because standard EBV serologies are not diagnostic and may not even be helpful, other markers of infection have been looked for. A decrease in the EBNA-1 to EBNA-2 ratio (Henle *et al.*, 1987), the absence of antibody to K antigen (Miller *et al.*, 1985, 1987), and the lack of antibodies to EBV-specific DNase or DNA polymerase (Jones *et al.*, 1988) have been reported but are unable to identify a significant proportion of CFS patients. EBV VCA-specific IgG$_3$ has been found in the vast majority of CFS patients studied by one investigator but the clinical utility of this test remains unproven (Linde *et al.*, 1987). The results of blood and throat cultures and EBV *in situ* hybridization of lymphocytes and throat washings have also been unrewarding (Gold *et al.*, 1990).

Although most patients report that their fatigue started after an acute flu-like illness, strong evidence for infectious etiologies is lacking. One recent study of CFS patients has demonstrated higher antibody titers to several members of the herpes virus family, implying a nonspecific immune activation (Holmes *et al.*, 1987). Two studies report evidence suggesting enteroviruses as an etiologic agent (Halpin and Wessely, 1989; Yousef *et al.*, 1988); one found circulating antigen and IgM complexes in the majority of patients with virus isolation in 22% (Yousef *et al.*, 1988). Moreover, enteroviral nucleic acid has been found more frequently in muscle cells of CFS patients than in control subjects (Archard *et al.*, 1988). We and others have found no evidence of retrovirus infection with HTLV-1, HIV or other retroviruses (Aoki *et al.*, 1987; Komaroff, unpublished; Komaroff and Buchwald, unpublished; Lloyd *et al.*, 1989; Prieto *et al.*, 1989). In addition, it has been postulated but remains unproven that a large number of other infectious agents may be involved, including human herpesvirus-6, adenoviruses, borrelia or lyme disease, Coxsackie B, toxoplasma and mycoplasma (Holmes *et al.*, 1987; Komaroff *et al.*, 1988b; Salit, 1985; Wakefield *et al.*, 1988).

It has been speculated that individuals who respond with usual vigor to infectious antigens may also have a heightened reactivity to allergens. In fact, allergies are a common feature of patients with CFS (Jones *et al.*, 1985; Jones and Straus, 1987; Straus *et al.*, 1985, 1988). Several investigators have explored this association and found increased cutaneous reactivity to allergens and increased levels of circulating IgE- and IgE-bearing T and B cells (Olson *et al.*, 1986a). Greater lymphocyte responsiveness to allergens and increased numbers of EBNA-bearing B cells in response to stimulation with specific antigens have also been noted (Olson *et al.*, 1986b). At present, the mechanisms linking allergy and CFS remain unknown.

Muscle studies of post-viral fatigue syndrome have demonstrated the absence of elevated muscle enzymes in 50 patients (Behan *et al.*, 1985) and anti-acetylcholine receptor antibodies in 20 patients (Jamal and Hansen, 1985). The majority of patients had muscle biopsies showing type II fiber atrophy or necrosis, and tubular and mitochondrial structural abnormalities (Behan *et al.*, 1985; Warner *et al.*, 1989), and 75% had abnormal single fiber electromyography (Jamal and Hansen, 1985). Excessive intracellular acidosis by nuclear magnetic resonance spectroscopy (Arnold *et al.*, 1984; Behan *et al.*, 1985) has also been reported. In contrast, another study examining metabolic and enzymatic markers of muscle activity in CFS found no evidence of a defect in the intermediary energy pathway (Byrne and Trounce, 1987). Likewise, other investigations have used a variety of techniques to document normal muscle strength, endurance and recovery (Lloyd *et al.*, 1988b; Stokes *et al.*, 1988) and normal cardiac function at rest (Montague *et al.*, 1989). However, on graded exercise testing patients with CFS have a markedly limited exercise capacity characterized by an inability to achieve the target heart rate, a lower exercise heart rate and an abbreviated exercise duration (Montague *et al.*, 1989).

For many patients, cognitive and neurologic problems are a major feature of this illness. We have begun to pursue these complaints with formal psychometric testing in the Lake Tahoe patients. Approximately 40% of patients scored at least two standard deviations below the mean on one of 12 tests. A smaller group performed terribly and 40% showed laterality of deficit, suggesting an organic etiology (Komaroff and Buchwald, unpublished).

Magnetic resonance imaging scans were also obtained on a large number of patients. The majority have multiple subcortical areas of high signal (Komaroff and Buchwald, unpublished). It must be emphasized that these scans were done on a highly selected group of patients and the significance of these findings is uncertain. In contrast, in two other studies only 7% of patients had similar lesions noted (Gold *et al.*, 1990; Warner *et al.*, 1989).

Some of these patients have also had lumbar punctures. In our patients, the most interesting findings are low numbers of mononuclear cells in the cerebrospinal fluid and an elevated opening pressure. Glucose, protein and culture results have been unremarkable (Komaroff and Buchwald, unpublished). Others have found elevated protein in 38%, increased immunoglobulin synthesis in 50% and an elevated cell count in 15% of patients (Warner *et al.*, 1989).

Taken together, the laboratory abnormalities observed in patients with CFS are diverse, sometimes conflicting, frequently modest in degree and of unclear clinical and pathophysiological importance. Although the significance of these abnormalities would be more convincing if they reflected changes in the clinical course, the immunologic aberrations in particular support the hypothesis of an underlying organic etiology in some patients with CFS.

ACKNOWLEDGEMENTS

This work was supported by grant R01A126788 from the National Institute of Allergy and Infectious Diseases and by a Young Investigator Award from the National Alliance for Research on Schizophrenia and Depression.

REFERENCES

Altman, C., Larratt, K., Golubjatnikov, R., Kirmani, N. and Rytel, M. (1988) *Clinical Research*, **36**, 845A.

Aoki, T., Usuda, Y., Miyakoshi, H., Tamura, K. and Herberman, R. B. (1987) Low natural killer syndrome: Clinical and immunologic features. *Natural Immunity and Cell Growth Regulation*, **6**, 116–128.

Archard, L. C., Bowles, N. E., Behan, P. O., Bell, E. J. and Doyle, D. (1988) Postviral fatigue syndrome: persistence of enterovirus RNA in muscle and elevated creatine kinase. *Journal of the Royal Society of Medicine*, **81**, 326–329.

Arnold, D. L., Bore, P. J., Radda, G. K., Styles, P. and Taylor, D. J. (1984) Excessive intracellular acidosis of skeletal muscle on exercise in a patient with a post-viral exhaustion/fatigue syndrome. *Lancet*, **i**, 1367–1369.

Behan, P. O., Behan, W. M. H. and Bell, E. J. (1985) The postviral fatigue syndrome—an analysis of the findings in 50 cases. *Journal of Infection*, **10**, 211–222.

Borysiewicz, L. K., Haworth, S. J., Cohen, J., Mundin, J., Rickinson, A. and Sissons, J. G. P. (1986) Epstein–Barr virus-specific immune defects in patients with persistent symptoms following infectious mononucleosis. *Quarterly Journal of Medicine*, **58**, 111–121.

Buchwald, D., Sullivan, J. L. and Komaroff, A. L. (1987) Frequency of 'chronic active Epstein–Barr virus infection' in a general medical practice. *Journal of the American Medical Association*, **257**, 2303–2307.

Byrne, E. and Trounce, I. (1987) Chronic fatigue and myalgia syndrome: mitochondrial and glycolytic studies in skeletal muscle. *Journal of Neurology, Neurosurgery and Psychiatry*, **50**, 743–746.

Caligiuri, M., Murray, C., Buchwald, D., Levine, H., Cheney, P., Peterson, D., Komaroff, A. L. and Ritz, J. (1987) Phenotypic and functional deficiency of natural killer cells in patients with chronic fatigue syndrome. *Journal of Immunology*, **139**, 3306–3313.

Cheney, P. R., Dorman, S. E. and Bell, D. S. (1989) Interleukin-2 and the chronic fatigue syndrome. *Annals of Internal Medicine*, **110**, 321.

DuBois, R. E. (1986) Gamma globulin therapy for chronic mononucleosis syndrome. *AIDS Research*, **2**, S191–S195.

DuBois, R. E., Seeley, J. K., Brus, I., Sakamoto, K., Ballow, M., Harada, S., Bechtold, T. A., Pearson, G. and Purtilo, D. T. (1984) Chronic mononucleosis syndrome. *Southern Medical Journal*, **77**, 1376–1382.

Gold, D., Bowden, R., Sixbey, J. *et al.* (1990) Chronic Fatigue. A prospective clinical and virologic study. *Journal of the American Medical Association*, **264**, 48–53.

Halpin, D. and Wessely, S. (1989) VP-1 antigen in chronic postviral fatigue syndrome. *Lancet*, **i**, 1028–1029.

Hamblin, T.J., Hussain, J., Akbar, A.N., Tang, Y.C., Smith, J.L. and Jones, D.B. (1983) Immunological reason for chronic ill health after infectious mononucleosis. *British Medical Journal*, **287**, 85–8.

Hellinger, W.C., Smith, T.F., Van Scoy, R.E., Spitzer, P.G., Forgacs, P. and Edson, R. S. (1988) Chronic fatigue syndrome and the diagnostic utility of antibody to Epstein–Barr virus early antigen. *Journal of the American Medical Association*, **260**, 971–973.

Henle, W., Henle, G., Andersson, J., Ernberg, I., Klein, G., Horwitz, C. A., Marklund, G., Rymo, L., Wellinder, C. and Straus, S. E. (1987) Antibody responses to Epstein–Barr virus-determined nuclear antigen (EBNA)-1 and EBNA-2 in acute and chronic Epstein–Barr virus infection. *Proceedings of the National Academy of Sciences of the USA*, **84**, 570–574.

Holmes, G. P., Kaplan, J. E., Stewart, J. A., Hunt, B., Pinsky, P. F. and Schonberger, L. B. (1987) A cluster of patients with a chronic mononucleosis-like syndrome: Is Epstein–Barr virus the cause? *Journal of the American Medical Association*, **257**, 2297–2302.

Horwitz, C. A., Henle, W., Henle, G., Rudnick, H. and Latts, E. (1985) Long-term serological follow-up of patients for Epstein–Barr virus after recovery from infectious mononucleosis. *Journal of Infectious Diseases*, **151**, 1150–1153.

Hotchin, N. A., Read, R., Smith, D. G. and Crawford, D. H. (1989) Active Epstein–Barr virus infection in post-viral fatigue syndrome. *Journal of Infection*, **18**, 143–150.

Ho-Yen, D. O., Carrington, D. and Armstrong, A. A. (1988) Myalgic encephalitis and alpha-interferon. *Lancet*, **i**, 125.

Jamal, G. A. and Hansen, S. (1985) Electrophysiological studies in the post-viral fatigue syndrome. *Journal of Neurology, Neurosurgery and Psychiatry*, **48**, 691–694.

Jones, J. F. and Straus, S. E. (1987) Chronic Epstein–Barr virus infection. *Annual Review of Medicine*, **38**, 195–209.

Jones, J. F., Ray, G., Minnich, L. L., Hicks, M. J., Kibler, R. and Lucas, D. O. (1985) Evidence for active Epstein–Barr virus infection in patients with persistent, unexplained illnesses: elevated anti-early antigen antibodies. *Annals of Internal Medicine*, **102**, 1–7.

Jones, J. F., Williams, M., Schooley, R. T., Robinson, C. and Glaser, R. (1988) Antibodies to Epstein–Barr virus-specific DNAs and DNA polymerase in the chronic fatigue syndrome. *Archives of Internal Medicine*, **148**, 1957–1960.

Kaslow, J. E., Rucker, L. and Onishi, R. (1989) Liver extract-folic acid-cyanocobalamin vs. placebo for chronic fatigue syndrome. *Archives of Internal Medicine*, **149**, 2501–2503.

Kibler, R., Lucas, D. O., Hicks, M. J., Poulos, B. T. and Jones, J. F. (1985) Immune function in chronic active Epstein–Barr virus infection. *Journal of Clinical Immunology*, **5**, 46–54.

Komaroff, A. L., Geiger, A. M. and Wormsley, S. (1988a) IgG subclass deficiencies in chronic fatigue syndrome. *Lancet*, **i**, 1288–1289.

Komaroff, A. L., Saxinger, C., Buchwald, D., Geiger, A. and Gallo, R. C. (1988b) A chronic 'post-viral' fatigue syndrome with neurologic features: serologic association with human herpesvirus-6. *Clinical Research*, **36**, 743A.

Kroenke, K., Wood, D. R., Mangelsdorff, A. D., Neier, N. J. and Powell, J. B. (1988) Chronic fatigue in primary care: prevalence, patient characteristics, and outcome. *Journal of the American Medical Association*, **260**, 929–934.

Lamy, M. E., Favart, A. M., Cornu, C., Mendez, M., Segas, M. and Burtonboy, G. (1982) Study of Epstein–Barr virus (EBV) antibodies: IgG and IgM anti-VCA, IgG anti-EA and Ig anti-EBNA obtained with an original microtiter technique: Serological criterions of primary and recurrent EBV infections and follow-up of infectious mononucleosis; Seroepidemiology of EBV in Belgium based on 5178 sera from patients. *Acta Clinica Belgica*, **37**, 281–298.

Lane, T. J., Manu, P. and Matthews, D. A. (1988) Prospective diagnostic evaluation of adults with chronic fatigue. *Clinical Research*, **36**, 714A.

Linde, A., Andersson, J., Lundgren, G. and Wahren, B. (1987) Subclass reactivity to Epstein–Barr virus capsid antigen in primary and reactivated EBV infections. *Journal of Medical Virology*, **21**, 109–121.

Linde, A., Hammarstrom, L. and Smith, C. I. E. (1988) IgG subclass deficiency and chronic fatigue syndrome. *Lancet*, **i**, 885–886.

Lloyd, A., Abi Hanna, D. and Wakefield, D. (1988a) Interferon and myalgic encephalomyelitis. *Lancet*, **i**, 471.

Lloyd, A. R., Hales, J. P. and Gandevia, S. C. (1988b) Muscle strength, endurance and recovery in the post-infection fatigue syndrome. *Journal of Neurology, Neurosurgery and Psychiatry*, **51**, 1316–1322.

Lloyd, A. R., Wakefield, D., Boughton, C. R. and Dwyer, J. M. (1989) Immunological abnormalities in the chronic fatigue syndrome. *Medical Journal of Australia*, **151**, 122–124.

Miller, G., Grogan, E., Fischer, D. K., Niederman, J. C., Schooley, R. T., Henle, W., Lenoir, G. and Liu, C. R. (1985) Antibody responses to two Epstein–Barr virus nuclear antigens defined by gene transfer. *New England Journal of Medicine*, **312**, 750–755.

Miller, G., Grogan, E., Rowe, D., Rooney, C., Heston, L., Eastman, R., Andiman, W., Niederman, J., Lenoir, G., Henle, W., Sullivan, J., Schooley, R., Vossen, J., Straus, S. and Issekutz, T. (1987) Selective lack of antibody to a component of EB nuclear antigen in patients with chronic active Epstein–Barr virus infection. *Journal of Infectious Diseases*, **156**, 26–31.

Montague, T. J., Marrie, T. J., Klassen, G. A., Berwick, D. J. and Horacek, B. M. (1989) Cardiac function at rest and with exercise in the chronic fatigue syndrome. *Chest*, **95**, 779–784.

Morag, A., Tobi, M., Ravid, Z., Revel, M. and Schattner, A. (1982) Increased (2'–5')-oligo-synthetase activity in patients with prolonged illness associated with serological evidence of persistent Epstein–Barr virus infection. *Lancet*, **i**, 744.

Morte, S., Castilla, A., Civeira, M.-P., Serrano, M. and Prieto, J. (1988) Gamma-interferon and chronic fatigue syndrome. *Lancet*, **ii**, 623–624.

Murdoch, J. C. (1988) Cell-mediated immunity in patients with myalgic encephalomyelitis syndrome. *New Zealand Medical Journal*, **101**, 511–512.

Olson, G.B., Kanaan, M. N., Gersuk, G. M., Kelley, L. M. and Jones, J. F. (1986a) Correlation between allergy and persistent Epstein–Barr virus infections in chronic-active Epstein–Barr virus infected patients. *Journal of Allergy and Clinical Immunology*, **78**, 308–314.

Olson, G. B., Kanaan, M. N., Kelley, L. M. and Jones, J. F. (1986b) Specific allergen-induced Epstein–Barr nuclear antigen-positive B cells from patients with chronic-active Epstein–Barr virus infections. *Journal of Allergy and Clinical Immunology*, **78**, 315–320.

Prieto, J., Subira, M. L., Castilla, A. and Serrano, M. (1989) Naloxone-reversible monocyte dysfunction in patients with chronic fatigue syndrome. *Scandinavian Journal of Immunology*, **30**, 13–20.

Read, R., Spickett, G., Harvey, J., Edwards, A. J. and Larson, H. E. (1988) IgG1 subclass deficiency in patients with chronic fatigue syndrome. *Lancet*, **i**, 241–242.

Roubalová, K., Roubal, J., Skopovy, P., Fucikova, T., Domorazova, E. and Vonka, V. (1988) Antibody response to Epstein–Barr virus antigens in patients with chronic viral infection. *Journal of Medical Virology*, **25**, 115–122.

Salit, I.E. (1985) Sporadic postinfectious neuromyasthenia. *Canadian Medical Association Journal*, **133**, 659–663.

Stokes, M. J., Cooper, R. G. and Edwards, R. H. T. (1988) Normal muscle strength and fatigability in patients with effort syndromes. *British Medical Journal*, **297**, 1014–1017.

Straus, S. E., Tosato, G., Armstrong, G., Lawley, T., Preble, O. T., Henle, W., Davey, R., Pearson, G., Epstein, J., Brus, I. and Blaese, R. M. (1985) Persisting illness and fatigue in adults with evidence of Epstein–Barr virus infection. *Annals of Internal Medicine*, **102**, 7–16.

Straus, S. E., Dale, J. K., Wright, R. and Metcalfe, D. D. (1988) Allergy and the chronic fatigue syndrome. *Journal of Allergy and Clinical Immunology*, **81**, 791–795.

Subirá, M., Castilla, A., Cireira, M. and Prieto, J. (1989) Deficient display of CD3 on lymphocytes of patients with chronic fatigue syndrome. *Journal of Infectious Diseases*, **160**, 165–166.

Tobi, M., Morag, A., Ravid, Z., Chowers, I., Weiss, V. F., Michaeli, Y., Ben-Chetrit, E., Shalit, M. and Knobler, H. (1982) Prolonged atypical illness associated with serological evidence of persistent Epstein–Barr virus infection. *Lancet*, **i**, 61–64.

Tosato, G., Straus, S., Henle, W., Pike, S. E. and Blaese, R. M. (1985) Characteristic T cell dysfunction in patients with chronic active Epstein–Barr virus infection (chronic infectious mononucleosis). *Journal of Immunology*, **134**, 3082–3088.

Wakefield, D., Lloyd, A. and Dwyer, J. (1988) Human herpesvirus 6 and myalgic encephalomyelitis. *Lancet*, **i**, 1059.

Warner, C.L., Cookfair, D., Meffuer, R., Bell, D., Ley, D. and Jacobs, L. (1989) Neurologic abnormalities in the chronic fatigue syndrome. *Neurology*, **39** (suppl.), 420.

Waters-Peacock, N., Wray, B. B. and Ades, E. W. (1988) A prospective study: Evaluation of the antibody-dependent cell mediated cytotoxicity assay in chronic active Epstein–Barr syndrome. *Journal of Clinical and Laboratory Immunology*, **27**, 11–12.

Weinstein, L. (1987) Thyroiditis and 'chronic infectious mononucleosis'. *New England Journal of Medicine*, **317**, 1225–1226.

Yousef, G. E., Bell, E. J., Mann, G. F., Murugesan, V., Smith, D. G. McCartney, R. A. and Mowbray, J. F. (1988) Chronic enterovirus infection in patients with postviral fatigue syndrome. *Lancet*, **i**, 146–147.

Immunology—general sources

Balkwell, F. R. (1989) Interferons. *Lancet*, **i**, 1060–1063.

Claman, H. N. (1987) The biology of the immune response. *Journal of the American Medical Association*, **258**, 2834–2840.

deShazo, L. P., Lopez, M. and Salvaggio, J. E. (1987) Use and interpretation of diagnostic immunologic laboratory tests. *Journal of the American Medical Association*, **258**, 3011–3011.

Frank, M. M. (1987) Current concepts. Complement in the pathophysiology of human disease. *New England Journal of Medicine*, **316**, 1525–1530.

Frank, M. M. (1989) Complement: A brief review. *Journal of Allergy and Clinical Immunology*, **84**, 411–420.

Johnston, R. B. Jr (1988) Current concepts: immunology. Monocytes and macrophages. *New England Journal of Medicine*, **318**, 747–752.

Klimas, N. G., Salvato, F. R., Morgan, R. and Fletcher, M. A. (1990) Immunologic abnormalities in chronic fatigue syndrome. *Journal of Clinical Microbiology*, **28**, 1403–1410.

Nossal, G. J. V. (1987) The basic components of the immune system. *New England Journal of Medicine*, **316**, 1320–1325.

O'Garra, A. (1989) Interleukins and the immune system 1. *Lancet*,**i**, 943–946.

O'Garra, A. (1989) Interleukins and the immune system 2. *Lancet*, **i**,1003–1005.

Stites, D. P., Stobo, J. D. and Wells, J. V. (1987) *Basic and Clinical Immunology*, 6th edn. Appleton and Large, Norwalk, CT, Los Altos, CA.

7

Pathological Changes in Skeletal Muscle in ME: Implications for Management

T. J. Peters and V. R. Preedy

King's College Hospital, London, UK

As patients with ME and its related disorders usually complain bitterly of skeletal muscle-related symptoms, it is not surprising that their muscles have recently been the object of intensive study using a variety of techniques. The aim of this chapter is therefore to assess these findings, at both the structural and functional levels, and to discuss them with special reference to their therapeutic implications.

MUSCLE HISTOPATHOLOGY

Although clinical examination of muscle bulk is usually normal in ME patients, particularly in the early stages of the disorder, histological assessment of both open and closed muscle biopsy specimens has claimed a variety of apparent abnormalities. It should be pointed out that muscle bulk and, in particular, muscle fibre histology is rapidly affected by immobility. Thus if a leg is immobilised, either experimentally or as a consequence of injury, muscle bulk is rapidly lost (Jaffe *et al.*, 1978; Gibson *et al.*, 1987). Similarly, in severe nutritional (protein–calorie) deficiency, in cachetic conditions, e.g. malignancy, and in elderly subjects, loss of muscle bulk is readily discernible even to the untrained observer. It is therefore important to distinguish any histological abnormalities found in ME patients (and other myopathies) which are primary to the disease from those secondary to immobility or to neurological abnormalities. It is noteworthy that centres frequently reporting histological abnormalities in ME patients are tertiary referral centres and are thus more likely to be seeing patients with longstanding complaints.

Post-viral Fatigue Syndrome. Edited by R. Jenkins and J. Mowbray
© 1991 John Wiley & Sons Ltd

Therefore these selected patients are more likely to have secondary changes in contrast to reports from centres specifically studying early cases.

Another important consideration is the processing of the biopsy samples. Unless care is taken during and following the biopsy procedure, artefacts may occur and will be confused with true histopathological findings. It is also important to use detailed histochemical methods to distinguish between type I (aerobic, slow twitch, red muscle fibres) and type II (anaerobic, fast twitch, white muscle fibres) and, if possible, to use objective quantitative measures of fibre diameters and other parameters (Slavin *et al.*, 1982).

In one of the earliest histopathological studies of muscle biopsies in patients with ME, abnormalities were claimed to be a consistent finding (Behan *et al.*, 1985). In a series of 50 patients they performed muscle biopsies (site unspecified) in 20 and all were abnormal. In 15 patients, single, widely scattered, necrotic fibres were seen, without any inflammatory response. The *in vivo* significance of the necrosis is uncertain but may have reflected an impaired immune system which was also demonstrated by these authors. A predominance of type II fibres was also reported but no quantitative information was provided. Histological studies of muscle biopsies from two patients with chronic ME were reported by Byrne *et al.* (1985). One subject showed type II fibre atrophy with no additional microscopic abnormalities and in the second subject type IIb fibre atrophy was noted as the sole lesion.

A recent study (Teahon *et al.*, 1988) of 30 patients with ME, referred directly by their general practitioners and thus likely to have the disease at an earlier stage, showed no consistent histological abnormalities. Detailed histo-morphometric studies were performed on type I and type II fibres in all subjects. No subject showed any evidence of type I fibre atrophy but five subjects showed evidence of hypertrophy which was marked in three subjects. Four biopsies showed type II fibre atrophy but in only one was it marked. Five subjects showed evidence of type II fibre hypertrophy, four of whom also showed type I muscle fibre hypertrophy. The absence of type I fibre atrophy is against any degree of disuse atrophy and it is noteworthy that only one of the 30 patients showed type II fibre atrophy. The importance of the fibre hypertrophy is not fully understood. In chronic alcoholic skeletal muscle myopathy, in which severe type IIb fibre atrophy is a cardinal sign, it may be seen in type I fibres in early or mild cases and is believed to represent a compensatory response to damage to the type II fibres (Martin *et al.*, 1985). The observation that in ME apparent hypertrophy of both type I and type II fibres occurs in 15% of subjects is currently unexplained.

A variety of histochemical stains for enzymes defective in varoius forms of genetic myopathy, e.g. myophosphorylase, myoadenylate kinase, phosphofructokinase and lactate dehydrogenase, are consistently normal and would seem to exclude a major defect in glycolysis in these patients. Normal lactate production in response to anaerobic forearm exercise is a general finding, again suggesting normal muscle glycolysis (Wagenmakers *et al.*, 1988).

ULTRASTRUCTURAL STUDIES

Reports of electron microscopic (EM) abnormalities have been noted in patients with ME. The study by Byrne *et al.* (1985) noted abnormal mitochondria with paracrystalline inclusions in one of two subjects. Behan *et al.* (1985) reported abnormalities in the sarcoplasmic reticulum but in neither of the studies were the lesions illustrated or quantified. They are, however, consistent with certain biochemical findings in the patient's muscle biopsies.

SERUM MUSCLE BIOCHEMISTRY

Assay of skeletal muscle cytoplasmic enzymes in the serum, most notably creatine kinase, is a highly sensitive index of muscle damage, particularly to the sarcolemma. Uniformly this activity and, where assayed, such enzymes as lactate dehydrogenase and aspartate aminotransferase, are consistently within the normal range in patients with ME (Teahon *et al.*, 1988). A raised level in patients suspected of having ME should lead to a serious questioning of the diagnosis.

Recent observations that alcoholic myopathy (Duane and Peters, 1988) and possibly other forms of proximal metabolic myopathy (Bando *et al.*, 1986) are associated with a decrease in plasma carnosinase activity is a useful non-invasive investigation for muscle fibre atrophy. Assays in the series of ME patients referred to above (Teahon *et al.*, 1988) have yielded normal values in all but two of 30 patients, consistent with the very occasional finding of muscle fibre atrophy.

MUSCLE METABOLIC STUDIES

A case reported by Arnold *et al.* (1984) generated considerable interest. In a single male patient they found, using ^{31}P nuclear magnetic spectroscopy to measure intracellular muscle fibre pH, excess acidification following prolonged ischaemic exercise presumed to be due to excessive lactate formation. During anaerobic exercise the calculated pH fell from 7.0 to 6.7 after two minutes and to 6.2 after four minutes. In contrast, normal subjects had similar resting levels, showed no significant fall after two minutes of isc-haemic exercise and only decreased to 6.5 after eight minutes. Recovery was essentially normal in the patient, suggesting that aerobic lactate metabolism and/or elimination was normal. Other unexplained abnormalities were present in the patient, including a markedly reduced ADP level after ex-ercise and an impaired recovery rate for phosphocreatine following the exercise protocol. Impaired muscle adenylate and creatine kinase activities are possibly implicated but no information on these points was provided. Although Behan *et al.* (1985) imply that similar findings were observed in six of their patient series, no subsequent publications have emerged on the topic. A personal communication from Professor G. Radda indicates that the abnormally high acidification seen in this subject is not a consistent finding in patients suspected of having ME.

MUSCLE MITOCHONDRIAL FUNCTION IN ME

One of the EM studies referred to above suggested ultrastructural abnor-malities in muscle mitochondria in a patient with ME. Edwards and his colleagues (Wagenmakers *et al.*, 1987) have reported muscle mitochondrial enzyme assays and mitochondria functional studies in patients with effort syndrome (Table 1). The relationship between effort syndrome patients and those with ME has been convincingly demonstrated at the psychiatric level by Wessely and Powell (1989) but studies of their muscle biochemistry are not necessarily synonymous. The results (Table 1) clearly indicate impaired mitochondrial function in effort syndrome patients. However, their inter-pretation is that these defects are entirely secondary to impaired muscle use and that, intrinsically, mitochondria (and other neuromuscular functions) are normal in these subjects. The decrease in mitochondrial activities is consistent with observations that type I, mitochondria-rich fibres are more susceptible to disuse atrophy than type II fibres (Gibson *et al.*, 1987).

Table 1 Muscle mitochondrial enzyme activities in muscle pain and control subjects

	Controls (14)	Muscle pain (20)
Cytochrome *c* oxidase	50 ± 9	32 ± 10[†]
Succinate dehydrogenase	7.7 ± 1.5	4.3 ± 1.6[†]
Citrate synthase	13.7 ± 3.5	10.1 ± 4.6[*]

Mean $\pm$ SD (μmol per min per g tissue) for *n* subjects.
Statistical analyses: [*] $p < 0.05$; [†] $p < 0.001$.
Data from Wagenmakers *et al.* (1988).

MUSCLE PROTEIN SYNTHESIS

As part of our study of muscle biopsies from patients with ME, tissue analyses for DNA, RNA and protein were performed. The results are shown in
Table 2. The patients show a significant 17% decrease in total RNA per cell.
The decrease in protein per cell does not reach statistical significance. This
observation suggested that a decrease in ribosomal RNA, which comprises
84% of muscle RNA compared with 13% for tRNA and mRNA (Young,
1970), must have occurred. It was concluded that biopsies from these patients showed impaired protein synthetic machinery, an observation consistent with the ultrastructural report of Byrne *et al.* (1985). This observation is
also consistent with the demonstration of a persistent RNA virus in muscle
tissues in ME patients (Bowles *et al.*, 1987). In order to investigate whether
these RNA alterations had any functional significance, *in vivo* rates of whole
body protein synthesis and quadriceps muscle protein synthesis were investigated by [^{13}C]leucine incorporation techniques (Halliday *et al.*, 1988). The
preliminary results (Pacy *et al.*, 1988) (Table 3) show reductions in muscle
protein synthesis consistent with the small decrease in muscle fibre protein
content in the biopsies. Rates of whole body protein synthesis were also
apparently reduced. This implies that there may be nonskeletal muscle involvement in the disorder. Alternatively, the contribution of the changes in
skeletal muscle may have been sufficiently large to affect whole body protein turnover. The pathogenic mechanisms for this decrease remain to be

Table 2   Quadriceps biopsy in control subjects and ME patients

	Controls (26)	ME (22)
RNA (mg/mg DNA)	0.64 ± 0.03	$0.54 \pm 0.03^+$
Protein (mg/mg DNA)	144 ± 7	$130 \pm 7^*$

Mean ± SE for *n* subjects.
Statistical analyses: $^* p < 0.1$; $^+ p < 0.05$.

Table 3   Protein synthesis in ME patients and in controls

	Whole body leucine flux (μmol/kg per h)	Whole body leucine oxidation (μmol/kg per h)	Protein synthesis	
			Whole body (μmol/h per kg)	Quadriceps (%/h)
Controls (6)	116 ± 12	15 ± 4	101 ± 10	0.046 ± 0.008
ME patients (6)	$83 \pm 7^\ddagger$	$13 \pm 8^*$	$68 \pm 8^\ddagger$	$0.034 \pm 0.008^+$

Mean ± SD for *n* subjects.
Statistical analysis: $^* p > 0.5$; $^+ p < 0.05$; $^\ddagger p < 0.001$.
Data from Pacy *et al.* (1988).

determined but the results are consistent with a decreased ability of the muscle to repair itself, a finding in accord with the clinical observation that excessive physical exercise leads to a relapse. Recent interest in the possible role of interleukins in the muscle symptomatology (Ho-Yen *et al.*, 1988) is noteworthy and is consistent with an effect of these and other mediators on muscle function, particularly protein synthesis and degradation rates (Baracos *et al.*, 1983; Clowes *et al.*, 1983; Charters and Grimble, 1989).

IMPLICATIONS FOR TREATMENT

The diagnosis of ME is a combination of exclusion of other forms of muscle pathology in conjunction with a constellation of one or more symptoms consistent with the ME syndrome. Muscle studies, including neurological examination, neurophysiological studies and biochemical and muscle biopsy examination, are usually aimed at excluding other muscle diseases. Unfortunately, as yet, no routine diagnostic histopathological tests are available to confirm a suspected diagnosis of ME. Other forms of muscle pathology seen in patients referred with possible ME and which may cause weakness and fibre atrophy are hypothyroidism, occult alcohol abuse, nutritional, especially vitamin D, deficiencies, diabetes mellitus, glucocorticoid excess (Cushing's syndrome) and hypokalaemia due to various causes. Disuse atrophy, various inherited muscle enzyme deficiencies, systemic connective tissue disorders and psychiatric syndromes, particularly depression, may be found in patients suspected of having ME. As patients frequently present with a self-diagnosed label which becomes increasingly reinforced with time, it is important to exclude any of the above disorders at an early stage: this is an essential function of a specialist referral centre.

A key question is whether the muscles in patients with the ME syndrome are normal or abnormal. The patients themselves are deeply and genuinely convinced that their muscles are at fault and strongly resent suggestions that there is nothing wrong with their muscles. Supporting the view that the muscles themselves are normal is the proposal from Edwards and colleagues that the fatigue is central rather than peripheral in origin (Edwards, 1988; Stokes *et al.*, 1988). In contrast to this conclusion, studies from the Edwards group have clearly shown reduced mitochondrial enzyme activities in patients with effort and associated syndromes, consistent with impaired muscle energy metabolism. The observations of a decreased muscle RNA content with reduced protein synthesis also indicate impaired muscle functional capacity and possibly a reduced response to injury. Lloyd *et al.* (1988) recently showed that recovery after an endurance protocol was impaired in patients with ME, consistent with the above observations. It thus appears that, although routine muscle histology and biochemical, immunological and neurophysiological studies in patients with ME are usually normal, more sophisticated investigations frequently show differences from controls in some of these areas. However, the precise aetiological and pathogenic role of these findings in the ME syndrome remain to be determined.

A recent letter by a former member of the Edwards group (Coakley, 1989) clearly states that 'muscle fatigue . . . does not exist' in patients with ME. Unfortunately, these views have been transmitted to the patients themselves, making their treatment considerably more difficult. This conflict between the patient's and their attending physician's attitudes to their disease and the patient's treatment expectancies for their problem is increasingly observed in a variety of disorders. For example, we have previously investigated these parameters in alcohol abusers and in their nursing and medical attendants. Thus, compared with hospital medical and nursing staff, alcoholics admitted to a district general hospital for assessment and re-education preferred a more organic approach to treatment and considered themselves to have a medical rather than a psychosocial disorder (Potamianos *et al.*, 1985a). Similar conclusions were reached in a study of perception of alcoholism by patients and their medical attendants, including general practitioners (Potamianos *et al.*, 1985b). This information has provided invaluable in the treatment of alcohol abusers, particularly in the initial patient–doctor interactions. Similar studies have not apparently been performed in ME patients and their medical advisers but it is highly likely that a similar and probably a more striking disparity occurs. Many physicians and neurologists state that the medical model of ME perceived by the patients is erroneous but at least in the initial interactions between doctor and patient a better therapeutic relationship is likely to be achieved if the attending physician is aware of and sympathetic to the disparity. Generation of patient–doctor conflict is unlikely to be beneficial to either party.

The observation that ME patients show evidence of impaired mitochondrial function in muscle biopsies, the demonstration of reduced muscle RNA and protein content and the impaired muscle protein synthesis clearly show organic defects in the muscle. These findings are consistent with the impaired recovery from exercise, demonstrated by objective testing and evident to patients themselves who frequently note that strenuous exercise is followed by a significant relapse. The impaired mitochondrial activity is believed to reflect a partial disuse atrophy of muscle in ME patients and thus a programme of graded exercises is recommended (Edwards, 1986). This should limit further atrophy and, if it can be adequately sustained, lead to decreased fatiguability. The level of exercise possible varies considerably but we have found swimming as a symmetrical non-weight-bearing form of graded exercise helpful to some patients. The concept of a positive feedback cycle of 'lethargy–inactivity–lethargy' will respond to an exercise programme, particularly if a depressive/anxiety element in the symptomatology can be interrupted (Edwards *et al.*, 1988). Impaired muscle protein synthesis is a common response to both acute (Preedy and Peters, 1988) and chronic (Preedy and Peters, 1989) toxic muscle injury. Thus patients should avoid exposure to any potential mytotoxins, including alcohol, take a well-balanced nutritionally adequate diet and maintain full mobility.

ACKNOWLEDGEMENT

We are grateful to Ms Rosamund Greensted for expert secretarial assistance.

REFERENCES

Arnold, D. L., Bore, P. J., Radda, G. K., Styles, P. and Taylor, D. J. (1984) Excessive intracellular acidosis of skeletal muscle on exercise in a patient with a post viral exhaustion/fatigue syndrome. *Lancet*, **i**, 1367–1369.

Bando, K., Ichihara, K., Shimotsuki, T., Toyoshima, H., Koda, K., Hayashi, C. and Kiyai, K. (1986) Reduced serum carnosinase activity in hypothyroidism. *Annals of Clinical Biochemistry*, **23**, 190–194.

Baracos, V., Rodemann, P., Dinarello, C. A. and Goldberg, A. L. (1983) Stimulation of muscle protein degradation and prostaglandin E_2 release by leukocytic pyrogen (Interleukin-1). *New England Journal of Medicine*, **308**, 553–558.

Behan, P. O., Behan, W. M. H. and Bell, E. J. (1985) The post viral fatigue syndrome—an analysis of the findings in 50 cases. *Journal of Infection*, **10**, 211–222.

Bowles, N. E., Archard, L. C., Behan, W. M. H., Doyle, D., Bell, E. J. and Behan, P. O. (1987) Detection of Coxsackie B virus-specific RNA in skeletal muscle biopsies of patients with a post viral fatigue syndrome. *Annals of Neurology*, **22**, 126.

Byrne, E., Trounce, I. and Dennett, X. (1985) Chronic relapsing myalgia (? post-viral): Clinical, histological and biochemical studies. *Australian and New Zealand Journal of Medicine*, **15**, 305–308.

Charters, Y. and Grimble, R. F. (1989) Effect of recombinant tumour necrosis factor on protein synthesis in liver, skeletal muscle and skin of rats. *Biochemical Journal*, **258**, 493–497.

Clowes, G. H. A., George, B. C., Villee, C. A. and Saravis, C. A. (1983) Muscle proteolysis induced by a circulating peptide in patients with sepsis or trauma. *New England Journal of Medicine*, **308**, 545–552.

Coakley, J. H. (1989) Myalgic encephalomyelitis and muscle fatigue. *British Medical Journal*, **298**, 1711–1712.

Duane, P. and Peters, T. J. (1988) Serum carnosinase activities in patients with alcoholic chronic skeletal muscle myopathy. *Clilnical Science*, **75**, 185–190.

Edwards, R. H. T. (1986) Muscle fatigue and pain. *Acta Medica Scandinavica*, **711**, 179–188.

Edwards, R. H. T. (1988) Hypothesis of peripheral and central mechanisms underlying occupation muscle pain and injury. *European Journal of Applied Physiology*, **57**, 275–281.

Gibson, J. N. A., Halliday, D., Morrison, W. L., Stoward, P. J., Hornsby, G. A., Watt, R. W., Murdoch, G. and Rennie, M. J. (1987) Decrease in human quadriceps muscle protein turnover consequent upon leg mobilization. *Clinical Science*, **72**, 503–509.

Halliday, D., Pacy, P. J., Cheung, K. N., Dworzak, F., Gibson, N. A. and Rennie, M. J. (1988) Rate of protein synthesis in skeletal muscle of normal man and patients with muscular dystrophy: a reassessment. *Clinical Science*, **74**, 237–240.

Ho-Yen, D. O., Carrington, D. and Armstrong, A. A. (1988) Myalgic encephalomyelitis and alpha-interferon. *Lancet*, **i**, 125.

Jaffe, D. M., Terry, R. D. and Spiro, A. J. (1978) Disuse atrophy of skeletal muscle. *Journal of Neurological Science*, **35**, 189–200.

Lloyd, A. R., Hales, J. P. and Gandevia, S. C. (1988) Muscle strength, endurance and recovery in the post-infection fatigue syndrome. *Journal of Neurology Neurosurgery and Psychiatry*, **51**, 1316–1322.

Martin, F., Ward, K., Slavin, G., Levi, J. and Peters, T. J. (1985) Alcoholic skeletal myopathy, a clinical and pathological study. *Quarterly Journal of Medicine*, **218**, 233–251.

Pacy, P. J., Read, M., Peters, T. J. and Halliday, D. (1988) Post-absorptive whole body leucine kinetics and quadriceps muscle protein synthetic rate (MPSR) in the post-viral syndrome. *Clinical Science*, **75**, 36–37.

Potamianos, G., Gorman, D. M. and Peters, T. J. (1985a) Attitudes and treatment expectancies of patients and general hospital staff in relation to alcoholism. *British Journal of Medical Psychology*, **58**, 63–66.

Potamianos, G., Winter, D., Duffy, S. W., Gorman, D. M. and Peters, T. J. (1985b) The perception of problem drinkers by general hospital staff, general practitioners and alcoholic patients. *Alcoholism*, **2**, 563–566.

Preedy, V. R. and Peters, T. J. (1988) Acute effects of ethanol on protein synthesis in different muscles and muscle protein fractions of the rat. *Clinical Science*, **74**, 461–466.

Preedy, V. R. and Peters, T. J. (1989) The effect of chronic ethanol ingestion on synthesis and degradation of soluble contractile and stromal protein fractions of skeletal muscles from immature and mature rats. *Biochemical Journal*, **259**, 261–266.

Preedy, V. R., Paska, L., Sugden, P. H., Schofield, P. S. and Sugden, M. C. (1988) The effect of surgical stress and short term fasting on protein synthesis *in vivo* in diverse tissues of the mature rat. *Biochemical Journal*, **250**, 179–188.

Slavin, G., Sowter, C., Ward, P. and Paton, K. (1982) Measurement of striated muscle fibre diameters using interactive computer aided microscopy. *Journal of Clinical Pathology*, **35**, 1268–1271.

Stokes, M. J., Cooper, R. G. and Edwards, R. H. T. (1988) Normal muscle strength and fatiguability in patients with effort syndromes. *British Medical Journal*, **297**, 1014–1016.

Teahon, K., Preedy, V. R., Smith, D. G. and Peters, T. J. (1988) Clinical studies of the post-viral fatigue syndrome (PVFS) with special reference to skeletal muscle function. *Clinical Science*, **75**, 45.

Wagenmakers, A. J. M., Kaur, N., Coakley, J. H., Griffiths, R. D. and Edwards, R. H. T. (1987) Mitochondrial metabolism in myopathy and myalgia. *Advances in Myochemistry*, **1**, 219–230.

Wagenmakers, A. J. M., Coakley, J. H. and Edwards, R. H. T. (1988) The metabolic consequences of reduced habitual activities in patients with muscle pain and disease. *Ergonomics*, **31**, 1519–1527.

Wessely, S. and Powell, R. (1989) Fatigue syndromes: a comparison of chronic 'post-viral' fatigue with neuromuscular and affective disorders. *Journal of Neurology, Neurosurgery and Psychiatry*, **52**, 940–948.

Young, V. R. (1970) The role of skeletal and cardiac muscle in the regulation of protein metabolism. In H. N. Munro (ed.) *Mammalian Protein Metabolism*, Vol. 4, pp. 586–674. Academic Press, New York.

8

Persistent Virus Infection of Muscle in Patients with Post-viral Fatigue Syndrome

Neil E. Bowles* and Leonard C. Archard†

*Université de Genève, Genève, Switzerland
†Charing Cross and Westminster Medical School, London, UK

INTRODUCTION

The post-viral fatigue syndrome (PVFS), sometimes called myalgic encephalomyelitis (ME), is a chronic or relapsing disorder which develops after a diagnosed or apparent virus infection (Behan *et al.*, 1985). The syndrome is characterized by a broad and variable range of symptoms, but particularly by excessive muscle fatiguability and exhaustion after exercise (Calder *et al.*, 1987; Holmes *et al.*, 1988). Myalgia, sleep disturbances and psychogenic symptoms are reported by some patients. Diagnosis is essentially by exclusion of other causes of chronic fatigue, e.g. malignancy, drug abuse or psychiatric disease. Reports both of epidemics and sporadic cases of PVFS have appeared over the past 50 years.

The lack of objective clinical signs and the observation that the syndrome is diagnosed particularly frequently among medical or hospital service staff and certain socio-economic classes led to the proposition that hysteria was a major factor (McEvedy and Beard, 1970). However, more recent data, combining improved diagnostic criteria with new laboratory techniques, have revealed organic abnormalities in some patients (Behan *et al.*, 1985). Single fibre electromyography (EMG) investigations have shown that some patients exhibit prolonged jitter values, indicative of abnormalities of conduction at neuromuscular junctions (Jamal and Hansen, 1985). Similar single fibre EMG abnormalities had been observed previously in patients with acute viral infections (Friman *et al.*, 1977). Investigations of muscle metabolism by nuclear magnetic resonance (NMR) spectroscopy have shown that muscle of some PVFS patients undergoes premature intracellular acidosis

Post-viral Fatigue Syndrome. Edited by R. Jenkins and J. Mowbray
© 1991 John Wiley & Sons Ltd

during exercise and has a prolonged recovery period (Arnold *et al.*, 1984; Archard *et al.*, 1988a). These data indicate dysfunction of muscle respiratory metabolism, particularly of the glycolytic pathway, in some patients.

Serological and epidemiological studies have implicated various infectious agents as aetiological agents of PVFS, but particularly enteroviruses (McCartney *et al.*, 1986; Yousef *et al.*, 1988) and herpes viruses (Tobi *et al.*, 1982; Arnold *et al.*, 1984).

This chapter describes data obtained in various studies, especially those using virus-specific molecular hybridization probes, which associate persistent virus infection of muscle with post-viral fatigue syndrome.

ENTEROVIRUSES

Enteroviruses are members of the family Picornaviridae and consist of more than 70 serotypes, including Coxsackie A and B viruses, echoviruses and the polio viruses. Although they are frequent agents of trivial or subclinical enteric disease, this group of viruses has been associated with more serious disease, ranging from upper respiratory tract infection and aseptic meningitis to paralytic poliomyelitis, congestive heart failure and fulminating multisystem infection of the neonate (Melnick, 1982). These viruses appear to have a particular tropism for muscle and nervous tissue.

The enteroviruses are small icosohedral particles, approximately 27 nanometres in diameter, and have a single-stranded, positive sense RNA genome, about 7.4 kilobases (kb) in length. The virus genome has mRNA function (i.e. positive polarity) and will prime cell-free protein synthesis. After infection of cultured cells *in vitro*, cellular protein synthesis is selectively inhibited and virus-specific protein synthesis predominates. The viral genome is translated as a monocistronic message yielding a 260 kilodalton precursor polyprotein, which is cleaved subsequently into the individual proteins by virus-encoded proteases. The virus genome is replicated by a virus-coded RNA-dependent RNA polymerase via a complementary negative sense or template strand. Following assembly of the virus structural proteins and encapsidation of a single copy of the virus genome in each progeny virus, the cell is lysed and many infectious particles are released.

Initially, the link between PVFS and enterovirus infection was provided by epidemiological studies. During a poliomyelitis outbreak in Los Angeles in 1934, many medical staff developed PVFS-like symptoms (Gilliam, 1938). A similar epidemic occurred in Akureyri, Iceland, in 1948 which subsequently protected the population from polio virus infection, suggesting that they had been infected with a related virus at that time (Sigurdsson and Gudmundsson, 1956). Two more recent serological studies of patients with PVFS suggest a role for enteroviruses, particularly the Coxsackie B viruses, as pathogenetic agents. Elevated neutralization antibody titres against Coxsackie B viruses have been detected in 50% of PVFS patients compared with 17% of healthy controls (Behan *et al.*, 1985). More significantly, Coxsackie B virus-specific IgM (indicating recent or persistent infection) was detected in 31% of patients compared with 9% of controls: virus-specific IgM responses in sequential sera from some PVFS patients persisted for one year or longer, suggesting virus persistence (McCartney *et al.*, 1986).

The detection of the enterovirus structural protein VP1 in immune complexes from the serum of PVFS patients has been described (Yousef *et al.*, 1988). This antigen was detected in 44 of 87 (51%) of patients compared with none of 36 controls: of those positive, 39 (89%) were still positive four months later. After acid dissociation of neutralizing antibodies, virus was isolated from the stools of 15 to 74 patients but none of 28 controls: the same serotype of virus was isolated from five of the 15 patients when retested one year later.

These data implicate persistent enterovirus infection in the pathogenesis of PVFS. The fact that virus persists in the gut of a proportion of patients may account for the serological observations described above but does not explain the aberrations of muscle metabolism and electrophysiology. Attempts to demonstrate infectious virus or virus-specific antigens in muscle samples from such patients had been consistently unsuccessful (Behan and Behan, 1988). This situation was comparable to heart muscle disease (myocarditis or dilated cardiomyopathy) associated with enterovirus infection in which virus could not be isolated after the early stages of disease, but serological data suggested persisting enterovirus infection (Morgan-Capner *et al.*, 1984). The use of molecular hybridization probes capable of detecting enterovirus genomic RNA in the affected tissue demonstrated that, in a proportion of patients, virus RNA could be detected in the myocardium for years after the onset of symptoms (Bowles *et al.*, 1986, 1989). Enterovirus-specific hybridization probes were used similarly to investigate muscle biopsy samples to determine whether a similar situation occurred in PVFS patients (Archard *et al.*, 1988a).

EPSTEIN–BARR VIRUS AND OTHER HERPES VIRUSES

The herpes viruses, including Epstein–Barr virus and Varicella-Zoster (chicken-pox) virus, have also been implicated in the pathogenesis of PVFS. Epstein–Barr virus (EBV) is a ubiquitous human pathogen with which most of the population becomes infected subclinically during childhood (Epstein and Morgan, 1983). If primary infection occurs during adolescence, infectious mononucleosis (glandular fever) usually results and may last for several years (Horowitz *et al.*, 1975). Varicella-Zoster virus infection leads to the vesicular skin lesions characteristic of chicken-pox and may then establish a latent infection of dorsal ganglia: reactivation causes shingles (Mims and White, 1984).

The genome of EBV is a 170-kb double-stranded DNA molecule which has been cloned and sequenced (Baer *et al.*, 1984). Only B lymphocytes and epithelial cells have been shown to have specific receptors for EBV (Epstein and Morgan, 1983; Sixbey *et al.*, 1987). Infection of lymphocytes results in B cell differentiation, polyclonal activation and immunoregulatory disturbances (Mims and White, 1984).

Several studies of patients with symptoms similar to those of PVFS found serological evidence of persistent EBV infection, irrespective of a clinical history of infectious mononucleosis (Tobi *et al.*, 1982; Straus *et al.*, 1985). There was no obvious clinical feature which distinguished these patients from those diagnosed as having PVFS due to enterovirus infection. One PVFS patient shown by NMR spectroscopy to have abnormal respiratory metabolism of muscle had developed symptoms of chronic muscle fatiguability after an episode of chicken-pox (Arnold *et al.*, 1984).

EBV-specific hybridization probes have been used to demonstrate the presence of EBV DNA sequences in muscle biopsy samples from PVFS patients (Archard *et al.*, 1989; Bowles *et al.*, 1990).

MOLECULAR HYBRIDIZATION IN VIRAL DIAGNOSIS

The contradiction of data from conventional clinical virological diagnostic techniques in patients with PVFS required other investigative procedures to solve this enigma. One such technique is molecular hybridization employing virus-specific hybridization probes to detect virus genetic material in the affected tissue.

Nucleic acid hybridization is the annealing of a labelled single-stranded nucleic acid probe to complementary target sequences through the formation of hydrogen bonds. Hybrid stability depends on the degree of sequence homology between the probe and target sequence: variables such as the temperature of hybridization, the presence of helix-destabilizing agents (e.g. formamide) or salt concentration also affect hybrid formation. The probes are labelled usually by incorporation of nucleotide radiolabelled (with ^{32}P, ^{35}S or ^{3}H) or modified (with biotin or digoxigenin) into its sequence. Hybrids formed with radiolabelled probes can be detected either by autoradiography or by scintillation counting whereas non-radioactively labelled probes are usually detected by the formation of an insoluble coloured product in an enzyme reaction, as in conventional immunocytochemistry. For example, probes labelled with biotin are detected using avidin or streptavidin, which have a high affinity for biotin, conjugated to an enzyme such as alkaline phosphatase or horseradish peroxidase (Leary *et al.*, 1983).

In the studies of the involvement of enteroviruses and EBV in PVFS, cloned DNA, cDNA, cRNA and synthetic oligonucleotides have been used as hybridization probes.

The detection of DNA viruses such as EBV may be performed by DNA–DNA hybridization using cloned virus DNA fragments. One problem has been that certain regions of herpes virus genomes have some homology to cellular DNA sequences (Peden *et al.*, 1982) and can give rise to spurious hybridization signals. The use of cloned DNA fragments from unique regions of the virus genome overcomes this problem. Virus genomic DNA is cloned by cleavage of the isolated DNA using restriction endonucleases and ligation of the fragments into a vector (either a bacterial plasmid or bacteriophage DNA) for subsequent propagation in a bacterial host. The amplified recombinant vector is then separated from the bacterial DNA.

The analogous approach to the detection of genomes of RNA viruses, such as the enteroviruses, is the use of complementary DNA (cDNA) sequences. The cDNA is synthesized by reverse transcription of the RNA genome by priming either with an oligo (dT) sequence complementary to the 3' polyadenylated terminus of the genome or with an oligonucleotide primer complementary to a defined region of the genome. Complementary DNA synthesized in this way can be ligated into a clonal vector and propagated as described above.

Cloned probes are generally labelled by one of two methods. In the first (nick translation), random single-stranded nicks are introduced into the DNA by the enzyme DNase I and then the exonucleose and polymerase activities of DNA polymerase I sequentially remove nucleotides and re-synthesize the DNA strand (Rigby *et al.*, 1977). In the second (random hexanucleotide primer extension), random primers are annealed to a denatured (i.e. single-stranded) DNA sequence and the complementary strand is synthesized using the Klenow (large) fragment of DNA polymerase I (Feinberg and Vogelstein, 1984). In each case, the probe is labelled by addition of a labelled deoxyribonucleotide to the reaction: this may be labelled radioactively or chemically. Probes of higher specific activity can be prepared by random primer extension.

An alternative is the cRNA probe (riboprobe) synthesized from a DNA template by a DNA-dependent RNA polymerase (Melton *et al.*, 1984). A cloned DNA or cDNA sequence is subcloned downstream of a promoter, such as that for the RNA polymerases encoded by phage SP6, T3 or T7. In the case of enteroviruses, we cloned cDNA in both orientations so that probes capable of detecting either the sense (genomic or positive) strand of the anti-sense (template or negative) strand could be synthesized independently. Thus cRNA probes can be used selectively to detect either strand of virus RNA or DNA (Rotbart *et al.*, 1988; Cunningham *et al.*, 1990). They also have the advantage that RNA–RNA duplexes are intrinsically more stable than RNA–DNA duplexes, which in turn are more stable than DNA–DNA hybrids, allowing higher stringency washes and reducing background hybridizations.

Synthetic oligonucleotide probes are synthesized on commercially available DNA synthesizers and are generally between 15 and 50 nucleotides in length. They are generally labelled with ^{32}P by the enzyme T4 kinase (Maniatis *et al.*, 1982) but can alternatively be labelled with an enzyme, such as alkaline phosphatase, during synthesis (Ruth, 1984). The major factors are that the target sequence must be known (although this allows probes directed against defined regions of the genome to be synthesized) and their relatively low specific activity.

THE USE OF ENTEROVIRUS-SPECIFIC HYBRIDIZATION PROBES

Polio virus type 1 was the first enterovirus genome to be cloned and sequenced (Kitamura *et al.*, 1981) but several other serotypes have been partially or completely cloned since then (Hyypia *et al.*, 1984; Kandolf and Hofschneider, 1985; Tracy, 1985; Bowles *et al.*, 1986). Hybridization to RNA immobilized on solid supports (Hyypia *et al.*, 1984) shows that the sequences of the 5' and 3' non-translated regions and sequences encoding non-structural proteins of the virus, such as the RNA-dependent RNA polymerase, are highly conserved. In practice, probes corresponding to the P1 region, encoding the virus structural proteins, are essentially serotype-specific, whereas probes from other regions are enterovirus group-specific (Figure 1) (Rotbart *et al.*, 1985; Zhang *et al.*, 1988). The nucleotide sequences of several serotypes of enterovirus have been published (Toyoda *et al.*, 1984; Lindberg *et al.*, 1987): this has confirmed the sequence homologies predicted by hybridization.

Slot blot hybridization with an enterovirus group-specific probe was used to investigate whether enterovirus RNA could be detected in muscle from patients with PVFS (Archard *et al.*, 1988a). RNA was isolated from muscle biopsy specimens from the quadriceps of patients or control tissue and blotted onto duplicate membranes. One filter was hybridized with a radiolabelled enterovirus group-specific cDNA probe (derived from Coxsackie B2 virus genomic RNA and complementary to sequences encoding the RNA-dependent RNA polymerase and the 3' non-translated region: Bowles *et al.* (1986)) and the other with a similarly labelled control probe (β-tubulin cDNA: Hall *et al.* (1983)) to quantitate the total RNA immobilized from each sample. After hybridization, the filters were washed to high stringency and autoradiographed, and the autoradiographic development of the film was quantitated by scanning densitometry. The signal generated with the virus-specific probe was expressed as a ratio to the strength of the signal with the

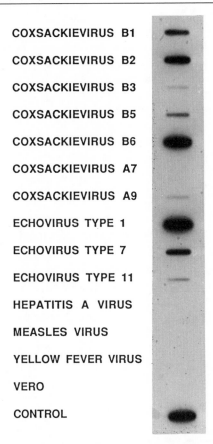

COXSACKIEVIRUS B1

COXSACKIEVIRUS B2

COXSACKIEVIRUS B3

COXSACKIEVIRUS B5

COXSACKIEVIRUS B6

COXSACKIEVIRUS A7

COXSACKIEVIRUS A9

ECHOVIRUS TYPE 1

ECHOVIRUS TYPE 7

ECHOVIRUS TYPE 11

HEPATITIS A VIRUS

MEASLES VIRUS

YELLOW FEVER VIRUS

VERO

CONTROL

Figure 1 Autoradiograph showing the group specificity of the hybridization probe derived from the 3'-terminal sequences of Coxsackie B2 virus, corresponding to part of the RNA polymerase coding sequence and the 3' non-translated region. The probe was hybridized to virus RNA isolated from infected cell lines, to cellular RNA from non-infected cells (vero) or to purified Coxsackie B2 virus genomic RNA (control)

control probe (Figure 2). In an initial series of 96 PVFS patients, 20 (21%) were found to have biopsy samples positive for enterovirus RNA (hybridization ratios > mean plus 3 × SD of controls: Archard *et al.*(1988a).

The duration of disease among the enterovirus-positive group ranged from two months to 20 years (Table 1) and indicates that enteroviruses are capable of persisting in muscle for many years. Coxsackie B virus-specific IgM assays suggest that only in patients with recent onset of symptoms is there a continuing humoral immune response against normal viral antigens. However, some patients may be infected with different enterovirus serotype, detected by molecular hybridization with the group-specific probe but not in a Coxsackie B virus-specific neutralization antibody or IgM assay.

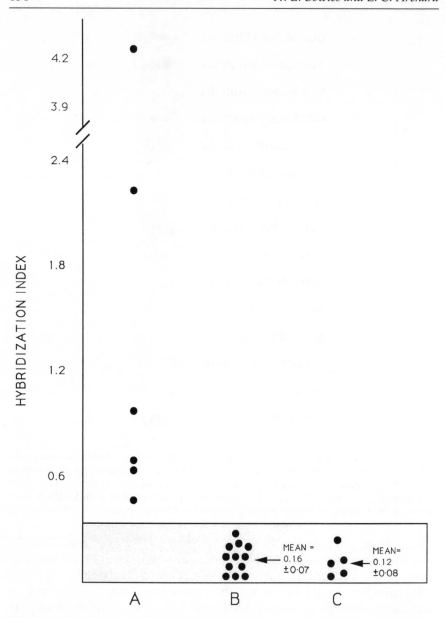

Figure 2 Detection of enterovirus RNA in skeletal muscle needle biopsy specimens. Groups A and B are samples from patients with post-viral fatigue syndrome and samples in group C are from controls. The hybridization index (HI) is the ratio for each sample of the autoradiographic signal (quantitated by scanning densitometry) with the virus-specific probe to that of the control probe. Samples in the shaded area (groups B and C) are negative for enterovirus RNA (less than $3 \times SD$ more than the mean HI of control group) and the remainder, group A, are positive

Table 1 Patient details and laboratory investigations of patients with muscle biopsy samples positive for enterovirus RNA

Patient	Age	Sex	Duration of disease (years)	Coxsackie B antibody titre		Serum CK units/ml*	Muscle biopsy pathology†	Single fibre electromyography
				IgM	NA			
1	33	F	2/12	B2,3,5	B3 (1024)	300	Positive	Positive
2	48	F	2.5/12	Negative	nd	<150	Positive	Negative
3	21	F	3/12	nd	Negative	<150	Positive	Negative
4	49	F	6/12	B4	nd	400	Positive	Negative
5	24	M	7/12	Negative	B4 (512)	<150	Negative	Negative
6	18	F	1	Negative	nd	<150	Negative	Positive
7	39	F	1	Negative	B4 (512)	<150	Negative	Negative
8	41	F	1	Negative	B2 (256)	210	Negative	Positive
9	49	M	1	Negative	nd	<150	Positive	Negative
10	40	F	1.5	nd	nd	<150	Positive	Negative
11	60	F	2	nd	B2 (256)	<150	Positive	Positive
12	40	F	2	B4	nd	<150	Positive	Negative
13	18	F	3	Negative	nd	310	Positive	Positive
14	44	F	4	Negative	Negative	265	Negative	Positive
15	39	M	4.5	nd	nd	<150	Positive	Positive
16	34	F	5	Negative	B4 (1024)	270	Negative	Negative
17	50	F	>10	Negative	Negative	260	Positive	Positive
18	52	M	15	nd	Negative	170	Positive	Negative
19	37	M	20	Negative	Negative	180	Negative	Positive
20	69	F	20	Negative	Negative	<150	Negative	Positive

* Normal value for CK = 150 units/ml.
† Nonspecific changes.
NA = Neutralizing antibody.
nd = Not done.

There was a strong correlation between elevated serum creatine kinase (CK) concentration and the detection of enterovirus RNA in this series of PVFS patients. This enzyme is a marker of muscle damage and large elevations in serum CK concentration have been reported in patients with various myopathies, including polymyositis. CK concentrations of up to two times normal levels have been reported in PVFS patients (Schwartz *et al.*, 1978). Of the 20 patients with muscle samples positive for enterovirus RNA, nine had constantly elevated CK; in comparison, only two of the 76 that appeared negative had elevated serum CK. Therefore, over 80% of the patients in whom continuing muscle damage was indicated by elevated serum CK had a persisting enterovirus infection of muscle.

There was no significant difference in histological or histochemical investigations of muscle biopsy samples between the groups positive or negative for enterovirus RNA in this study. There were a number of nonspecific changes, primarily scattered atrophic fibres, type II fibre hypertrophy and occasional single fibre necrosis. Such histopathological changes are compatible with the observation of mildly elevated serum CK in some patients.

Nine of the 20 patients whose biopsy samples were positive for enterovirus RNA showed abnormally prolonged jitter on examination by single fibre electromyography. One patient, positive for enterovirus RNA and who has symptoms for more than 10 years, had abnormal histology, exhibited prolonged jitter on single fibre EMG, had elevated serum CK and also showed NMR spectroscopy abnormalities of the type described previously (Arnold *et al.*, 1984).

To date, we have studied muscle biopsy samples from a total of 140 PVFS patients and 34 (24%) were positive for enterovirus RNA. Enterovirus RNA was not detected in any of 152 control samples of human muscle. This figure is likely to be an underestimate of the occurrence of enterovirus RNA in muscle of PVFS patients because of sampling errors arising from the study of a portion of a single muscle biopsy sample from each patient. Our analogous studies of enterovirus-induced heart muscle disease have revealed foci of infection by enteroviruses (Archard *et al.*, 1988b). Multiple samples of muscle from each patient would be required to provide a more accurate figure for the frequency of virus involvement.

THE DETECTION OF EPSTEIN–BARR DNA IN MUSCLE BY MOLECULAR HYBRIDIZATION

As homology between regions of EBV DNA and human genomic DNA have been reported (Peden *et al.*, 1982), a probe which gave minimal cross-hybridization and representing coding sequences likely to be conserved between isolates was selected (Archard *et al.*, 1989). This probe corresponds to a non-repetitive part of the coding region of the EBV nuclear antigen 1 (EBNA-1) (Arrand *et al.*, 1981). Antibodies to EBNA-1, as well as other EBV-specific antigens, have been described in patients with PVFS (Tobi *et al.*, 1982; Straus *et al.*, 1985). DNA was isolated from additional portions of muscle biopsy samples of 72 of the 96 patients with PVFS, described above, plus four further patients, and blotted onto duplicate nitrocellulose membranes (Archard *et al.*, 1989). One filter was hybridized with the EBV-specific probe and the second with a control probe (γ-actin cDNA) (Gunning *et al.*,1983): after autoradiography and scanning densitometry the results were expressed as above. As before, the hybridization signals of the samples from PVFS patients fell into two groups. Sixty-eight of the test samples were statistically indistinguishable from the control group of 48 samples (Figure 3: groups A and B). However, eight samples from PVFS patients gave positive signals, exceeding the mean plus 3 × SD of control samples.

All eight patients with muscle biopsy samples positive for EBV had typical PVFS and had serological evidence of EBV infection (Table 2). The duration of disease ranged between four months and 12 years. Six of the eight had nonspecific abnormalities of muscle histology of the type described above. Six of the eight were tested by single fibre EMG and five showed abnormally prolonged jitter. Two of the eight patients positive for EBV DNA in muscle were examined by NMR spectroscopy: one was normal while the other showed an abnormally low intracellular pH at rest and abnormal changes in the concentration of intracellular muscle phosphates on recovery after exercise.

By comparison of the hybridization signal from the virus-specific probe with that of the control probe it was estimated that EBV nuclear antigen-specific sequences were present at between five and 50 copies per cell equivalent. Microscopic examination of muscle samples does not reveal a lymphocytic infiltrate, suggesting that the EBV sequences are present in muscle fibres and not in lymphocytes.

To date, we have studied muscle biopsy samples from a total of 86 PVFS patients for EBV sequences and eight (9%) were positive. No muscle biopsy sample was positive for both EBV and enterovirus genomic sequences.

These data are the first demonstration that EBV can be detected in muscle: since B lymphocytes are the only cell type known to continually express the cell surface structure used as a virus receptor (Epstein and Morgan, 1983), infection of muscle may be comparable to EBV infection of epithelial cells which display virus-specific receptors only during an early stage of differentiation (Sixbey *et al.*, 1987). Alternatively, EBV-infected lymphocytes may fuse with non-susceptible cells (Shapiro and Volsky, 1983). Transfection of EBV DNA into cells can result in limited expression of genes but may not result in a complete replication cycle (Shapiro and Volsky, 1983; Shapiro *et al.*, 1982).

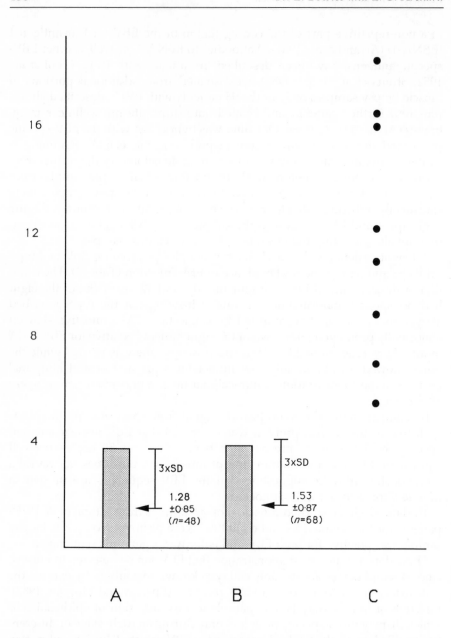

Figure 3 Detection of Epstein–Barr virus DNA in skeletal muscel needle biopsy specimens. Groups B and C are samples from patients with post-viral fatigue syndrome. Samples in group A are from controls. Samples in groups A and B are negative for EBV DNA (less than 3 × SD more than the mean HI of control group) and the remainder, group C, are positive

Table 2 Patient details and laboratory investigations of patients with muscle biopsy samples positive for Epstein–Barr virus DNA

Patient	Age	Sex	Duration of disease (year)	EBV serology		Muscle biopsy pathology	Single fibre electromyography
1	58	F	4/12	EBNA EA VCA	1/160 1/8 1/60	Type II fibre predominance	Abnormal: prolonged jitter
2	34	F	6/12	EBNA EA VCA	1/160 1/8 1/160	Normal	Normal
3	43	M	1	EBNA EA VCA	1/160 1/8 1/256	Type II fibre excess: some fibre necrosis	nd
4	54	F	2	EBNA EA VCA	<1/5 Negative Negative	Normal	nd
5	50	M	4	EBNA EA VCA	1/160 1/20 1/60	Abnormal fibre size: no fat	Abnormal: prolonged jitter
6	25	F	8	EBNA EA VCA	1/80 1/5 1/32	Nonspecific changes	Abnormal: prolonged jitter
7	41	F	10	EBNA EA VCA	1/160 1/16 1/64	Nonspecific changes	Abnormal: prolonged jitter
8	63	M	12	EBNA EA VCA	1/80 1/16 1/160	Nonspecific changes	Abnormal: prolonged jitter

EBNA = Epstein–Barr virus neclear antigen.
EA = Epstein–Barr virus early antigen.
VCA = Epstein–Barr virus capsid antigen.
nd = Not done.

DEFECTIVE ENTEROVIRUS STRAINS ASSOCIATED WITH PERSISTENCE

The specificities of cRNA probes are essentially as reported for cDNA probes but cRNA probes offer at least a 10-fold increase in sensitivity (Cova et al., 1988). Replication of the enterovirus genome occurs via the synthesis of an anti-sense (template or negative) strand by the virus-encoded RNA-dependent RNA polymerase (Perez-Bercoff,1978). This strand acts as a template for the preferential synthesis of the sense (genomic or positive) strand which is either translated to yield the virus-specific polyprotein or packaged into the virus capsid and eventually released from the cell. As cRNA probes are single-stranded and can be prepared complementary to either polarity of enterovirus RNA, they allow the relative abundance of the sense strand and the anti-sense strand to be determined. During cytolytic infections of cells cultured in vitro the sense strand predominates over the anti-sense by between 40 : 1 (Rotbart et al., 1988) and 100 : 1 (our unpublished data). We also observed a similar preponderance of positive, genomic strand of enteroviral RNA in muscle from CD-1 mice with an experimental Coxsackie B1-induced polymyositis (Strongwater et al., 1984) where fibre necrosis and infiltration by inflammatory cells indicates active virus replication.

We have applied such probes to the study of RNA isolated from muscle biopsy samples from patients with PVFS: in all cases tested which were positive for enterovirus RNA, the sense and anti-sense strands were present in approximately equimolar amounts (Cunningham et al., 1990). Representative data are shown here in Figure 4: the control probe is cDNA complementary to the cell-cycle independent mRNA species 7B6 (Kaczmarek et al., 1985). These data suggest that persistence of enterovirus RNA in muscle is associated with the selection of virus defective in the control of virus genomic RNA replication. The molecular basis of this defect is unknown but could result from changes in the polymerase itself or of its recognition sequences in viral RNA.

PROGNOSTIC SIGNIFICANCE OF ENTEROVIRUS PERSISTENCE

The significance of persistent enterovirus infection of myocardium in patients with chronic non-inflammatory heart muscle disease (dilated cardiomyopathy) has been studied (Archard et al., 1990). This disease is believed to be a sequela of an enterovirus-induced myocarditis, resulting from persistence of enterovirus RNA sequences in the myocardium (Goodwin, 1983; Archard et al., 1988b). The proportion of those patients with persisting enterovirus RNA in myocardium that developed congestive cardiac failure (and had undergone transplantation or died) was four times greater than those of clinically similar patients who were enterovirus

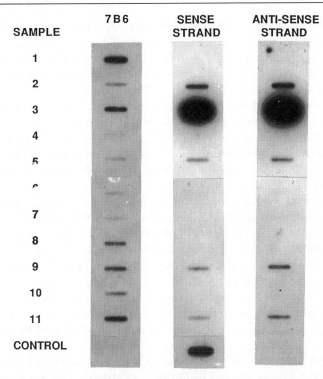

Figure 4 Hybridization of the 7B6 control riboprobe or the enterovirus group-specific riboprobes, detecting either the sense (genomic) strand or the anti-sense (template strand), to RNA isolated from muscle biopsy specimens of patients with post-viral fatigue syndrome (samples 1–11) or to purified Coxsackie B2 virus genomic RNA (control). The 7B6 probe quantitates the total RNA immobilized from each muscle sample (Kaczmarek *et a.*, 1985). In all cases where enterovirus RNA sequences are detected in muscle samples the amounts of sense and anti-sense strands are approximately equivalent

negative. The demonstration of a persistent enterovirus infection of myocardium is now the strongest available prognostic indicator for the development of end-stage dilated cardiomyopathy.

The prognostic significance of persistent enterovirus RNA in the muscle of patients with PVFS is unknown. However, some PVFS patients recover spontaneously while others go through periods of remission and relapse and this may be related to presence of enterovirus sequences in muscle.

PATHOGENESIS OF PERSISTENT VIRUS INFECTION IN PVFS

The studies described above have demonstrated that a proportion of patients with PVFS have a persistent virus infection of muscle for up to several years after the onset of symptoms. The failure to demonstrate a continuing humoral or cellular immune response against normal viral antigens suggests that immune-mediated pathogenetic mechanisms are not important. The only evidence available so far relating to pathological changes of muscle comes from single fibre EMG and from NMR spectroscopy studies which have indicated defects in muscle metabolism in some patients. Although the mechanism of such changes are unknown, the perturbation of normal cellular functions by persistent virus infection has been described (Oldstone, 1989) and we have proposed that PVFS is an acquired metabolic myopathy induced by persistent virus infection (Archard et al., 1988a).

This proposal would account for the symptoms of muscle fatiguability and myalgia and for the prolonged time for recovery after exercise experienced by most PVFS patients. The neurological or psychogenic symptoms are more difficult to relate to persistent virus infection. In some patients, infection of the central nervous system may occur since enteroviruses are also associated with neurological disease, such as poliomyelitis or aseptic meningitis. Another possibility is that, in response to virus infection, immune mediators such as the interferons or interleukins are released, resulting in the further symptoms described by some PVFS patients.

Data from heart muscle disease suggest that dilated cardiomyopathy is a sequela of a virus-induced inflammatory disease (myocarditis). By extrapolation, it may be that PVFS is a sequela of a transient viral myositis, such as polymyositis or dermatomyositis. The demonstration of enterovirus RNA sequences in the muscle of patients with polymyositis/dermatomyositis or PVFS supports this hypothesis (Bowles et al., 1987; Archard et al., 1988a). However, while enterovirus and, possibly to a lesser extent, EBV, are probably aetiological, it seems likely that a range of persisting viruses may be capable of inducing this syndrome.

ACKNOWLEDGEMENTS

We are very grateful to Louise Cunningham for the use of unpublished data, to Michael Mackett for the EBV probes, to Kathy Barrett for the 7B6 riboprobe construct, to Peter Behan and Russell Lane for allowing us to study tissue from their patients and to Eleanor Bell, David Doyle and Doris Taylor for serology, histology and NMR spectroscopy results, respectively.

REFERENCES

Archard, L. C., Behan, P. O., Bell, E. J., Doyle, D. and Bowless, N. E. (1988a) Postviral fatigue syndrome: persistence of enterovirus RNA in muscle and elevated creatine kinase. *Journal of the Royal Society of Medicine*, **81**, 326–329.

Archard, L. C., Freeke, C. A., Richardson, P. J. *et al.*, (1988b) Persistence of enterovirus RNA in dilated cardiomyopathy: a progression from myocarditis. In: H.-P. Schultheis (ed.) *New Concepts in Viral Heart Disease*, pp. 347–362, Springer-Verlag, Berlin.

Archard, L. C., Peters, J. L., Behan, P. O., Doyle, D., Mackett, M. and Bowles, N. E. (1989) Post viral chronic fatigue syndrome: Persistence of Epstein–Barr virus DNA in muscle. In D. V. Ablashi *et al.* (eds) *Eptstein–Barr Virus and Human Disease II*, pp. 439–444, Humana Press, Clifton, NJ.

Archard, L. C., Bowles, N. E., Cunningham, L. *et al.* (1990) Enterovirus RNA sequences in hearts with dilated cardiomyopathy: a pathogenetic link between virus infection and dilated cardiomyopathy. In: G. Baroldi, F. Camerini and J. F. Goodwin (eds) *Advances in Cardiomyopathies*. Springer-Verlag, Berlin, pp. 194–198.

Arnold, D. L., Radda, G. K., Bore, P. J., Styles, P. and Taylor, D. L. (1984) Excessive intracellular acidosis of skeletal muscles on exercise in a patient with postviral exhaustion/fatigue syndrome. *Lancet*, **i**, 1367–1369.

Arrand, J. R., Rymo, L., Walsh, J. E., Bjorck, E., Lindahl, T. and Griffin, B. E. (1981) Molecular cloning of the complete Epstein–Barr virus genome as a set of overlapping restriction endonuclease fragments. *Nucleic Acids Research*, **9**, 2999–3014.

Baer, R., Bankier, A. T., Biggin, M. D. *et al.* (1984) DNA sequence and expression of the B95-8 Epstein–Barr virus genome. *Nature*, **310**, 207–211.

Behan, P. O. and Behan, W. M. H. (1988) The postviral fatigue syndrome. *CRC Critical Reviews in Neurobiology*, **4**, 157–178.

Behan, P. O., Behan, W. M. H. and Bell, E. J. (1985) The postviral fatigue syndrome—an analysis of the findings in 50 cases. *Journal of Infection*, **10**, 211–222.

Bowles, N. E., Richardson, P. J., Olsen, E. G. J. and Archard, L. C. (1986) Detection of Coxsackie-B-virus-specific RNA sequences in myocardial biopsy samples from patients with myocarditis and dilated cardiomyopathy. *Lancet*, **i**, 1120–1123.

Bowles, N. E., Dubowitz, V., Sewry, C. A. and Archard, L. C. (1987) Dermatomyositis, polymyositis and coxsackie-B-virus infection. *Lancet*, **i**, 1004–1007.

Bowles, N. E., Rose, M. L., Taylor, P., Banner, N. R., Morgan-Capner, P., Cunningham, L., Archard, L. C. and Yacoub, . H. (1989) End-stage dilated cardiomyopathy: persistence of enterovirus RNA in myocardium at cardiac transplantation and lack of immune response. *Circulation*, **80**, 1128–1136.

Bowles, N. E., Peters, J. L., Behan, P. O., Doyle, D., Mackett, M. and Archard, L. C. (1990) Persisting Epstein–Barr virus DNA in muscle of patients with postviral fatigue syndrome. *Epidemiology and Infection* (submitted).

Calder, B. D., Warnock, P. J., McCartney, R. A. and Bell, E. J. (1987) Coxsackie B viruses and the post-viral fatigue syndrome: a prospective study in general practice. *Journal of the Royal College of General Practitioners*, **37**, 11–14.

Cova, L., Kopecka, H., Aymard, M. and Girard, M. (1988) Use of cRNA probes for the detection of enteroviruses by molecular hybridization. *Journal of Medical Virology*, **24**, 11–18.

Cunningham, L., Bowles, N.E., Lane, R. J. M., Dubowitz, V. and Archard, L. C. (1990) Persistence of enterovirus RNA in chronic fatigue syndrome is associated with the abnormal production of equal amounts of positive and negative stands of enteroviral RNA. *Journal of General Virology*, **71**, 1399–1402.

Epstein, M. A. and Morgan, A. J. (1983) Clinical consequences of Epstein–Barr virus infection and possible control by an anti-viral vaccine. *Clinical and Experimental Immunology*, **53**, 257–271.

Feinberg, A. P. and Vogelstein, B. (1984) A technique for radiolabelling DNA restriction endonuclease fragments to high specific activity. *Analytical Biochemistry*, **137**, 266–267.

Friman, G., Schiller, H. H., Schwartz, M. S. (1977) Disturbed neuromuscular transmission in viral infections. *Scandinanvian Journal of Infectious Diseases*, **9**, 99–103.

Gilliam, A. G. (1938) *Epidemiological study of an epidemic, diagnosed as poliomyelitis, occurring among the personnel of the Los Angeles County General Hospital during the summer of 1934.* United States Public Health Bulletin No. 240, pp. 1–90.

Goodwin, J. F. (1983) Myocarditis as a possible cause of cardiomyopathy. In H. Just and H. P. Schuster (eds) *Myocarditis—Cardiomyopathy*, pp. 7–11, Springer-Verlag, Berlin.

Grist, N. R. and Bell, E. J. (1974) A six year study of Coxsackie virus B infections in heart disease. *Journal of Hygiene*, **73**, 165–172.

Gunning, P., Ponte, P., Okayama, H., Engel, J., Blau, H. and Kedes, L. (1983) Isolation and characterization of full length cDNA clones for human α-, β-, and γ-Actin mRNAs: Skeletal but not cytoplasmic actins have an amino-terminal cysteine that is subsequently removed. *Molecular and Cellular Biology*, **3**, 787–795.

Hall, J. L., Dudley, L., Dobner, P. R., Lewis, C. A. and Cowan, N. J. (1983) Identification of two human beta-tubulin isotypes. *Mollecular and Cellular Biology*, **3**, 854–862.

Holmes, G. P., Kaplan, J. E., Gantz, N. M. *et al.* (1988) Chronic fatigue syndrome: a working case definition. *Annals of Internal Medicine*, **108**, 387–389.

Horowitz, C. A., Henle, W., Henle, G. and Schmitz, H. (1975) Clinical evaluation of patients with infectious mononucleosis and development of antibodies to the R component of the Epstein–Barr virus-induced early antigen complex. *American Journal of Medicine*, **58**, 330–338.

Hyypia, T., Stålhandske, P., Vainiopaa, R. and Pettersson, U. (1984) Detection of enteroviruses by spot hybridization. *Journal of Clinical Microbiology*, **19**, 436–483.

Jamal, G. A. and Hansen, S. (1985) Electrophysiological studies in patients with postviral fatigue syndrome. *Journal of Neurology, Neurosurgery and Psychiatry*, **48**, 691–694.

Kaczmarek, L., Calabrett, B. and Baserga, R. (1985) Expression of cell-cycledependent genes in phytohemagglutinin stimulated human lymphocytes. *Proceedings of the National Academy of Sciences of the USA*, **82**, 5372–5379.

Kandolf, R. and Hofschneider, P. H. (1985) Molecular cloning of the genome of a cardiotropic coxsackie B3 virus: full-length reverse-transcribed recombinant cDNA generates infectious virus in mammalian cells. *Proceedings of the National Academy of Sciences of the USA*, **82**, 4818–4822.

Kitamura, N., Semler, B. L., Rothberg, P. G. *et al.* (1981) Primary structure, gene organization and polypeptide expression of poliovirus RNA. *Nature*, **291**, 547–553.

Leary, J. J., Bright, D. J. and Ward, D. C. (1983) Rapid sensitive colorimetric method for visualising biotin-labeled probes hybridised to DNA or RNA immobilised on nitrocellulose: Bio-blots. *Proceedings of the National Academy of Sciences of the USA*, **80**, 4045–4049.

Lindberg, A. M., Stålhandske, P. O. K. and Pettersson, U. (1987) Genome of coxsackievirus B3. *Virology*, **156**, 50–63.

Maniatis, T., Fritsch, E. F. and Sambrrok, J. (1982) *Molecular Cloning*. Cold Spring Harbor Laboratory, Cold Spring Harbor.

McCartney, R. A., Banatvala, J. E. and Bell, E. J. (1986) Routine use of μ-antibody capture ELISA for the serological diagnosis of Coxsackie B virus infections. *Journal of Medical Virology*, **19**, 205–212.

McEvedy, C. P. and Beard, P. W. (1970) Royal Free epidemic of 1955: a reconsideration. *British Medical Journal*, **1**, 7–11.

Melnick, J. L. (1982) Enteroviruses. In A. S. Evans (ed.) *Viral Infections of Humans*, pp. 187–251. Plenum, New York.

Melton, D. A., Krieg, P. A., Rebagliati, M. R., Maniatis, T., Kinn, K. and Green, M. R. (1984) Efficient *in vitro* synthesis of biologically active RNA and RNA hybridization probes from plasmids containing a bacteriophage SP6 promoter. *Nucleic Acids Research*, **12**, 7035–7056.

Mims, C. A. and White, D. O. (1984) *Viral Pathogenesis and Immunology*, Blackwell Scientific, Oxford.

Morgan-Capner, P., Richardson, P. J., McSorley, C., Daly, K. and Pattison, J. R. (1984) Virus investigations in heart muscle disease. In H. D. Bolte (ed.) *Viral Heart Disease*, pp. 95–115. Springer Verlag, Berlin.

Oldstone, M. B. A. (1989) Viral alteration of cell function. *Scientific American*, **261**(2), 34–40.

Peden, K., Mounts, P. and Hayward, G. S. (1982) Homology between mammalian cell DNA sequences and human herpesvirus genomes detected by a hybridization procedure with high-complexity probe. *Cell*, **31**, 71–80.

Perez-Bercoff, R. (1978) Replication of viral RNA. In R. Perez-Bercoff (ed.) *The Molecular Biology of Picornaviruses*, pp. 293–318. Plenum, New York.

Rigby, P. W. J., Dieckmann, M., Rhodes, C. and Berg, P. (1977) Labeling deoxyribonucleic acid to high specific activity by nick translation with DNA polymerase I. *Journal of Molecular Biology*, **113**, 237–251.

Rotbart, H. A., Levin, M. J., Villarreal, L. P., Tracy, S. M., Semler, B. L. and Wimmer, E. (1985) Factors affecting the detection of enteroviruses in cerebrospinal fluid with coxsackievirus B3 and poliovirus 1 cDNA probes. *Journal of Clinical Microbiology*, **22**, 220–224.

Rotbart, H. A., Abzug, M. J., Murray, R. S., Murphy, N. L., Levin, M. J. (1988) Intracellular detection of sense and antisense enteroviral RNA by in situ hybridization. *Journal of Virological Methods*, **22**, 295–301.

Ruth, J. L. (1984) Chemical synthesis of non-radioactively-labeled DNA hybridization probes. *DNA*, **4**, 123–128.

Schwartz, M. S., Swash, M. and Gross, M. (1978) Benign postinfection polymyositis. *British Medical Journal*, **2**, 1256–1257.

Shapiro, I. M. and Volsky, D. J. (1983) Infection of normal human epithelium cells by Epstein–Barr virus. *Science*, **219**, 1225–1228.

Shapiro, I. M., Volsky, D. J., Saemundsen, A. K., Anisimova, E. and Klein, G. (1982) Infection of the human T-cell-derived leukaemia line Molt-4 by Epstein–Barr virus (EBV): induction of EBV-determined antigens and virus reproduction. *Virology*, **120**, 171–181.

Sigurdsson, B. and Gudmundsson, K. R. (1956) Clinical findings six years after outbreak of Akureyri disease. *Lancet*, **i**, 766–767.

Sixbey, J. W., Davis, D. S., Young, L. S., Hutt-Fletcher, L., Tedder, T. F. and Rickinson, A. B. (1987) Human epithelial cell expression of an Epstein–Barr virus receptor. *Journal of General Virology*, **68**, 805–811.

Straus, S. E., Tosato, G., Armstrong, G. *et al.* (1985) Persisting illness and fatigue in adults with evidence of Epstein–Barr virus infection. *Annals of Internal Medicine*, **102**, 7–16.

Strongwater, S. L., Dorovini-Zis, K., Ball, R. D. and Schnitzer, T. J. (1984) A murine model of polymyositis induced by Coxsackievirus B1 (Tucson strain) *Arthritis and Rheumatism*, **27**, 433–442.

Tobi, M., Morag, A., Ravid, Z. *et al.* (1982) Prolonged atypical illness associated with serological evidence of persistent Epstein–Barr virus infection. *Lancet*, **i**, 61–64.

Toyoda, H., Kohara, M., Kataoka, Y., Suganuma, T., Omata, T., Imura, N. and Nomoto, A. (1984) Complete nucleotide sequences of all three poliovirus serotype genomes. *Journal of Molecular Biology*, **174**, 561–585.

Tracy, S. (1985) Comparison of genomimc homologies in the coxsackievirus B group by use of cDNA:RNA dot-blot hybridization. *Journal of Clinical Microbiology*, **21**, 371–374.

Yousef, G. E., Bell, E. J., Mann, G. F., Murugusen, V., Smith, D. G., McCartney, R. A. and Mowbray, J. F. (1988) Chronic enterovirus infection in patients with postviral fatigue syndrome. *Lancet*, **i**, 146–150.

Zhang, H. Y., Yousef, G. E., Bowles, N. E., Archard, L. C., Mann, G. F. and Mowbray, J. F. (1988) Detection of enterovirus RNA in experimentally infected mice by molecular hybridization: specificity of sybgenomic probes in quantitative slot blot and in situ hybridization. *Journal of Medical Virology*, **26**, 375–386.

9

Neurophysiological Findings in the Post-viral Fatigue Syndrome (Myalgic Encephalomyelitis)

Goran A. Jamal
University of Glasgow, Glasgow, UK

INTRODUCTION

Muscle fatigability and myalgia are the most dominant and constant features of the post-viral fatigue syndrome (PVFS). Their importance is such that the diagnosis should not be entertained without them. In PVFS there is a clear absence of conspicuous muscle cell damage when investigated by traditional methods. It is, however, beyond any doubt that muscles are involved in this syndrome with both metabolic and ultrastructural abnormalities (Arnold *et al.*, 1984, 1985; Archard *et al.*, 1988). Presence of viral particles in muscles of patients with this syndrome has recently been reported, thus raising the possibility of a persistent viral infection as the underlying cause (Yousef *et al.*, 1988; Archard *et al.*, 1988). Such persistent viral particles may render the muscle cells unable to carry out their specialised functions. It is therefore not surprising that skeletal muscles should be involved in PVFS and that traditional neurophysiological or morphological methods may not show evidence of such abnormality.

A question which would be relevant to the pathophysiology of PVFS is whether or not persistent viral infection can cause any abnormality of skeletal muscle. Muscle involvement with prominent neurophysiological abnormalities is well known to occur in acute viral infections (Schwartz *et al.*, 1978) and a variety of muscle enzyme abnormalities and subtle ultrastructural mitochondrial damage have also been reported following viral infections (Astrom *et al.*, 1976). Myalgia is a frequent feature of acute infectious illnesses, particularly influenza, in which pain in the muscles of the leg and lower back is characteristic. It usually improves rapidly but may be intense

Post-viral Fatigue Syndrome. Edited by R. Jenkins and J. Mowbray
© 1991 John Wiley & Sons Ltd

for several days and serum creatine kinase concentration may be slightly raised during this time (Middleton *et al.*, 1970; Friman, 1976). Fatiguability is also a common feature in acute viral infection and Friman (1977) reported a slight weakness soon after resolution of the acute illness in such patients. In a later study Friman *et al.* (1977) reported transient changes in neuromuscular transmission in the acute phase of viral infections even in patients without myalgia and such changes were verified by sophisticated neurophysiological techniques. There have also been several reports of more severe muscle involvement complicating viral infections (Chou and Gutman, 1970; Mejlszenkier *et al.*, 1973; Fukuyama *et al.*, 1977; Schwartz *et al.*, 1978). Distinct neurophysiological abnormalities are usually present in these patients (Schwartz *et al.*, 1978).

The reported neurophysiological findings in this chapter are from patients in whom the diagnosis of PVFS was very well scrutinised and who were identified following structured criteria for case definition. This case definition was restricted by intention to maximise accuracy of the diagnosis. The patients included had fulfilled all of the following four major criteria:

(a) Very prominent persistent or relapsing muscle fatiguability and myalgia of at least six months duration present at rest but made worse with little exercise. This should have been accompanied by negative neurological examination and in particular absence of evidence of muscle weakness.

(b) Other clinical conditions, especially those that may produce similar symptoms, were excluded in all patients by thorough evaluation based on careful clinical history, physical examination, conventional neurophysiological (electromyography and nerve conduction) studies and other appropriate laboratory examinations. Special emphasis was put on excluding cervical radiculopathy, neuropathy, nerve trauma, known myopathies, diabetes mellitus or other endocrine diseases, chronic pulmonary cardiac, hepatic, renal and haematological disorders, chronic psychiatric illnesses or any other concurrent problem in the neuromuscular system. Patients with excessive alcohol ingestion or those on any neurotoxic drugs were also excluded. Concentric needle EMG and nerve conduction studies were performed to exclude any neurogenic or frank myopathic abnormality. Neuromuscular junction defects were excluded in all patients by repetitive stimulation studies and acetylcholine receptor antibody estimation.

(c) All patients had clear evidence of a recent viral infection by laboratory methods.

(d) All patients had two or more abnormal findings when subjected to the following immunological and/or morphological findings: *in vitro* lymphocyte function (as estimated by lymphocyte protein synthesis), lymphocyte subset examination, helper/inducer lymphocyte ratio, immune complex and complement studies. A large number of these patients were also subjected to muscle biopsy with both light and electron microscopic examination and the majority of these patients showed ultrastructural abnormalities. Muscle biopsy studies also served to exclude any known neurogenic or myopathic disorders in these patients.

ELECTROENCEPHALOGRAPHY

It is our experience and that of others (Pampiglione *et al.*, 1978) that about 80–90% of patients with PVFS show some EEG changes. These are usually modest and of a discrete nature. The changes comprise an excess of irregular slow-wave activity with a patchy distribution appearing on one or the other side of the brain without any constant focal features. No sharp waves, spikes or complexes are seen at any stage of the disease or during recovery. The changes seen are, therefore, not dissimilar to those seen in some cases of multiple sclerosis. The severity, distribution and character of these EEG changes bear no similarity to those EEG abnormalities seen in cases of acute encephalitis or encephalopathies of metabolic, endocrine or toxic aetiologies. The severity and extent of EEG changes in PVFS appear to be unrelated to the severity of symptoms (Pampiglione *et al.*, 1978).

CONCENTRIC NEEDLE ELECTROMYOGRAPHY AND NERVE CONDUCTION STUDIES

Several of these conventional neurophysiological studies have failed to demonstrate any evidence of definite neurogenic or myopathic abnormality in patients with PVFS (Richardson, 1956; Jamal and Hansen, 1985, 1988, 1989; Thomas, 1987). Nerve conduction studies, including those of motor and sensory fibres, produce normal results in all cases. As these studies only test the large-diameter peripheral nerves (Jamal *et al.*, 1987), 30 patients with the diagnosis of PVFS were examined in our laboratory using the technique of thermal threshold measurement of Jamal *et al.* (1985) which provides a very sensitive objective assessment of the small fibre pathway, including the unmyelinated and the thinly myelinated nerve fibres, and these produced entirely normal results. There is thus no evidence from these studies of any neurogenic lesion in these patients either in the large myelinated or in the small peripheral nerve fibre populations.

Conventional concentric needle electromyogram (EMG) also shows normal results in patients with PVFS with no evidence of neurogenic changes or muscle fibre degeneration. Some authors have reported occasional irregular fasciculations, especially during the early stages of the disease (Richardson,

1956). However, examination of a very large number of patients in our laboratory did not show any spontaneous activity. Examination of motor unit potentials produced some controversial findings, including disturbances of volition (Richardson, 1956), but these disturbances have been interpreted by some authors as non-organic (McEvedey and Beard, 1970; Thomas, 1987). Richardson (1956) reported 'grouping of motor unit potentials' where many motor unit potentials occurred in groups interrupted by periods of relative silence in between and these were reported to occur particularly during the recovery phase. Each group was reported to be about 45–50 ms in duration and coming at a frequency of 5–10 per second. In a short letter to the *Lancet*, Thomas (1987) reported that the muscle weakness in patients with PVFS is of a 'volitional' type with poorly sustained fluctuating effort which is capable of improvement by encouragement. He also reported that EMG demonstrated a low firing rate on maximum volition and that this was accompanied by 'grouping of motor unit activity'. Thomas (1987) stated that in some patients simultaneous activation of agonist and antagonist muscles was also demonstrable, thus raising the possibility of simulation of symptoms. We have seen in our laboratory a reduced recruitment pattern during maximal volition in about half of the patients and in about a quarter of these we have observed the phenomenon of grouping of the motor unit potentials. However, individual motor units within these groups or in patients with reduced recruitment patterns all have parameters entirely within the normal limits. Such observations are not necessarily organic in nature (McEvedey and Beard, 1970; Jamal and Hansen, 1985; Thomas, 1987). In the patients who have recovered, full and normal interference patterns are restored. We have performed some of the studies reported by Thomas (1987) on several patients with PVFS. We have not found evidence of simultaneous activation of agonist and antagonist muscles except very occasionally, namely in one or two patients. The vast majority of patients are capable of maintaining a steady firing rate in the individual motor unit during the examination with single fibre electromyography. We do not therefore agree that there is evidence of simulation of symptoms in the vast majority of patients with PVFS.

In general the concentric needle EMG and nerve conduction studies show some controversial results which are not necessarily organic. The conventional needle EMG provides a good overall picture of the structure and function of individual motor units and the concerted action of these units at a given level of effort. It does not, however, discriminate between potentials from different muscle fibres within the motor unit, all of which fire almost synchronously. It is possible that these conventional studies might not be of adequate sensitivity and might therefore miss dysfunction of a relatively low grade in the motor unit or in the individual muscle fibres. A variety of methods are available to study the individual muscle fibre physiology and among these the technique of single fibre electromyography has proved to be the most valuable, not only to study the pathophysiology of the motor unit at individual muscle fibre level, but also to provide accurate and sensitive quantification of the function of the motor unit in general (Jamal, 1989).

SINGLE FIBRE ELECTROMYOGRAPHY

The technique of single fibre electromyography (SF-EMG) is designed to investigate the motor unit and its components in a much more sensitive way than the conventional neurophysiological methods. This technique has also proved to be useful for the detection of abnormalities and for the characterisation of the functional status of the motor unit as well as for assessing the degree of stability of the neuromuscular junction (Jamal, 1989). Several parameters of function can be measured in SF-EMG. These are outlined below.

Jitter

In measuring this parameter the special SF-EMG electrode is positioned carefully inside the muscle while this is put to minimal voluntary activation. The needle is then carefully manipulated until it comes to a position where it records potentials derived from two single muscle fibres which belong to the same motor unit. By fixing one potential on the screen the time relationship of the two potentials can then be studied accurately. Though apparently time locked, the interpotential interval of the two single fibre potentials shows little variation in consecutive discharges so that the second potential appears on the screen at a variable time after the first one. Jitter is this fluctuation of the interpotential interval. An impulse which activates the two muscle fibres of the same unit is propagated along the axon of the unit. It then splits along the individual intramuscular axonal branches to each of the muscle fibres before crossing the neuromuscular junction and travelling along the muscle fibres to reach the point of detection by the SF-EMG electrode. The variability of the interpotential interval (i.e. jitter) can therefore only arise beyond the point where the initial single discharge along the main axon follows two different pathways to reach the point of recording. The part of the motor unit proximal to the branching of the motor axon is not implicated in the production of jitter. The source of jitter is from one or more of the following components of the peripheral part of the motor unit: the intramuscular axonal branches, the neuromuscular junction or the muscle fibres. In SF-EMG jitter measurement, a pair of single fibre potentials is identified and their jitter is measured from a very large number (100–500) of consecutive discharges. The measurement is repeated for other pairs of single fibres so that jitter values for a number of paired potentials are obtained. Abnormality of jitter studies is then identified in one of two ways: firstly, if 10% or more of the single fibre potential pairs showed abnormal jitter values, and secondly, if the mean overall jitter value for all the pairs measured exceeded a certain limit (Stalberg and Trontelj, 1979). In the studies reported below we have adopted much stricter criteria to identify abnormalities of jitter. Jitter studies were regarded to be abnormal only when 40% or more of the potential pairs showed increased values *and* when overall mean jitter values were abnormally high.

Jitter measurements in patients with PVFS produced abnormal values in not less than 75% of patients even with the application of these very strict criteria. Two controlled studies have been published from our laboratory (Jamal and Hansen, 1985, 1989) and since then many other patients have been examined with similar results (Figure 1).

Values of individual pair jitter may be as high as 400–500 μs in certain cases (i.e. 10 times the upper limit of normal). Following these initial studies several patients have been examined in our laboratory with other psychiatric diagnoses and these produced results within the normal limits.

Impulse blocking

If the delay of the second potential is long enough then it may fail to appear altogether, a phenomenon called blocking (Stalberg and Tronelj, 1979; Jamal, 1989). This blocking is usually due to inadequate neurotransmitter release and is therefore commonly seen in defects of neuromuscular junction transmission. In these disorders, such as myasthenia gravis, blocking occurs when jitter values exceed 80–100 μs (Stalberg and Trontelj, 1979). No impulse blocking was observed in any of the patients examined in our laboratory despite very high jitter values (sometimes reaching five or six times this threshold level). The phenomenon of concomitant (or paired) blocking, where two or more single fibre potentials always block and reappear simultaneously, is neurogenic in origin (Stalberg and Trontelj, 1979). This may happen when recording is made from three or more single muscle fibres. In this case the block must be in an axonal branch which is common to the muscle fibres, the potentials of which block simultaneously (Stalberg and Trontelj, 1979; Jamal, 1989). Concomitant blocking has not been observed in any of the patients that we have examined.

Fibre density

Fibre density (FD) is a measure of the mean number of single muscle fibre potentials of a motor unit detected simultaneously from within the uptake area of the SF-EMG electrode and is highly correlated to the number of single muscle fibres contained in the motor unit (Stalberg and Trontelj, 1979;

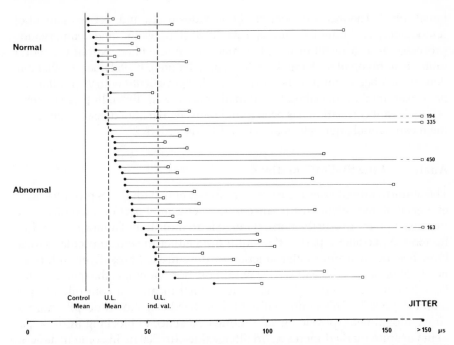

Figure 1 Jitter values of the right extensor digitorum communis muscle for 40 patients with the post-viral fatigue syndrome. Control values are indicated by vertical lines showing (from left to right): mean jitter (23.4 µs), the upper limits of mean overall jitter (34 µs) and the upper limit of jitter for a single pair (55 µs). Each patient is represented by a horizontal line. The solid dot (●) at the left end of the line represents the mean overall jitter excluding the pair with the highest jitter. The squares (□) at the right end of the line represent the pair with the highest jitter. The second highest values for two patients are represented by triangles (▲) indicating that they have abnormal jitter because of two pairs with values greater than 55 µs. Reproduced with permission from the publisher: Jamal and Hansen (1985) *Journal of Neurology, Neurosurgery and Psychiatry*, **48**, 691–694

Jamal, 1989). To measure the FD, the SF-EMG electrode is randomly inserted in the muscle and the needle is then manipulated so that a single fibre potential is optimally recorded and maximised. The number of simultaneously occurring time-locked single fibre potentials for a time interval of at least 5 ms is then counted. At least 20 such estimates are made from different recording sites. The average of these is then taken as the FD (Stalberg and Trontelj, 1979; Jamal, 1989). In 60% of the recording sites in a normal muscle the needle records only one potential, in 35% of the sites it records two potentials, and three or more time-locked potentials are recorded very occasionally. The normal mean FD of 20 insertions thus ranges from 1.3 to 1.8 in most muscles in normal subjects (Stalberg and Trontelj, 1979;

Jamal, 1989). The measurement of FD provides useful indirect assessment of remodelling of the motor unit as a result of denervation and reinnervation processes or as a result of rearrangement of muscle fibres within the motor unit due to myopathic changes (Stalberg and Trontelj, 1979; Jamal, 1989). Fibre density has been found to be normal in all the patients with PVFS that we have examined in this laboratory (Jamal and Hansen, 1989). In these patients no significant correlation has been found between the fibre density values and the mean overall jitter values (Jamal and Hansen, 1989).

Analysis of the SF-EMG findings

The abnormality of jitter measurement in patients with PVFS provides solid evidence of an organic disturbance in the peripheral part of the motor unit. Increased jitter outside the normal range is an indicator of abnormal conduction in the peripheral part of the motor unit, either the intramuscular axonal branches, the neuromuscular junction or the muscle fibres. Even in the minority of patients who had values within the normal range, the mean overall jitter has always been higher than the normal mean of a controlled population (Figure 1). This abnormality of jitter has been shown despite normal conventional neurophysiological findings. Absence of blocking in these patients despite marked increases in jitter values (to 500 μs in some instances) makes the neuromuscular junction an unlikely site of involvement, as blocking is expected to occur frequently with jitter values above 100 μs in cases of neuromuscular junctional defects (Stalberg and Trontelj, 1979; Jamal, 1989). Similarly, absence of concomitant blocking in any of the patients that we have tested would make the intramuscular axonal branches an unlikely candidate for the increased jitter values in PVFS patients. Increased fibre density occurs in neurogenic and myopathic disorders in which there is a rearrangement and/or an increase in the number of muscle fibres contained in the motor unit. Fibre density is a very sensitive index of muscle fibre splitting, of general muscular atrophy with shrinkage of muscle fibres and of collateral sprouting (Stalberg et al., 1975; Stalberg and Trontelj, 1979; Jamal, 1989). Normal FD in patients with the PVFS therefore suggests lack of collateral sprouting or muscle fibre splitting in this syndrome. This is also in accordance with the absence of blocking or concomitant blocking on SF-EMG studies. Therefore abnormalities of muscle fibre propagation are the most likely cause of increased jitter in these patients. It is not known yet whether or not there is additional impairment of excitation/contraction coupling in the T-tubules or sarcoplasmic reticulum in patients with PVFS. Failure of impulse propagation within the T-tubules would not necessarily be detected when recording is made from the muscle fibre surface.

It has been speculated that the jitter abnormality without impulse blocking is not related to the pathogenesis of fatigue (Lloyd et al., 1988;

Stokes *et al.*, 1988). This claim is discounted by the fact that a substantial proportion of patients with myasthenia gravis and undisputed fatigue show increased jitter without impulse blocking as the only neurophysiological abnormality (Stalberg and Trontelj, 1979). Since jitter findings in PVFS are prominent at the beginning of symptoms and during the acute phase of a viral illness (Jamal and Hansen, 1985), is it very unlikely that they are due to disuse as suggested by some authors (Stokes *et al.*, 1988). Studies of strength and endurance have generally failed to show significant abnormality in patients with effort or chronic fatigue syndromes many of whom had no positive virological or immunological changes (Lloyd *et al.*, 1988; Stokes *et al.*, 1988). In some patients added 'force' was demonstrated through the application of superimposed electrical stimulation during fatiguing voluntary contraction (Stokes *et al.*, 1988). This was interpreted by the authors to suggest incomplete muscular activation and to indicate a non-muscular component to the fatigue. These techniques, like the other neurophysiological techniques, test large numbers of motor units or the whole muscle and may therefore be unable to detect subtle physiological abnormality at individual muscle fibre level. Thus, the demonstration of added amplitude to externally applied electrical stimuli does not necessarily rule out subtle physiological deficit which may operate during the patient's attempt of volition while undetected by externally applied electrical stimulation.

The muscle fibre abnormality in the SF-EMG studies is supported by several non-neurophysiological findings. Muscle biopsies in patients with PVFS show a variety of nonspecific changes, including subtle and patchy muscle fibre necrosis, scattered atrophic fibres and abnormality of type II muscle fibres. Electron microscopic studies show intramuscular tubular aggregates and mitochondrial abnormalities in some patients. Examination of patients by the ^{31}P-NMR technique shows evidence of an abnormal early intramuscular acidosis following exercise which is out of proportion to the associated changes in high-energy phosphates (Arnold *et al.*, 1984, 1985; Grosse *et al.* 1988; Miller *et al.*, 1988). This is assumed to represent excessive lactic acid formation arising from a disorder of regulation of muscle metabolism involving the relative contributions of aerobic versus anaerobic processes. It is believed that this abnormality is related to ultrastructural damage of the muscle fibre and may be reponsible for the muscle fibre membrane disorder. These changes are probably related to the symptom of fatigue. Miller and Milner-Brown (1984) found evidence of impairment of impulse propagation along the muscle fibre membrane following fatigue in healthy individuals. The authors found that the magnitude of this impairment depended on the degree and duration of fatigue as well as on the intrinsic properties of individual muscles. It remains to be seen whether the muscle propagation abnormalities reported in patients with PVFS would become even more prominent following much more excessive exercise than that seen in normal individuals. Mukherjee *et al.* (1987) recently reported evidence of abnormality and dysfunction of the red blood cell membrane in patients with PVFS. Wakefield and Lloyd (1987) suggested that this and the neurophysiological findings may reflect a generalised membrane dysfunction, the brunt of which probably falls on the muscle fibre membrane, and that this may lead to excessive fatiguability which is the hallmark of the disease. An interesting recent finding has been the demonstration of abnormal local lymphokine response in patients with PVFS (Strauss *et al.*, 1985; Ho-Yen *et al.*, 1988). Increased local interferon or lymphokine reactions may be elicited from the local cell-mediated immune response to intracellular pathogens in muscles and other tissues and this is not necessarily reflected in circulating lymphokine levels (Ho-Yen *et al.*, 1988). Abnormal local lymphokine response has been found to be present in acute viral infection and patients with these acute infections show the same pattern of neurophysiological findings as in PVFS even when they do not have associated myalgias (Friman *et al.*, 1977). This abnormal local lymphokine reaction may arise from a persistent viral infection which has been demonstrated to occur in patients with PVFS (Youself *et al.*, 1988). Archard *et al.* (1988) have demonstrated the presence of abnormal enterovirus-specific RNA in skeletal muscles of a substantial number of patients with PVFS up to 20 years after onset of the disease, thus seriously raising the possibility of an aetiological role of persistent viral infection in this syndrome. It will be interesting to find out whether or not such local abnormal lymphokine response is related to the neurophysiological and metabolic abnormalities in the skeletal muscle. Abnormalities of muscle cell membrane potentials have been found to be induced by lymphokines such as tumour necrosis factor (Tracey *et al.*, 1986) and these lymphokines are also known to induce altered cellular energy metabolism both *in vitro* and *in vivo* (Morag *et al.*, 1982).

SIGNIFICANCE OF THE NEUROPHYSIOLOGICAL FINDINGS

In a critical reappraisal of the syndrome and various studies performed on PVFS, David *et al.* (1988) stated that the SF-EMG neurophysiological findings are 'the most persuasive evidence for muscle dysfunction in this syndrome to date'. Although the neurophysiological findings reported here do not form characteristic patterns to provide specific diagnosis of the syndrome, they supply solid evidence for the organic nature of the syndrome and provide valuable information concerning transmission of impulses in the peripheral part of the motor unit. The changes tend to illustrate the functional disturbances and the possible associated ultrastructural morphological changes in the muscle fibres. These neurophysiological studies should play an important role in any case definition criteria for PVFS.

The EEG changes in PVFS suggest a discrete and patchy disturbance of cerebral function with variable intensity and distribution. These changes, though definite, are nonspecific in nature and are of little help in the diagnosis of the syndrome.

REFERENCES

Archard, L. C., Bowles, N. E., Behan, P. O. *et al.* (1988) Post viral fatigue syndrome: Persistence of enterovirus RNA in muscle and elevated creatine kinase. *Journal of the Royal Society of Medicine*, **81**, 326–329.

Arnold, D. L., Radda, G. K., Bore, P. J. *et al.* (1984) Excessive intracellular acidosis of skeletal muscles on exercise in a patient with a post viral exhaustion/fatigue syndrome. *Lancet*, **1**, 1367–1369.

Arnold, D. L., Bore, P. J., Radda, G. K. *et al.* (1985) Enhanced intramuscular acidosis during exercise by patients with post viral exhaustion/fatigue syndrome. *Neurology (Cleveland)*, **35** (Suppl. 1), 165.

Astrom, E., Friman, G. and Pilstrom, L. (1976) Effects of viral and mycoplasma infections on ultrastructure and enzyme activities in human skeletal muscle. *Acta Pathologetica Microbiolica Scandinavica*, **84**, 113.

Chou, S. M. and Gutman, L. (1970) Picornavirus—like crystals in subacute polymyositis. *Neurology (New York)*, **20**, 205–213.

David, A. S., Wessley, S. and Pelosi, A. (1988) Post viral fatigue syndrome: time for a new approach. *British Medical Journal*, **296**, 696–699.

Friman, G. (1976) Serum creatine phosphokinase in epidemic influenza. *Scandinavian Journal of Infectious Diseases*, **8**, 13–20.

Friman, G. (1977) Effect of acute infectious disease on isometric muscle strength. *Scandinavian Journal of Clinical and Laboratory Investigation*, **37**, 303–308.

Friman, F., Schiller, H. and Schwartz, M. (1977) Disturbed neuromuscular transmission in viral infections. *Scandinavian Journal of Infectious Diseases*, **9**, 99–103.

Fukuyama, Y., Ando, T. and Yokota, J. (1977) Acute fulminant myoglobinuric polymyositis with picornavirus-like crystals. *Journal of Neurology, Neurosurgery and Psychiatry*, **40**, 775–781.

Gross, B., Glasberg, M., Kensora, T., Smith, M. B. and Welch, K. M. A. (1988) ^{31}P NMR spectroscopy and histochemical study of benign myalgic and fatigue syndrome. *Neurology (New York)*, **38** (Suppl. 1), 410.

Ho-Yen, D. O., Carrington, D. and Armstrong, A. A. (1988) Myalgic encephalomyelitis and alpha-interferon. *Lancet*, **i**, 125.

Jamal, G. A. (1989) Update: Singe fibre electromyography. Principles and applications. *Journal of Electrophysiological Technology*, **52**, 99–106.

Jamal, G. A. and Hansen, S. (1985) Electrophysiological studies in the post viral fatigue syndrome. *Journal of Neurology, Neorosurgery and Psychiatry*, **48**, 691–694.

Jamal, G. A. and Hansen, S. (1988) Post viral fatigue syndrome. *British Medical Journal*, **296**, 1067–1068.

Jamal, G. A. and Hansen, S. (1989) Post viral fatigue syndrome: Evidence for underlying organic disturbance in the muscle fibre. *European Neurology*, **29**, 273–276.

Jamal, G. A., Hansen, S., Weir, A. I. and Ballantyne, J. P. (1985) An improved automated method for the measurement of thermal thresholds. 1. Normal subjects. *Journal of Neurology, Neurosurgery and Psychiatry*, **48**, 354–360.

Jamal, G. A., Hansen, S., Weir, A. I. and Ballantyne, J. P. (1987) The neurophysiologic investigation of small fibre neuropathies. *Muscle and Nerve*, **10**, 537–545.

Lloyd, A. R., Hales, J. P. and Gandevia, S. C. (1988) Muscle strength, endurance and recovery in the post-infection fatigue syndrome. *Journal of Neurology, Neurosurgery and Psychiatry*, **51**, 1316–1322.

McEvedy, C. P. and Beard, P. W. (1970) Royal Free epidemic of 1956: a reconsideration. *British Medical Journal*, **1**, 7–11.

Mejlszenkier, J. D., Safran, A. P., Healy, J. J., Embree, L. and Oullette, E. M. (1973) The myotosis of influenza. *Archives of Neurology*, **29**, 441–443.

Middleton, P. H., Alexander, R. M. and Szymanski, M. T. (1970) Severe myotosis during recovery from influenza. *Lancet*, **2**, 533–535.

Miller, R. G. and Milner-Brown, S. (1984) Impulse propagation along the muscle membrane is impaired during muscle fatigue. *Neurology (Cleveland)*, **34**, (Suppl. 1), 131.

Miller, R. G., Boska, M. D., Moussari, R. S., Carson, P. J. and Weiner, M. W. (1988) ^{31}P nuclear magnetic resonance studies of high energy phosphates and pH in human muscle fatigue. *Journal of Clinical Investigation*, **81**, 1190–1196.

Morag, A., Tobi, M., Ravid, Z., Revel, M. and Schattner, A. (1982) Increased (2'–5') Oligo-A-synthetase activity in patients with prolonged illness associated with serological evidence of persistent Epstein–Barr virus infection. *Lancet*, **1**, 744.

Mukherjee, T. M., Smith, K. and Marcos, K. (1987) Abnormal red blood cell morphology in myalgic encephalomyelitis. *Lancet*, **2**, 328–329.

Pampiglione, G., Harris, R. and Kennedy, J. (1978) Electroencephalographic investigations in myalgic encephalomyelitis. *Postgraduate Medical Journal*, **54**, 752–754.

Richardson, A. T. (1956) Some aspects of the Royal Free Hospital epidemic. *Annals of Physical Medicine*, **3**, 81–89.

Schwartz, M., Swash, M. and Gross, M. (1978) Benign postinfection polymyositis. *British Medical Journal*, **2**, 1256–1257.

Stalberg, E. and Trontelj, J. V. (1979) *Single Fibre Electromyography*. Mirvalle Press, Old Woking.

Stalberg, E., Schwartz, M. S. and Trontelj, J. V. (1975) Single fibre electromyography in various processes affecting the anterior horn cell. *Journal of Neurological Sciences*, **24**, 403–415.

Stokes, M. J., Cooper, R. G. and Edwards, R. H. T. (1988) Normal muscle strength and fatigability in patients with effort syndromes. *British Medical Journal*, **297**, 1014–1017.

Strauss, S., Josato, C., Armstrong, C. *et al.* (1985) Persisting illness and fatigue in adults with evidence of Epstein Barr virus infection. *Annals of Internal Medicine*, **102**, 7–16.

Thomas, P. K. (1987) Post viral fatigue syndrome. *Lancet*, **1**, 218–219.

Tracey, K., Lawry, S., Beutler, B. *et al.* (1986) Cahchetin tumor necrosis factor mediates changes of skeletal muscle membrane potential. *Journal of Experimental Medicine*, **164**, 1368–1373.

Wakefield, D. and Lloyd, A. (1987) Pathophysiology of myalgic encephalomyelitis. *Lancet*, **1**, 125.

Yousef, G. E., Bell, E. J., Mann, G. F. *et al.* (1988) Chronic enterovirus infection in patients with post viral fatigue syndrome. *Lancet*, **1**, 146–150.

10

Cognitive Changes in Myalgic Encephalomyelitis

Andrew Smith

University of Wales College of Cardiff, Cardiff, UK

INTRODUCTION

The post-viral fatigue syndrome or myalgic encephalomyelitis (ME) has been widely studied during recent years and this has led to a clearer definition of the features of the illness. The distinguishing characteristic is muscle fatigue, which is often made worse by exercise. However, other symptoms, including behavioural abnormalities, are almost invariably present and these have not been examined in detail. The symptoms usually develop after an apparent viral infection and the most consistent psychological problem is mild depression, often accompanied by anxiety, intense introspection and hypochondriasis. These features have led to considerable debate about whether this illness is due to a viral infection, or whether it is really a psychiatric disorder. This issue will not be discussed in detail here although it must be pointed out that there is now clear evidence (described later in the chapter) that *some* ME patients do have chronic viral infections, muscle damage and immunological abnormalities.

ME patients often report problems of attention, memory and language and the main aim of the present chapter is to review some recent research on these features of the illness. Many people with ME report that they cannot concentrate as well as they did, are not as incisive in their thought, have a decreased ability to learn and have a poor memory. They also report increased visual sensitivity, finding fluorescent lighting and complex patterns very disturbing. Another feature of the illness is the inability to remember names. The patients also report disturbed or irregular sleep, and some have an inordinate desire to sleep which may be indistinguishable from narcolepsy.

Post-viral Fatigue Syndrome. Edited by R. Jenkins and J. Mowbray
© 1991 John Wiley & Sons Ltd

It should be stressed that all of the above behavioural problems are based on the subjective reports of the patients, and that these have not been recorded in a systematic way. This means that it is essential to collect data on these topics using standardised measuring instruments, and also to confirm subjective impressions with objective measurement of mental functions. The majority of this chapter is concerned with preliminary studies which have adopted these approaches. However, before these are described some previous research on the effects of viral infections and immune responses on behaviour is described. This is preceded by a brief review of the evidence for muscle damage in ME, viral infections and ME, and ME and immunological disorders.

Myalgic encephalomyelitis and muscle disorders

Jamal and Hansen (1985) have found that single fibre electromyography confirms muscle damage (prolonged jitters) in 75% of ME patients tested. Arnold *et al.* (1984), using ^{31}P nuclear magnetic resonance, have also demonstrated that ME patients have a derangement in muscle energy metabolism with abnormally early intracellular acidosis, out of proportion to the associated changes in high-energy phosphates. In other words, we now have strong evidence that some ME patients do have muscle damage, which can be detected by objective tests.

Evidence for chronic viral infections in ME

Research by Behan and his colleagues (e.g. Behan *et al.*, 1985; Fegan *et al.*, 1983) has established that some ME patients have significantly increased anti-Coxsackie antibodies. Two recent reports also implicate Coxsackie and other enteroviruses in the illness. First, Bowles *et al.* (1987) have used viral nucleic acid probes to identify Coxsackie viral genome in skeletal muscle biopsies of a group of these patients. Second, Yousef *et al.* (1988) have shown that some patients not only excrete enteroviruses long after disease onset but also have identifiable virus in circulating immune complexes, together with raised specific IgM antibody titres.

Other studies (e.g. Isaacs, 1948) suggest that the Epstein–Barr virus (EBV) can be the pathogenic agent in ME. Behan and Behan (1985) have also reviewed studies showing that influenza A and B, herpes zoster, rubella and hepatitis B viruses can all produce acute myositis. In other words, there is a great deal of evidence suggesting that chronic viral infections may be involved in ME.

Immunological disorders and ME

If ME is due to a chronic viral infection one would expect to find immunological abnormalities; this is certainly the case in other persistent viral infections (see Southern and Oldstone, 1986). Behan *et al.* (1985) have already reported immunological abnormalities in 50 ME patients. Immunoglobulin concentrations (IgG, IgA and IgM) were normal but three different immune complex assays revealed positive results in 58 of the 100 samples taken. Detectable abnormalities in the suppressor/cytotoxic lymphocyte subsets were also observed, with the suppressor/cytotoxic percentage being significantly decreased in patients with acute ME. In patients who had been ill for a longer period it was the helper/inducer lymphocytes that were decreased.

Recent research has examined whether ME patients have abnormalities in the production and release of lymphokines and cytokines, such as interleukin-1 and -2 and the interferons. Direct measurement of the interferon levels of ME patients shows that they often have higher levels than do matched controls (Ho-Yen *et al.*, 1988). It has also been shown that prolonged administration of interferon leads to excessive fatigue and depression (MacDonald *et al.*, 1987) which suggests that an abnormal interferon system (induced by chronic infection) could be responsible for some of the symptoms of ME. Interferons also induce changes in cognitive function and these are described in a following section.

Recent research (Behan, personal communication) has shown that certain ME patients often have extremely high levels of interleukin-1-beta. This cytokine is known to trigger fever (via its effect on the hypothalamus), act on nerve and muscle cells, decrease the white cell count, cause sleepiness and appetite loss, act on the liver to upset protein production and affect sugar metabolism. Again, it appears likely that this cytokine could be responsible for many of the symptoms of ME.

To summarise the above sections, we can now say that there is objective evidence that certainly some ME patients have a chronic viral infection, muscle damage and immune system abnormalities. We must now consider some recent research on viral infections and behaviour to see whether there is evidence that infection influences CNS function and performance efficiency.

Effects of respiratory virus infections on performance

One of the problems of studying acute viral infections is that they are hard to predict and it is often difficult to determine which virus produced the illness. In order to overcome these problems recent research has examined the effects of experimentally induced colds and influenza on performance. These studies, carried out at the MRC Common Cold Unit, have clearly demonstrated under controlled conditions that respiratory viruses (colds and influenza) have central nervous system (CNS) effects (even though the viruses do not get into the CNS).

Early results (e.g. Smith *et al.*, 1987a,b, 1988b) demonstrated that colds and influenza have selective effects on performance, with influenza impairing detection of targets occurring at uncertain times or in unknown locations, and colds impairing hand–eye co-ordination (see Smith (1989) for a review). We have also shown that subclinical infections influence performance, and that the performance impairments remain after the clinical symptoms have gone (Smith et al., 1989). Indeed, there is considerable evidence to show that even acute infections can produce post-viral effects. Wood (1989) has reviewed the post-influenza syndrome and reached the following conclusions:

(a) Influenza is capable of producing muscle changes which resemble benign polymyositis (Schwartz et al., 1978).
(b) Psychiatric problems often increase after an influenza epidemic.
(c) Grant (1972) studied a group of skilled professionals who had returned to work following an attack of influenza. All of these made frequent technical errors without realising, and believed that they were functioning properly. This shows that there are 'after-effects' of influenza and these provide a clear demonstration of acute post-viral effects.

The mechanism underlying the CNS effects of influenza is known and is described in the following section.

Effects of alpha-interferon on performance

When a person develops influenza, alpha-interferon is endogenously produced. Smith et al. (1988a) injected normal volunteers with alpha-interferon and those receiving 1.5 Mu of interferon developed symptoms which closely resembled influenza. They also showed identical changes in performance to those shown by people with influenza, with some functions being impaired (e.g. slower reaction times to unexpected stimuli) but others (e.g. hand–eye co-ordination) remaining intact. Furthermore, after-effects of interferon challenge were observed even though the symptoms had disappeared. The fact that interferons (and other lymphokines and cytokines) have CNS effects suggests that the behavioural problems of ME may reflect abnormal lymphokine/cytokine systems.

To summarise the above sections, one may conclude that viral infections influence CNS functions and behaviour. The exact pattern appears to depend on the type of virus and it is essential, therefore, to determine which functions are impaired in ME patients with known viral infections. In the case of influenza, the behavioural effects can plausibly be explained by interferon production. This may also be the mediator responsible for the impairments reported in ME, and future research must consider the relationship between the state of the interferon systems and the CNS effects associated with ME.

The next part of the chapter considers recent research on the behavioural impairments associated with ME.

AN OVERVIEW OF THE RESEARCH PROGRAMME

Our research on behavioural problems associated with ME has three main aims:

(a) To provide a detailed profile of the behavioural abnormalities associated with ME.
(b) To examine the relationship between the behavioural problems, past medical history and current symptomatology.
(c) To determine whether abnormal lymphokine/cytokine systems are responsible for the impairments.

These topics are being studied (or are going to be studied) using the following methodologies:

(a) A questionnaire study of over 200 ME patients to assess the subjective reports of problems of memory, attention and motor function.
(b) Subjects from the above sample have carried out objective tests of memory, attention and perceptual-motor skills.
(c) It is of interest to compare the ME group with matched 'normal' controls. However, ME patients often report psychiatric symptoms and these may be responsible for certain impairments. It is essential, therefore, to compare the ME group with depressed patients. Other problems may be a direct function of the muscle damage and it is important to compare the ME patients with a group who have muscle damage produced in some other way (e.g. patients with polymyositis).
(d) In collaboration with Professor Behan, Glasgow University, we are currently examining whether these patients have abnormalities in the production and release of lymphokines and cytokines. It will be of major interest to examine the relationship between any performance abnormalities and the functioning of the interferon/interleukin systems.
(e) Many ME patients show marked changes in the severity of the illness. It is important, therefore, to carry out longitudinal studies to determine which impairments reflect the current state of the patient and which are largely independent of the severity of the symptoms.

Subjects

The majority of the subjects taking part in the research are members of the Mid-Sussex and Hailsham groups of the ME Association. Other people with ME have heard about the research and contacted us directly with a view to taking part. The studies of the relationship between lymphokine/cytokine function and performance are being carried out in Glasgow in collaboration with Professor Behan.

The questionnaire study

In order to assess the past medical history of the ME patients and to obtain a detailed description of current symptoms we have developed our own questionnaire. This is described in detail below. In addition to this questionnaire we have asked the ME patients to fill in a modified version of the Middlesex Hospital Questionnaire (Crown and Crisp, 1966), which measures anxiety, depression, somatic symptoms and obsessional symptoms. The patients also fill in the Cognitive Failures Questionnaire (Broadbent *et al.*, 1982) which measures failures of attention, memory and action. Other questionnaires measure perceived stress (Cohen *et al.*, 1983) and physical symptoms (Cohen and Hobermann, 1983).

The post-viral fatigue questionnaire provides the following information: (a) demographics, (b) history of the illness, (c) information on diagnoses, tests for the presence of viruses, tests for muscle damage, (d) current state of health, and (e) factors which change the person's condition.

Results of the survey

The survey was carried out by post and over 90% of the questionnaires were returned ($N = 232$). Thirty-six per cent of the sample had received a positive result regarding the presence of a viral infection, and a much smaller number had been shown to have abnormal muscle metabolism.

The results which are of major interest here are the cognitive failure scores. These, and the anxiety, depression and somatic symptoms scores, are shown for the ME patients and 100 controls in Table 1.

The above data show that ME patients report more cognitive failures than the control subjects, and that this was observed both for those who had been given a positive viral identification and for those who had either received a negative result or had not had a test. Certain types of problem were more frequently reported by the ME patients than others and these are shown in Table 2.

These results confirm previous reports which have suggested that ME patients have concentration problems, memory impairments, and suffer from anomia.

Table 1 also shows that the ME patients have higher levels of anxiety, somatic symptoms and depression than the control group. One of the problems of using questionnaires to assess impairments of memory, attention and action is that subjects who report a large number of these also have high neuroticism scores. The subjects in the present sample were subdivided into those with low and high neuroticism scores and it was found that high levels of psychopathology were associated with more problems of memory and attention. This is shown in Table 3.

One may summarise this section by concluding that the questionnaire survey revealed that ME patients had higher levels of cognitive failure than

Table 1 Mean scores from the Middlesex Hospital Questionnaire and Cognitive Failures Questionnaire for controls, patients who had a positive virus identification (ME+) and those who had a negative result or no assay (ME–)

	Anxiety	Somatic symptoms	Depression	Cognitive failures
Controls	4.3	3.3	3.3	42.2
N = 100	(2.9)	(2.3)	(2.5)	(11.7)
ME+	6.4	6.3	7.7	54.9
N = 83	(2.8)	(2.9)	(2.6)	(15.7)
ME–	7.0	7.1	8.1	52.7
N = 149	(3.4)	(3.4)	(2.8)	(19.3)

High scores = high levels of anxiety, etc. Standard deviations in parentheses

Table 2 Types of cognitive failure reported by ME group

Do you read something and find you haven't been thinking about it and must read it again?

Do you find you forget why you went from one part of the house to the other?

Do you fail to notice signposts on the road?

Do you find you forget whether you've turned off a light or a fire or locked the door?

Do you fail to listen to people's names when you are meeting them?

Do you fail to hear people speaking to you when you are doing something else?

Do you find yourself suddenly wondering whether you've used a word correctly?

Do you have trouble making up your mind?

Do you forget where you put something like a newspaper or a book?

Do you daydream when you ought to be listening to something?

Do you find you forget people's names?

Do you start doing one thing at home and get distracted into doing something else (unintentionally)?

Do you find you can't quite remember something although it's 'on the tip of your tongue'?

Table 3 Cognitive failures scores for ME patients with high and low neuroticism scores

	High neuroticism	Low neuroticism
ME+	62.6	47.7
	(14.0)	(16.7)
ME–	61.0	46.1
	(18.4)	(17.4)

ME+, patients who have had a positive result from a test for the presence of a virus; ME–, a negative result, or no test. Standard deviations in parentheses a control group, but that this largely reflected the higher levels of psychopathology.

The next stage in the research has used objective measures of performance to determine the extent of the reported deficits.

Assessment of performance impairments in ME patients

On the basis of the questionnaire results it was possible to select 18 ME patients who had received a positive result on the VP1 test or who had been shown to have high levels of EBV antibodies. These patients also had many of the clinical symptoms associated with ME.

The patients carried out a series of performance tests designed to measure visual sensitivity, motor function, and aspects of memory and attention. They were compared with a group of nine control subjects.

Psychomotor function

Many of the patients had problems walking or doing other types of physical activity. Two computerised tests were used to examine their speed of reaction. The first measured simple reaction time and the subject had to press a key on a computer keyboard when a spot appeared in the box in the centre of the computer monitor. The second task, the five choice serial reaction time task, involved self-paced serial responding. Five boxes were shown on the computer monitor and a spot appeared in one of the boxes. The subject had to press a key which corresponded to the box and the spot then appeared in another box, the subject pressed the key which corresponded to that box, and so on. This task lasted for four minutes. The data from these two tasks are shown in Table 4.

It can be seen that the ME group were considerably slower than the controls on both tasks. This result is not too surprising in that it probably reflects a direct effect of the muscle damage.

Table 4 Performance on psychomotor tasks

	Controls	ME Group
Simple reaction time	253 ms (40)	409 ms (112)
Five choice serial response task	315 responses in four minutes (59)	233 responses in four minutes (50)

Standard deviations in parentheses.

Visual sensitivity

Many ME patients report that they find certain patterns very disturbing. This was examined using the pattern shown in Figure 1, which is known to induce illusions of shape, colour and movement, and also discomfort.

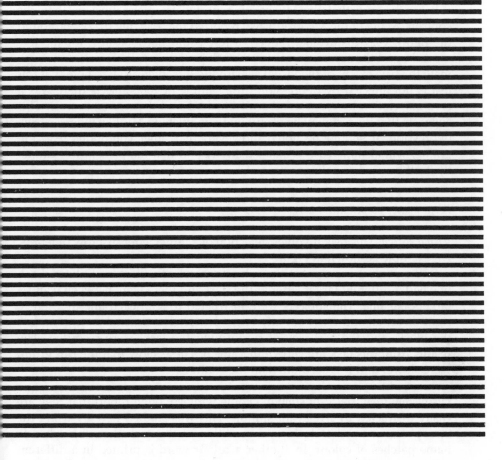

Figure 1 The pattern with spatial characteristics that produce illusions and visual discomfort

The subjects were instructed to look at the centre of the figure from a distance of 40 cm for five seconds. They then reported on a checklist which illusions (if any) occurred (red, orange, green, blue, yellow, blurring, bending of stripes, shimmering, flickering, shadowy shapes, or any other). The mean numbers of illusions reported by the ME group and the controls are shown in Table 5.

It can be seen that the ME group reported far more illusions than the controls. Many of the ME group also reported that they felt dizzy and found the figure very disturbing. Indeed, a few could not look at it for the five seconds, and the scores shown for the ME group may, therefore, underestimate the true extent of the visual sensitivity. It is interesting to note that this test is not affected by depression (in a sample of 100 subjects there was a zero correlation between number of illusions and depression scores). This suggests that the test may be useful in distinguishing ME-like illnesses from depression. It should be noted, however, that other conditions (e.g. migraine) will also increase visual sensitivity and that the present test cannot by itself be used as a diagnostic test.

Performance on attention tasks

Visual search. This task involves detection of a target letter in a row of letters. An example is shown in Figure 2.

In the present experiment the subjects searched a block of 12 lines. Each line had a different target letter at the start and there were between 0 and 3 targets per line. The subjects were instructed to scan each line in a left to right direction and cross out any target letters. The time taken to complete the block, and the accuracy of performing the task, were recorded. The results from this task are shown in Table 6. These show that the ME group were slower and less accurate than the controls.

Distraction from irrelevant stimuli. People with ME often report that they are easily distracted by irrelevant stimuli. This was studied here by using the Stroop colour-word task. In one condition of this task the subject has to name patches of colour. In another a colour word is printed in a different colour (e.g. RED printed in green ink) and the person has to name the colour

Table 5 Number of visual illusions reported

Controls	ME Group
1.3	3.38
(0.6)	(1.2)

Standard deviations in parentheses.

```
O  LJNETHSXUWMBGPRKZDYVREWSGBLVDYZHTUKPXJNOVSUZBDOPWYKLNGHEXMTJ

P  MHFYLDSXWIPEJKCONQZTKWHLICDFMTZESNUPYOJQILUEDSCMHQJPYFKONXWZ

T  DFISZAOJNBYHCXGRTKEVOFXATENGDCBZSKLIHYRVKLXEGNHDZIVJSRYOAFBC

X  OBKLFQMZADUGJVNTHISYVNGQZHUBSFIJKAOLMTYDOHNVBIMTLXYADGKSFUQZ

H  DWQJPLHYXSOKTVCZUIFNMLTDKYVUJWCZISNPOFXQDUYLNVQHFSOPKJCZMIWT

Z  TWIMFHBKOGSCXZYAJNPEBYOKTGFUJEPNAIMSXCWHNOUGTMPXCYFEAIKJHWSB

Y  NMXQCHBOZUIPDVJAELFRXDUCJBZFEPLINVHORAQMDXFHPZUCAQBRVOJIEYMN

F  GAQOVUSIMTFDCWBJYNRXUADTIWZCNBJOVYRFQSGXOCWFBNSTUQMGJIDAYXVZ

N  YPGMQRSWZFKLVHIOUBEDWQMYKDUPELRVIOHBSGZFYVNUSPHIGEZFBKWMORDL

U  UTVPNDSHQJWEBAGFMYKCWPQGNEBFJTMVCYDXAKSHCGMUJBTVWKNSPAYQEHXF

N  DIKCGPRLQEYSBTUWOFNJPECBDKFOLXRWJQGYSITUQGWDJUPKIBSTXEFOLCYN

C  XJZSNMKHORETPGDIBWUVRKGOJVSTUIPWNMDHCEZBVDKMGPCZJTXHOINWERBS
```

Figure 2   The visual search task. The subject has to scan each line and cross out any occurrences of the target letter shown to the left of the line

Table 6   Performance on the different types of attention task

	Controls	ME Group
Visual search		
Speed	119.3 s	172.8 s
	(36)	(50)
Accuracy	98% correct	86% correct
	(2)	(12)
Stroop interference (the difference between naming the colour of the irrelevant colour names and naming patches of colour)	34.0 s (13)	88 s (36)

Standard deviations in parentheses.

and ignore the word. This condition is performed more slowly than the simple colour-naming condition and the extent of the distraction from the irrelevant word was much greater in the ME group. This is shown in Table 6.

Sustained attention and memory for information in a story. Many ME patients report that they have difficulty attending to stories or watching films. In the present experiment subjects were played a short story (about 15 minutes) and then had to answer questions about the story. Some were designed to assess the extent to which the subject followed the theme of the story and others examined memory for detail. The results showed that the ME group had worse recall of both types of information, suggesting that they had general problems in maintaining attention. These results are shown in Table 7.

These results may not only reflect problems of sustained attention but may also be due to retrieval deficits. Memory problems associated with ME were also studied and these are described in the next section.

Memory tasks

The results up to now suggest that the ME patients are impaired on most tasks. However, a slightly different pattern was observed for the memory tasks.

Digit span. In this task the subject has to repeat in serial order a sequence of digits. If the subject is successful the length of the sequence is increased by one. The mean digit spans for the controls and ME group are shown in Table 8. The difference between the two groups was not significant.

Table 7 Recall of important information (relating to the theme of a story) and unimportant detail

	Controls		ME Group	
	Important	Unimportant	Important	Unimportant
% correct	71.9	56.3	56.8	23.9
	(16)	(33)	(22)	(24)

Standard deviations in parentheses.

Table 8 Performance on memory tasks

	Controls	ME Group
Digit span	6.3	6.0
	(0.6)	(1.4)
Free recall		
Primacy effect	83.3%	35.4%
	(14)	(18)
Recency effect	50.0%	41.7%
	(25)	(22)
Recognition memory		
Hits[*]	62%	70%
	(18)	(13)
False alarms[†]	10%	32%
	(1)	(3)

[*] Correct recognition of words shown before.
[†] Incorrect response to words not shown before.
Standard deviation in parentheses.

Free recall. In this task the subjects were shown a list of 20 words (each word being presented on the computer screen for two seconds) and then had to write down as many as they could remember in any order they liked. In this task one usually finds that the first few words are recalled well (the 'primacy effect') and so are the last few words (the 'recency effect'). This was observed in the control group and these results are shown in Table 8. The ME group were very poor at recalling the first few items but their recall of items later in the list nearly matched the controls.

Recognition memory. The subjects were shown a list of words and then carried out other performance tasks. Approximately 45 minutes later they were shown another list containing the original words and others which had not been shown before. The results showed that the ME group were better at detecting the words shown before than the controls. However, they only achieved this by making a large number of false alarms (responding 'Yes shown before' to words which had not been shown). These effects are shown in Table 8.

This pattern of results is extremely interesting and resembles results obtained with Korsakoff patients who have mamillary body damage.

Semantic memory tasks. Many aspects of memory do not require recall or recognition of material recently presented but involve recall from general knowledge. This 'semantic memory' was examined using two tasks. In the first subjects were shown sentences which were either true (e.g. 'Canaries have wings') or false (e.g. 'Dogs have wings'). The subjects had to complete as many of these as possible in three minutes. The results showed that the ME group completed fewer items than the controls, and the mean scores are shown in Table 9.

Another problem commonly reported by people with ME is the inability to find the correct word to use. This was examined by giving the subjects a list of category names, each followed by a letter, and the subjects had to produce an example of the category beginning with that letter (e.g. Animal–

Table 9 Performance on semantic memory tasks

	Controls		ME Group	
	D	ND	D	ND
Category instances: (number produced in 1.5 minutes)	22.7 (6.4)	17.7 (7.0)	14.6 (4.9)	10.5 (5.4)
Semantic processing: (number completed in 3 minutes)	125.5 (24)		90.3 (34)	

Standard deviations in parentheses.   D = dominant instances of categories.
ND = non-dominant instances.

D–Dog). Some of the lists were arranged so that good instances of the categories were likely to be produced, whereas others could only be completed by producing more obscure examples. The results from this test are shown in Table 9, and again it can be seen that the ME group produced fewer instances in both versions of the tasks.

Overall conclusions from these studies

The results obtained using objective measures of performance confirmed many of the subjective reports of behavioural problems. There was clear evidence of slower motor performance, visual sensitivity, impairments on attention tasks and various memory deficits. It is unlikely that these reflect a general impairment of intellectual function as the digit span performance of the two groups was very similar. The results also suggest that many of the behavioural impairments differ from those associated with depression. Obviously direct comparisons with depressed patients are now required, as are comparisons with patients with muscle damage produced in other ways. It is also necessary to carry out longitudinal studies to determine whether the effects change during the illness or are largely independent of the clinical condition of the patient. The ME subjects studied in the first experiment had quite severe physical impairments and generally felt that they were at the worse stage of the illness so far. In a subsequent study we have been able to examine patients with less severe disabilities. The results of the controls, severely impaired ME group and less severely impaired group are summarised in Table 10.

Table 10   A comparison of the performance of the controls with those with mild and severe impairments

	Controls	Mild impairment	Severe impairment
Simple reaction time	253 ms (40)	355 ms (70)	409 ms (112)
Five choice (responses in 4 minutes)	315 (59)	262 (61)	233 (50)
Illusions	1.3 (0.6)	3.2 (1.0)	3.4 (1.2)
Free recall			
Primacy	83.3% (14)	47.2% (16)	35.4% (18)
Rest of list	37.5% (25)	27.1% (20)	26.0% (22)
Digit span	6.3 (0.6)	6.4 (0.9)	6.0 (1.4)

Standard deviations in parentheses.

It is interesting to note that the pattern of results is very similar for both those with severe and those with mild impairments (although the extent of the impairments are reduced in the mild group). This suggests that our preliminary findings do have some generality and may be observed in people with differing degrees of symptomatology. It should be noted that the present samples were defined as ME cases on the basis of their symptoms and on a positive VP1 result (or, in a few cases, on the basis of high EBV antibodies). It is now essential to consider the behavioural impairments found in a well-studied group, where details of the extent of the muscle damage, immune system function, and CNS function are known. Such a study is now in progress (in collaboration with Professor Peter Behan) and the results will provide a clearer picture of what underlies the behavioural problems that are clearly such a major feature of ME.

REFERENCES

Arnold, D. L., Radda, G. K., Bore, P. J., Styles, P. and Taylor, D. J. (1984) Excessive intracellular acidosis of skeletal muscle on exercise in a patient with a post-viral exhaustion/fatigue syndrome. *Lancet*, 1367–1369.

Behan, W. M. H. and Behan, P. O. (1985) Immunological features of polymyositis/dermatomyositis. *Springer Seminars in Immunopathology*, **8**, 267.

Behan, P. O., Behan, W. M. H. and Bell, E. J. (1985) The postviral fatigue syndrome—an analysis of the findings in 50 cases. *Journal of Infection*, **10**, 211–222.

Bowles, N. E., Archard, L. C., Behan, W. M. H., Doyle, D., Bell, E. J. and Behan, P. O. (1987) Detection of Coxsackie B virus-specific RNA in skeletal muscle biopsies of patients with a postviral fatigue syndrome. *Annals of Neurology*, **22**, 126.

Broadbent, D. E., Cooper, P. J., FitzGerald, P. F. and Parkes, K. R. (1982) The Cognitive Failures Questionnaire (CFQ) and its correlates. *British Journal of Clinical Psychology*, **21**, 1–6.

Cohen, S. and Hoberman, H. (1983) Positive events and social supports as buffers of life change stress. *Journal of Applied Social Psychology*, **13**, 99–125.

Cohen, S., Kamarck, T. and Mermelstein, R. (1983) A global measure of perceived stress. *Journal of Health and Social Behaviour*, **24**, 385–396.

Crown, S. and Crisp, A. H. (1966) A short clinical diagnostic self-rating scale for psychoneurotic patients. *British Journal of Psychiatry*, **112**, 917–923.

Fegan, K. G., Behan, P. O. and Bell, E. J. (1983) Myalgic encephalomyelitis—report of an epidemic. *Journal of the Royal College of General Practitioners*, **33**, 335–337.

Grant, J. (1972) Post-influenzal judgement deflection among scientific personnel. *Asian Journal of Medicine*, **8**, 535–539.

Ho-Yen, D. O., Carrington, D. and Armstrong, A. A. (1988) Myalgic encephalomyelitis and alpha-interferon. *Lancet*, **1**, 125.

Isaacs, R. (1948) Chronic mononucleosis syndrome. *Blood*, **3**, 858.

Jamal, G. A. and Hansen, S. (1985) Electrophysiological studies in the post-viral fatigue syndrome. *Journal of Neurology, Neorosurgery and Psychiatry*, **48**, 691–694.

MacDonald, E. M., Mann, A. H. and Thomas, H. C. (1987) Interferons as mediators of psychiatric morbidity. *Lancet*, **ii**, 1175–1178.

Schwartz, M. S., Swash, M. and Gross, M. (1978) Benign post-infection polymyositis. *British Medical Journal*, **2**, 1256–1257.

Smith, A. P. (1989) A review of the effects of colds and influenza on human performance. *Journal of the Society of Occupational Medicine*, **39**, 65–68.

Smith, A. P., Tyrrell, D. A. J., Coyle, K. and Willman, J. S. (1987a) Selective effects of minor illnesses on human performance. *British Journal of Psychology*, **78**, 183–188.

Smith, A. P., Tyrrell, D. A. J., Al-Nakib, W., Coyle, K. B., Donovan, C. B., Higgins, P. G. and Willman, J. S. (1987b) Effects of experimentally-induced virus infections and illnesses on psychomotor performance. *Neuropsychobiology*, **18**, 144–148.

Smith, A. P., Tyrrell, D. A. J., Coyle, K. B. and Higgins, P. G. (1988a) Effects of interferon alpha on performance in man: A preliminary report. *Psychopharmacology*, **96**, 414–416.

Smith, A. P., Tyrrell, D. A. J., Al-Nakib, W., Coyle, K. B., Donovan, C. B., Higgins, P. G. and Willman, J. S. (1988b) The effects of experimentally-induced respiratory virus infections on performance. *Psychological Medicine*, **18**, 65–71.

Smith, A. P., Tyrrell, D. A. J., Al-Nakib, W., Barrow, G. I., Higgins, P. G., Leekam, S. and Trickett, S. (1989) Effects and after-effects of the common cold and influenza on human performance. *Neuropsychobiology*, **21**, 90–93.

Southern, P. and Oldstone, M. B. A. (1986) Medical consequences of persistent viral infection. *New England Journal of Medicine*, **314**, 359.

Wood, C. (1989) *The longer-term effects of influenza.* Unpublished report to the Influenza Monitoring and Information Bureau.

Yousef, G. E., Mann, G. F., Smith, D. G., Bell, E. J., Murugeson, V., McCartney, R. A. and Mowbray, J. F. (1988) Chronic enterovirus infection in patients with postviral fatigue syndrome. *Lancet*, **i**, 146–150.

11

Interferon in Viral Illness and Myalgic Encephalomyelitis

E. McDonald and A. Mann

Institute of Psychiatry, London, UK

Interferon has been postulated as a possible mediator of fatigue in the post-viral fatigue syndrome (McDonald *et al.*, 1987; Wakefield and Lloyd, 1987; Lever *et al.*, 1988). The aims of this chapter are to (1) describe what inter-ferons are, (2) describe their activity in viral infections and (3) discuss any role interferon may have in post-viral fatigue syndrome (PVFS).

INTERFERON

Interferon is the body's most rapidly produced defence against viruses. Inter-feron was discovered by Isaacs and Lindenmann in 1957 during a study of viral interference (Lindenmann, 1982). It was known for some time that if a cell or organism was infected with one virus then a second virus added subsequently would not be able to replicate as well as normal (Burke, 1985). Isaacs and Lindenmann in a simple experiment showed that an interfering substance was being formed in and released from infected cells. They showed that this substance was distinct from the virus and they named it interferon.

The initial paper by Isaacs and his colleagues was called 'The Interferon' as at that time a single substance was thought to be responsible for viral interference (Isaacs and Lindenmann, 1957). Tyrrell's work in 1959 gave the first clue that there was more than one interferon when he showed that interferon made in calf cells was inactive in chick cells and vice versa (Tyrell, 1959). Although the word interferon is often used in the singular, it is now known that the interferons are a family of at least 23 distinct proteins and glycoproteins (Rager-Zisman and Bloom, 1985).

Post-viral Fatigue Syndrome. Edited by R. Jenkins and J. Mowbray
© 1991 John Wiley & Sons Ltd

TYPES OF INTERFERONS

The interferons are heterogeneous populations of proteins and glycoproteins representing products of at least 23 different genes (Rager-Zisman and Bloom, 1985). There are three classes of interferon: alpha (α), beta (β) and gamma (γ). These types are also described by the cell type in which they are produced, i.e. α-IFN = leukocyte-IFN, β-IFN = fibroblast-IFN, and γ-IFN = immune-IFN. All the interferons exhibit antiviral, antiproliferative and immunoregulatory activities. However, alpha- and beta-interferon are more potent antiviral agents while gamma-interferon appears to have greater immunomodulatory properties.

PRODUCTION OF INTERFERONS

Viruses were the first recognised inducers of interferons but it is now known that a wide variety of natural and synthetic non-viral agents can induce interferons in animals and cell cultures. Alpha- and beta-interferon are induced by viruses, bacteria, mycobacteria, rickettsia, mycoplasma, chlamydia and a wide variety of protozoa. Some viruses are particularly good inducers of alpha-interferon (e.g. Sendai virus) while others are particularly poor (e.g. respiratory syncytial virus, which explains the occurrence of protracted upper and lower respiratory tract infections found in infants infected with this virus). Gamma-interferon is primarily produced by T lymphocytes following exposure to mitogens or specific antigens (Rager-Zisman and Bloom, 1985).

Transcription of a cellular gene has been found to be essential for production of interferon, and interferon genes have been found in all vertebrates, thus making the interferon system fairly old in evolutionary terms (Gillespie et al., 1984). The genes for human alpha- and beta-interferon reside on the short arm of chromosome 9, while that of gamma-interferon is on chromosome 12 (Derynck, 1983).

The first phase of interferon antiviral activity occurs when a virus or other inducer enters a cell or attaches to the cell membrane, leading to derepression of the interferon gene. Once the genes are activated, messenger RNA (mRNA) is produced and the interferon protein is formed by translation in the cytoplasmic ribosomes (Derynck, 1983). Messenger RNA synthesis starts within a short time after induction, and rises to a maximum two to eight hours later, and then the concentration falls away. Once interferon has been formed it is rapidly secreted from the cells into the surrounding areas. Interferon production is short-lived (one to four days) and is followed by a refractory state lasting five to 13 days during which time no further interferon is secreted.

Some systems fail to form interferon. This has been shown in some cases to be due to the presence of an interferon gene whose action is repressed in some way, as for example in teratocarcinoma cells. These are transformed stem cells and as they differentiate they become capable of producing interferon. This means that the interferon system is not used in the early embryo and may explain the damaging effects of viral infection in the first trimester of pregnancy (Burke, 1985).

Although interferon is a powerful antiviral agent, it has been found that certain viruses have anti-interferon effects. Certain viruses can block the antiviral state and inhibit the interferon-induced enzymes which are believed to play a role in the inhibition of viral growth.

INTERFERON ACTIVITY

Interferons have the ability to affect the regulation of a vast array of cellular functions. They have antiviral activities but also possess potent antiproliferative and immunoregulatory properties. They induce changes in the cell membrane (e.g. increasing the expression of HLA antigens), in cell size and in the cytoskeleton. Interferon also stimulates the production of prostaglandins and corticosteroids.

Interferons do not inactivate viruses but protect cells by producing a series of alterations to cellular metabolism which interfere with nucleic acid and protein synthesis and also with the assembly of virus particles. Interferons are active in very small amounts; only a few molecules per cell appear to be required to trigger the response.

The first step of interferon activity is the binding of interferon to receptors on the cell membrane. Interferon also enters the cell but it is not known whether this activity is essential for the establishment of antiviral activity. A second messenger is then produced which transmits a signal to the appropriate genes. Cyclic AMP has been proposed as a possible messenger. A number of cellular genes are activated and these can be detected by the presence of a series of new proteins in interferon-treated cells. Proteins of identified function include 2, 5A-synthetase, protein kinase, those of the major histocompatibility complex and indolamine-2, 3-dioxygenase.

There are three ways in which the viral particles are affected by the host cell coming into contact with interferon. Viral protein synthesis is inhibited and the transcription of some early virus genes is also inhibited. Release of viral particles from the infected cells is delayed and either the viruses accumulate underneath the plasma membrane, or the process continues but the released viruses are defective in some way, which decreases their infectivity.

INTERFERON IN HEALTH

Interferon cannot usually be detected in the serum of healthy individuals. However, Bocci (1981) has proposed that interferon is produced under normal physiological conditions (Bocci, 1981; Bocci et al., 1984).

A mixture of interferons may be produced spontaneously by lymphoid tissue in the gut. This lymphoid tissue is constantly being challenged by old and new antigens absorbed from the gut and it may be that interferon has a role in maintaining immunological homeostasis. Very small amounts of interferon may also be produced continuously in the lungs but this does not appear to enter the circulation.

INTERFERON IN DISEASE

Patients with acute viral illnesses have high levels of circulating interferon and, in 70%, their cells are in an antiviral state (Rager-Zisman and Bloom, 1985). Most viruses are good inducers of interferon but a few are conspicuously poor. These include acute hepatitis A and B, glandular fever and respiratory syncytial virus. Some hepatitis B carriers have a reduced capacity to produce alpha- and gamma-interferon (Ikeda et al., 1986) but can respond to exogenous alpha-interferon.

Interferon production in humans is not limited to acute virus infection. A variety of Gram-positive and Gram-negative bacteria, chlamydiae, mycoplasmas, rickettsiae and coxiella have been shown to induce interferon in vitro and in animals. Interferon has been demonstrated in the cerebrospinal fluid (CSF) of bacterial as well as aseptic meningitis patients (Haahr, 1968). It has also been found in the ear secretions of children with acute otitis media caused by haemophilus influenza (Homie et al., 1982). Circulating interferon has been identified in protozoan infections. Gamma-interferon has been found in the CSF of patients with acute herpes encephalitis, but it is not present in postinfectious encephalitis (Lebon et al., 1988).

Autoimmunity and immunodeficiency are often associated with the presence of circulating interferon. Many of the non-specific features of autoimmune diseases can be mimicked by injecting interferon. Interferons have been described in the sera of patients with systemic lupus erythematosus, rheumatoid arthritis, scleroderma, Sjogren's syndrome, vasculitis and Behcet's syndrome (Hooks et al., 1979, 1982; Ohno et al., 1982). An abnormal acid-labile interferon is present in the sera of patients with HIV infection (DeStefano et al., 1982).

Detectable levels of alpha-interferon have been found in the CSF (Libikova et al., 1979) and in the serum (Preble and Torrey, 1985) of schizophrenics. However, other workers have been unable to replicate these findings (Rimon et al., 1985).

INTERFERON AS A THERAPEUTIC AGENT

Since the discovery of interferon in the late 1950s much work has been done in investigating the therapeutic applications of interferon in viral infections and cancers. Recent advances in recombinant DNA technology have meant that sufficient quantities of pure alpha-interferon can be produced and made available for clinical trials. Prior to this, preparations of interferon were made from human blood buffy coat cells or lymphoblastoid cell lines. These methods of production are both costly and difficult so controlled trials could not be mounted.

In neoplastic diseases treatments with alpha- and beta-interferon have been undertaken and found to cause regression of certain tumours in individual patients. Several mechanisms may be involved in this process. Interferon slows the rate of tumour cell multiplication and this may lead to cell death. Interferon may induce changes in the cell surface, making tumour cells more sensitive to host defence mechanisms.

Interferons have been used in both prophylaxis and treatment of a number of human viral infections. Cells develop an antiviral state when treated with interferon. Time and RNA synthesis are required for this to occur. Interferon inhibits virus growth at the level of the uncoating of the virus, viral RNA and protein synthesis and virus maturation and release.

Interferon has been used in patients with chronic hepatitis B with considerable success. Interferon inhibits the hepatitis B virus replication, reducing infectivity and preventing the development of cirrhosis and hepatocellular carcinoma. Patients who benefit from interferon are those with active viral replication. Thrice weekly injections of alpha-interferon for three to six months has an overall response rate of 50% (Lever and Thomas, 1986).

Herpes simplex dendritic keratitis, varicella zoster in immunocomprised patients, cytomegalovirus and viral papillomas respond to interferon treatment. Colds and flus can be modified or prevented by prophylactic interferon. Interferon has also been used with some success in Kaposi's sarcoma (DeWit *et al.*, 1988) and trials are currently underway in patients who are HIV antigen positive.

SIDE EFFECTS OF INTERFERON

The reporting of side effects due to interferon therapy has been consistent. Purification of interferon does not decrease its toxicity and the toxicity is considered to be inherent to the interferons themselves (Scott *et al.*, 1981). The side effects are dose-related and therefore dose-limiting but are reversible on stopping treatment. Individual tolerance varies and tolerance is better with intermittent schedules of administration. Similar toxic effects have been reported for all three classes of interferon.

After a single i.m. injection of more than 10 units of alpha-interferon a symptom complex develops characterised by fever, headache, malaise and myalgia. These symptoms develop about three hours after injection and last for 12–20 hours. When patients are given daily doses of interferon the febrile response decreases and is usually gone within 10 days. These symptoms are followed by the onset of fatigue and this is the most frequent dose-limiting toxic effect.

Reversible gastrointestinal (anorexia, nausea, vomiting and diarrhoea), cardiovascular (hypotension, cardiac dysrhythmia and tachycardia) haematological (lymphopaenia and leucopenia) and renal (proteinuria) side effects have been reported. Hair loss has been observed after prolonged treatment.

Many researchers have drawn attention to the central nervous system (CNS) toxicity that accompanies interferon therapy. The toxicity is dose-related and dose-limiting and is reversible on stopping interferon. CNS disturbance is also more prevalent in older patients.

The most commonly reported neuropsychiatric symptoms are fatigue, psychomotor retardation, poor concentration, irritability, depression, anxiety, withdrawal, drowsiness, hypersomnia and lack of initiative and energy. Confusion, disorientation, agitation, visual hallucinations and increased slow-wave activity in encephalograms have also been reported (Mattson et al., 1983; Rohatiner et al., 1983; Farkkila et al., 1984; Renault et al., 1987; Adams et al., 1984; Smedley et al., 1983; McDonald et al., 1987).

The most important of these symptoms is fatigue as it is the most common side effect and the most common reason for interferon treatment to be stopped. Fatigue is reported in up to 100% of patients on alpha-interferon. There is individual variation in the level of fatigue experienced. Large doses of interferon are not required for the fatigue to occur.

No satisfactory explanation for the cause of the fatigue has emerged. It has been suggested that the intense fatigue may be a manifestation of a complex neurotoxicity, most suggestive of frontal lobe changes resulting in a neurasthenia syndrome (Adams et al., 1984). Human alpha-interferon preparations contain immunologically and biologically recognisable endorphin activities (Smedley et al., 1983). It binds to opiate receptors in vivo. When injected intracerebrally into mice it causes potent endorphin-like effects such as lack of spontaneous movement, catalepsy and analgesia (Blalock and Smith, 1981). These actions are prevented by and reversed by giving naloxone. It has been postulated that these effects may be related to the interferon-induced fatigue.

Wakefield and Lloyd postulate that interferon-induced dysfunction of the muscle membrane may be the pathophysiological basis of exercise-aggravated muscle fatigue in patients with ME (Wakefield and Lloyd, 1987).

INTERFERON AND FATIGUE IN PVFS

It has already been noted that fatigue is a very common feature in interferon therapy. Patients on interferon who suffer from this fatigue find that it is exacerbated by physical exercise. Some patients have to stop working, particularly those whose occupations have a largely physical component, while the majority report that their social functioning is impaired. Despite the agreement on the occurrence of fatigue as a side effect of interferon therapy, there is difficulty in comparing this with that occurring in PVFS because 'fatigue' is largely undefined in interferon studies. For example, the distinction is rarely made between mental and physical fatigue.

The other most common side effects of interferon treatment are poor concentration, irritability, loss of interest, anxiety and depression (McDonald *et al.*, 1987). These symptoms are also commonly reported in patients suffering from PVFS. This has prompted several investigators to look for evidence of abnormal interferon function in patients with PVFS.

INTERFERON ASSAYS IN CHRONIC FATIGUE

A number of different syndromes have been postulated to be related to chronic fatigue. The two referred to below are post-viral fatigue syndrome (PVFS) and postinfectious syndrome (PIFS). PVFS refers to chronic fatigue occurring in the presence of a chronic viral infection, whereas PIFS refers to chronic fatigue subsequent to an infectious illness.

Two studies investigating chronic illness and fatigue in patients with persistent Epstein–Barr virus infection found only one patient with circulating interferon out of 50 tested. This was in contrast to seven out of seven patients with acute infectious mononucleosis who were found to have circulating interferon (Jones *et al.*, 1985; Straus *et al.*, 1985).

Ho-Yen *et al.* (1988) tested blood from 15 patients, who were within seven days of an exacerbation of ME, and blood from 10 healthy controls. They found that, using a sensitive method that systematically measured alpha-interferon, levels are not particularly abnormal in patients with ME (Ho-Yen *et al.*, 1988). Lloyd *et al.* (1988) examined the sera of 52 patients who fulfilled their diagnostic criteria for PIFS and the sera from 20 healthy adults. Their results indicated that patients with PIFS do not have increased serum gamma-interferon levels (Lloyd *et al.*, 1988).

A study conducted in 1988 examined the sera of 45 patients attending the ME Association physician and found that there was again no evidence of circulating alpha-interferon (McDonald *et al.*, unpublished).

Lever *et al.* (1988) set about investigating virus-stimulated interferon levels following the lack of success of the above studies. They decided to study children with PVFS as they felt that it would be easier to distinguish genuine cases in this group. They investigated the *in vitro* interferon response of a sample of children from a school in Aberystwyth where an outbreak of PVFS among both children and some immediate family members was associated with positive neutralising antibody responses against Coxsackie B4 in all cases. Affected children produced significantly more alpha-interferon *in vitro* than controls. It is not clear whether these individuals have an excessive interferon response to viral stimulation either as a result of persistent infection or as a genetic characteristic.

Another approach to examining interferon activity is to measure the activity of 2,5-oligoadenylate synthetase, an enzyme specifically induced by interferon. In a study of 18 patients with persisting Epstein-Barr virus infection, the activity of 2,5-oligoadenylate synthetase was increased in five patients studied (Straus *et al.*, 1985).

Evidence of this activity has also been reported by Morag *et al.* (1982) in patients with serological evidence of persisting Epstein-Barr virus infection.

CONCLUSIONS

Interferon has a well-documented role in viral illness, particularly in acute viral illnesses such as influenza where it is believed to account for the pyrexia, myalgia and fatigue experience in the symptomatic period.

Fatigue produced by interferon is a well-documented phenomenon in patients receiving interferon as a therapeutic agent in chronic viral disease and malignancies.

It is disappointing then that no evidence of circulating interferon has been found in patients suffering from ME/PVFS/PIFS but as it is known that interferon is rapidly removed from the circulation it is not surprising that positive results have not been found.

There is, however, some encouragement to be gained from the findings of increased interferon production *in vitro* in response to viral stimulation in patients believed to have PVFS and of increased 2,5-oligoadenylate synthetase activity in patients with persisting Epstein–Barr virus infection.

REFERENCES

Adams, F., Quesada, J. and Gutterman, J. (1984) Neuropsychiatric manifestations of human leucocyte interferon therapy in patients with cancer. *Journal of the American Medical Association*, **252**, 262–264.

Blalock, J. E. and Smith, E. M. (1980) Human leukocyte interferon: Structural and biological relatedness to ACTH and endorphins. *Proceedings of the National Academy of Sciences of the USA*, **77** (10), 5972–5974.

Blalock, J. E. and Smith, E. M. (1981) Human leukocyte interferon: Potent endorphin-like opioid activity. *Biochemical and Biophysical Research Communications*, **101** (2), 472–478.

Bocci, V. (1981) Production and role of interferon in physiological conditions. *Biological Review*, **56**, 49–85.

Bocci, V., Muscettola, M., Paulesu, L. and Grasso, G. (1984) The physiological interferon response 11. *Journal of General Virology*, **65**, 101–108.

Burke, D. C. (1985) The interferons. *British Medical Bulletin*, **41** (4), 333–338.

Derynck, R. (1983) More about interferon cloning. In I. Gresser (ed.) *Interferon*, Vol. 5, pp. 181–203. Academic Press, London.

DeStefano, E., Friedman, R. M., Friedman-Kien, A. E., Goedert, J. J., Henriksen, D., Preble, O. T., Sonnabend, J. A. and Vilcek, J. (1982) Acid-labile leucocyte interferon in homosexual men with Kaposi's sarcoma and lymphadenopathy. *Journal of Infectious Diseases*, **146**, 451–455.

DeWit, R., Schnattenkerk, J. K., Boucher, C., Bakker, P., Veenhof, K. and Danner, S. A. (1988) Clinical and virological effects of high dose recombinant alpha-interferon in disseminated AIDS related Kaposi's sarcoma. *Lancet*, **ii**, 1214–1217.

Farkkila, M., Iivanainen, M., Roine, R., Niemi, M. L. and Cantell, K. (1984) Neurotoxic and other side-effects of high-dose interferon in amyotrophic lateral sclerosis. *Acta Neurologica Scandinavica*, **69**, 42–46.

Gillespie, D., Pequignot, E. and Carter, W. A. (1984) Evolution of interferon genes. In W. A. Came and W. A. Carter (eds) *Interferons and Their Applications*, pp. 45–63. Springer-Verlag, Berlin.

Haahr, S. (1968) The occurrence of interferon in the cerebrospinal fluid of patients with bacterial meningitis. *Acta Pathologica Microbiologica Scandinavica*, **73**, 264–274.

Homie, V., Pollard, R. B., Kleyn, K., Lawrence, B., Peskuric, T., Paucker, K. and Baron, S. (1982) Presence of interferon during bacterial otitis media. *Journal of Infectious Diseases*, **145**, 811–814.

Hooks, J. J. Mousopoulos, H. M., Geis, S., Stahl, N., Decker, J. and Notkins, A. L. (1979) Immune interferon in the circulation of patients with auto-immune disease. *New England Journal of Medicine*, **301**, 5–8.

Hooks, J. J., Jordan, G. W., Cupps, T., Mousopoulos, H. M., Fauci, A. S. and Notkins, A. L. (1982) Multiple interferons in the circulation of patients with SLE and vasculitis. *Arthritis and Rheumatism*, **25**, 396–400.

Ho-Yen, D. O., Carrington, D. and Armstrong, A. (1988) M. E. and alpha interferon. *Lancet*, **i**, 125.

Ikeda, T., Lever, A. Thomas, H. C. (1986) Evidence for a deficiency of interferon production in patients with chronic hepatitis B virus infection acquired in adult life. *Hepatology*, **6** (5), 962–965.

Isaacs, A. and Lindenmann, J. (1957) Virus interference. 1. The interferon. *Proceedings of the Royal Society of London*, **147**, 258–267.

Jones, J., Ray, G., Minnich, L., Hicks, M. J., Kibler, R. and Lucas, D. (1985) Evidence for active Epstein-Barr virus infection in patients with persistent unexplained illnesses: Elevated anti-early antigen antibodies. *Annals of Internal Medicine*, **102**, 1–7.

Lebon, P., Boutin, B., Dulac, O., Ponsot, G. and Arthuis, M. (1988) Interferon gamma in acute and sub-acute encephalitis. *British Medical Journal*, **296**, 9–11.

Lever, A. and Thomas, H. C. (1986) Treatment of chronic hepatitis B virus infection. *Clinics in Tropical Medicine and Communicable Diseases*, **1** (2), 377–393.

Lever, A., Lewis, D., Bannister, B., Fry, M. and Berry, N. (1988) Interferon production in post-viral fatigue syndrome. *Lancet*, **ii**, 101.

Levin, S. and Hahn, T. (1981) Evaluation of the human interferon system in viral disease. *Clinical and Experimental Immunology*, **46**, 475–483.

Libikova, H., Breier, S., Kocisova, M., Pogady, J., Stunzner, D. and Vjhazyova, D. (1979) Assay of interferon and viral anti-bodies in the cerebrospinal fluid in clinical neurology and psychiatry. *Acta Biologica Medica Germanica*, **38**, 879–93.

Lindenmann, J. (1982) From interference to interferon: a brief historical introduction. In D. A. J. Tyrrell and D. C. Burke (eds) *Interferon: Twenty Years on*, pp. 3–6. The Royal Society, London.

Lloyd, A., Abi-Hanna, D. and Wakefield, D. (1988) Interferon and myalgic encephalomyelitis. *Lancet*, **i**, 471.

Mattson, K., Niiranen, A., Iivanainen, M., Farkkila, M., Bergstrom, I., Holsti, L. R., Kauppinen, H. L. and Cantell, K. (1983) Neurotoxicity of interferon. *Cancer Treatment Reports*, **67** (10), 958–961.

McDonald, E. M., Mann, A. H. and Thomas, H. C. (1987) Interferons as mediators of psychiatric morbidity. *Lancet*, **ii**, 1175–1178.

Morag, A., Tobi, M., Ravid, Z., Revel, M. and Schnattner, A. (1982) Increased 2′-5′-oligoadenylate synthetase activity in patients with prolonged illness associated with serological evidence of Epstein–Barr virus infection. *Lancet*, **i**, 744.

Ohno, S., Kato, F., Matsuda, H., Fujii, N. and Minagawa, T. (1982) Detection of gamma interferon in the sera of patients with Behcets disease. *Infection and Immunity*, **36**, 202–208.

Preble, O. T. and Torrey, E. F. (1985) Serum interferon in patients with psychosis. *American Journal of Psychiatry*, **142**, 1184–1186.

Rager-Zisman, B. and Bloom, B. R. (1985) Interferons and natural killer cells. *British Medical Bulletin*, **41**, (1), 22–27.

Renault, P. F., Hoofnagle, J. H., Park, Y., Mullen, K. D., Peters, M., Jones, D. B., Rustgi, V. and Jones, A. (1987) Psychiatric complications of long term interferon alpha therapy. *Archives of Internal Medicine*, **147**, 1577–1580.

Rimon, R., Ahokas, A., Hintikka, J. and Heikkila, L. (1985) Serum interferon in schizophrenia. *Annals of Clinical Research*, **17**, 139–140.

Rohatiner, A. Z. S., Prior, P. F., Burton, A. C., Smith, A. T., Balkwill, F. R. and Lister, T. A. (1983) Central nervous system toxicity of interferon. *British Journal of Cancer*, **47**, 419–422.

Scott, G. M., Secher, D. S., Flowers, D., Bate, J., Cantell, K. and Tyrrell, D. A. J. (1981) Toxicity of interferon. *British Medical Journal*, **282**, 1345–1348.

Smedley, H., Katrak, M., Sikora, K. and Wheeler, T. (1983) Neurological effects of recombinant human interferon. *British Medical Journal*, **286**, 262–264.

Straus, S., Tosato, G., Armstrong, G., Cawley, T., Preble, O. T., Henle, W., Davey, R., Pearson, G., Epstein, J., Brus, I. and Blaese, R. M. (1985) Persisting illness and fatigue in adults with evidence of Epstein–Barr virus infection. *Annals of Internal Medicine*, **102**, 7–16.

Tyrell, D. A. J. (1959) Interferon produced by cultures of calf kidney cells. *Nature*, **184**, 452–453.

Wakefield, D. and Lloyd, A. (1987) Pathophysiology of myalgic encephalitis. *Lancet*, **ii**, 918–919.

12

Chronic Aspects of Akureyri Disease

Byron Hyde* and Sverrir Bergman†

*The Nightingale Research Foundation, Ottowa, Canada
†University of Iceland, Reykjavik, Iceland

SUMMARY

Since Sigurdsson published his 'six year after study' in 1956, there has been no mention in the literature of the chronic aspects of myalgic encephalomyelitis (ME). Ten victims of the 1948 epidemic were reviewed. The main findings were: after an initial period of marked disability, patients were successfully integrated into their respective social and work environments; a high incidence of both initial and late reccurrences of cardiac irregularities; evidence of minor ongoing motoneurone difficulties; a marked improvement in mental and cognitive abilities after the first several years; a marked improvement but definite physical limitation in the majority of the patients examined. The nature and the history of the disease is in keeping with a viral or infectious etiology. There was no evidence that these patients suffered from hysterical, depressive or psychiatric disease. A brief review of the literature concerning the Akureyri epidemic and a statement of one of the current scientific views of this illness are included.

INTRODUCTION

Myalgic encephalomyelitis (ME) appears to be a chronic viral disease involving the immune system (Behan and Behan, 1988; Behan et al., 1985), metabolic pathways of muscle tissue (Arnold et al., 1984) and injury to the spinal nervous system (Marinacci and Van Hagen, 1965; Marinacci, 1968; Jamal and Hansen, 1985). The affected individuals suffer from easy muscular

Post-viral Fatigue Syndrome. Edited by R. Jenkins and J. Mowbray
© 1991 John Wiley & Sons Ltd

fatigue with an extremely slow period of recuperation after the muscle is exercised. The patient frequently complains of fatigue and pain in the legs, arms and intercostal muscles, but the phenomenon is found equally in the voluntary and involuntary muscles of the eye and bladder with associated visual and urinary tract area problems. Rare is the patient who does not complain of head and spinal pain or discomfort that at times can be extreme. Rare is the patient who does not experience one of either gynecological, testicular or bladder symptoms. Patients frequently complain of irritability, easy mental fatigue, cognitive gaps and emotional lability.

Since 1680, when Thomas Sydenham first described this disease complex as occurring after an acute febrile episode, the medical world has been polarized as to the infectious or psychoneurotic origins of this illness. Recently there has been a real or apparent increase in the endemic frequency of this disease. Many researchers believe that ME is an endemic viral disease that periodically occurs in epidemic manifestations. There is considerable support for this view. Epidemics simply represent geographically and medically visible loci of increased disease activity in the community. Thus the epidemic in 1934 in the Los Angeles County Hospital was associated with a poliomyelitis epidemic involving large areas of California; the epidemic of 1948 in the town of Akureyri was associated with a major recurrent poliomyelitis epidemic in Iceland; the Royal Free Hospital epidemic in 1955 was associated with a widespread increase in ME sporadic activity involving all of England and Scotland in 1954–1955. All of these epidemic associations have been extensively recorded in the literature. The Lake Tahoe epidemic in 1984 was concurrent with a marked increase of ME activity starting in 1983 but peaking in 1984 in North America. This pandemic is well known by many of the workers in the field but has yet to be documented in the literature.

The viral cause of ME in the United States has, until recently, been considered to be the herpes family of viruses. For most of the last decade, the herpes virus known as Epstein–Barr virus (EBV) was reported to be the cause. The EBV etiology has recently met with disfavor and the current American hypothesis involves another herpes virus, HHV6 (Salahuddin *et al.*, 1986). HHV6 may well meet the same fate as EBV and also be rejected.

In Britain, Australia and New Zealand, most workers over the years have come to associate this disease with enterovirus infections. Canadian researchers have had split allegiances. Recent work would tend to support the enteroviral theory. Peter Behan notes that ME has been shown to follow in the wake of the majority of the enteroviruses, including Coxsackie B and A, polio virus and echovirus. He also notes that ME has followed after infectious hepatitis A, and that some virologists place it in the enterovirus group because of some of its physical properties. Behan also notes its occurrence after infection with certain of the herpes family such as EBV and varicellar zoster virus. Inoue in Japan has associated a similar disease complex with serological evidence of another herpes-like virus, Inoue–Melnick virus (Inoue, 1971). Behan mentions occurrences after rubella and influenza A, both RNA viruses.

THE AKUREYRI EPIDEMIC

Akureyri is a town in Iceland, situated at the extreme south end of a long fiord that opens into the Greenland Sea. In 1948 this town became the scene of what was believed at the time to be an unprecedented epidemic of 'a disease simulating poliomyelitis' (Sigurdsson *et al.*, 1950). The epicentre of the epidemic was in itself unusual as it was located in the main secondary school where students from the outlying district of Akureyri boarded. Schools were not usually affected by poliomyelitis. The school and residence are situated on a bluff that gives a magnificent view of the town and the fiord below. Behind the school are the high cliffs resembling low mountains that rise up to a plateau. Immediately to the south of the school is a small botanical garden of perhaps two acres. Akureyri's only hospital is beside the garden, about 500 feet from the school.

In July 1948, an epidemic of paralytic poliomyelitis broke out in Iceland. During the next four months, 42 persons fell ill. Then, in the single month of November 1948, in the town of Akureyri, 265 persons succumbed. Before the epidemic had ceased that winter, Sigurdsson *et al.* (1950) had recorded 476 cases in Akureyri and a total of 1121 victims in Iceland. Although no one doubted that many of the earlier cases were classical poliomyelitis, almost at once questions arose as to the true identity of what appeared to be a different disease.

It is not generally realized today, but epidemic poliomyelitis was then a relatively newly identified epidemic disease, having been first described by the Swedish physician Bergenholz only in 1881 (Wickman, 1913). After that date, the size, number and dispersion of poliomyelitis epidemics grew around the world. In 1905 the world's first mega-epidemic of poliomyelitis (Wickman, 1913) occurred in Stockholm, involving 1017 victims. The Icelandic epidemic of 1948 thus occurred only 43 years after this first major epidemic. Though much was known about poliomyelitis by that date, viral techniques had not been developed to any level of proficiency. The other paralytic enteroviruses, Coxsackie viruses and echoviruses, had first been discovered only in 1948 (Dalldof and Sickles, 1948). From the first recognized epidemic in 1881 until today, our concept of what poliomyelitis really encompasses has been in a state of flux. Not only were the accepted limits of poliomyelitis questioned, but poliomyelitis itself had also shown many dramatic changes over its short history. In many respects, poliomyelitis was not a constant. Yet, if the fact that 1121 victims had fallen ill in the Iceland epidemic of 1948–1949 was not unusual, there were several unique features of this epidemic.

During the six months of October 1948 to March 1949, 476 persons fell ill in the town of Akureyri out of a total population of 3200 (488 in the district of Akureyri). Sigurdsson *et al.* (1950) noted that the two patients who fell ill in October were severely paralysed and that these were definitely cases of poliomyelitis. However, when Byron Hyde interviewed one of these two patients, E. H., 40 years later she described having had certain features quite unlike classical poliomyelitis at the start of her illness. These included a ME-type pain syndrome, protracted convalescence, chronic fatigue syndrome, muscle weakness and eye signs. After these first two cases, however, there is consensus that the epidemic forgot to follow the rules. The following represent some of the findings typical of ME but considered unprecedented in a typical epidemic of poliomyelitis:

(a) 6.7% of the population of Akureyri fell ill.
(b) The epidemic lasted five to six months.
(c) There were no immediate deaths recorded.
(d) The incidence was significantly higher in women.
(e) The recorded incidence in young children was low.
(f) Multiple cases in households were common.
(g) The epidemic persisted into the fall–winter period.
(h) There was a high degree of nervousness, sweats, palpitations and fatigue. Loss of memory was also noted.
(i) Paresthesias were common.
(j) Significant hyperesthesia (hypersensitivity) or hypoalgesia was common in the afflicted limbs.
(k) Tenderness of the muscles was a conspicuous feature in 19 of the 25 cases quoted and sometimes this tenderness was confined to small spots in the muscles.
(l) Deep reflexes in both arms or legs were absent in 10 of the 25 cases quoted.
(m) Abdominal reflexes were absent in 14 of the 25 cases quoted.
(n) The period of convalescence tended to be very protracted even for apparently mild cases.
(o) Relapses occurred frequently.
(p) Aching pains and fatigue tended to persist in some cases for the extent of the period studied and past the period that paralysis or weakness lasted.
(q) Even in late stages of the disease, there were persistent or intermittent headaches.
(r) Patients frequently had visual impairment made worse by reading.

(s) Six of the 24 hospitalized patients showed subacute arthritis.
(t) There was a grouping of victims in one of the schools that involved both teachers and pupils.

Together, the findings described above were quite unlike the accepted view of poliomyelitis, but the fact that was most specifically different from poliomyelitis was the protracted and relapsing nature of the disease. In some cases the second instance of paresis, low fevers, or decreased or increased disturbances of sensation occurred as long as eight weeks after the initial attack and, in the case of muscle weakness, frequently reccurred in a previously unaffected limb. The concentration and spread in a school was considered highly unusual for poliomyelitis. Sigurdsson *et al.* (1950) noted that many of the subjective symptoms were considered functional. This functional concept undoubtedly was due in part (a) to the remitting nature of this apparently new disease, (b) to the concentration in women, (c) to the fact that the authors believed they were dealing with a variant of poliomyelitis, and (d) to the fact that the disease in Akureyri did not conform to the pattern expected in poliomyelitis. There were few cases reported in children under five years. Even after apparent recovery, fatigue occurred after minimal exertion irrespective of paresis.

FOLLOW-UP STUDIES OF THE AKUREYRI EPIDEMIC

Six years later, two of the original authors, Sigurdsson and Gudmundsson (1956), reviewed 39 patients from the Akureyri epidemic. It was found that only 31% of the patients examined were free from objective clinical signs and only 13% considered themselves completely recovered. A total of 72% of the sample still complained of nervousness and fatigue and 62% still complained of muscle pain. Only 20% continued to complain of loss of memory. Signs of paresis, hypoalgesia, and hypoaesthesia were common.

Seven years later, in 1955, a type 1 polio virus epidemic of poliomyelitis struck Iceland. Those areas that had previously been attacked by Akureyri disease showed very few cases of paralysis and so appeared to have resistance to this new poliomyelitis epidemic. However, in the original 1948 epidemic, although polio virus was searched for, no virus was recovered.

In 1956, when a trial poliomyelitis vaccination was tested in Iceland, Sigurdsson found that children from those regions struck by Akureyri disease in 1948 responded with a better antibody increase than individuals from those areas that had not been so infected (Sigurdsson *et al.* 1958). Because of these two observations, it was felt that Akureyri disease might have been caused by a virus related to polio virus. It is not mentioned in Sigurdsson's paper, but this resistance may have equally arisen from the poliomyelitis epidemics of 1945 and 1946–1947 that were quite widespread yet did not appear to provide any protection from the 1948 ME epidemic.

On the other hand, Sigurjonssen (1959) reviewed the 1945 and 1946–1947 poliomyelitis epidemics in Iceland. He described features similar to those noted in the Akureyri epidemic in 1948. There was no mention in this study of any carry-over, i.e. no patient who was infected in 1947 was shown to have fallen ill again in 1948.

EVIDENCE OF ENDEMICITY

There is a suggestion that, after 1948, the disease process became endemic in Iceland. At least patients continued to present and complain of a disease with similar features. We have not been able to discover the recording of any new disease after 1958. Hart (1969) mentions one American airman with Akureyri disease in 1958, returning invalided from Iceland to Pittsfield, Massachusetts. This epidemic was never published but it is mentioned by Henderson and Shelokov (1959) and by Behan and Behan (1980) as occurring in 1955–1956. The exact date is not important but it does illustrate that the disease was considered to be still active around that period in Iceland. This information is also consistent with the illness of J. I., who fell ill in Reykjavik in October 1955 and who was interviewed for this study.

This persistence of endemic disease is also consistent with the epidemic recorded by White and Burtch (1954) in Kingston, upper New York State, an area that continues to have an unusually large number of recent ME patients. It is impossible to know if these ongoing low-grade epidemics represent anything more than heightened awareness of a disease that may be endemic in all communities. The largely unnoticed North American pandemic of ME that struck in 1984 appears to have been preceded by a substantially smaller one in 1983, followed by ongoing new illness at a significantly lower rate (Hyde, in preparation). This peaking incidence in North America in 1984 has been observed by many workers studying ME. Over half of the 300 patients that I have reviewed in Ottawa with this disease fell ill in 1984. The Lake Tahoe epidemic also started in September 1984 and involved a large number of school teachers in Incline Village on the shores of Lake Tahoe.

This date is significant because, in Great Britain, the reputed epidemic peak was not in 1984 but in 1985 and, although no papers have yet been published concerning this, the impression is that of an unusually large number of new cases of ME occurring in that year. This opinion has been confirmed by Dr Eleanor Bell, one of Scotland's leading virologists, who has noted that for 20 years the level of Coxsackie virus titres and Coxsackie IgM in the general public remained stable, but that it rose sharply in 1985. The

IgM levels fell in the winter of 1987. The titres are slow to fall, and are expected to remain high until 1990, and then to return to baseline levels as noted up to 1986, where presumably they will remain until the next epidemic. Although these observations do not provide proof that the epidemic was provoked by Coxsackie viruses, it certainly is consistent with the enterovirus theory of cause.

A FOLLOW-UP EXAMINATION OF 10 PATIENTS 40 YEARS LATER

Methods

Ten patients were reviewed in May 1988, nine who had fallen ill in Akureyri in the winter of 1948 and another who had features of Akureyri disease but who had fallen ill in the Reykjavik area in October 1955. The patients varied in age from 58 to 84 with the exception of one woman who had fallen ill at the age of five and was 45 at the time of review. The sample consisted of eight women and two men. All patients were interviewed for approximately one to two hours by Byron Hyde. In most instances a neurologist was also present. All of these patients had had complete physical examinations and laboratory work-ups on numerous previous occasions and no other disease was found or suspected except for secondary medical conditions mentioned. These patients were chosen because they were readily available and known to the medical services. It is not known how rerepresentative these ten patients were, or, indeed, what proportion they were of all patients from the epidemic who had developed chronic sequelae and who were still alive. Further epidemiological analysis is required before we can acquire an understanding of the process of development of such longstanding chronicity.

Antecedent disease features

When the ten 1948 Akureyri patients were interviewed in May 1988, it was found that three had first fallen ill in 1947. In each case the disease was of a similar nature, with burning pain in one or more limbs, severe prostration, and profound muscular weakness. The illness was short-lived, lasting about two weeks, followed by an apparently complete recovery. In addition, the husband of one of these women had fallen ill with paralytic poliomyelitis in 1945. Sigurjonssen relates that these unusual features occurred in both the Icelandic poliomyelitis epidemic of 1945 and that of 1946–1947. The fact that a similar type of disease occurred in three of the ten patients the year before falling seriously ill in 1948 was quite unanticipated. One of these women was the gymnastics teacher in charge at the Akureyri school where so many of the 476 Akureyri patients fell ill. It is also perhaps significant that, in 1948, this woman's husband and at least two of her children also fell ill with Akureyri disease. Although the conjecture is not open to serious analysis, this woman would have been in an ideal position to have been the cause of dissemination of the 1948 disease.

Possible increased cardiac death risk

The ten patients interviewed were asked if they knew the cause of death of any other Akureyri disease patients. One patient, B. F., fell ill in 1948 at the age of 50, with Akureyri disease, followed in the same year with Parkinson's disease. He died of Parkinson's disease in 1960. This Parkinson relationship has also been observed by Dr John Richardson of the Newcastle-upon-Tyne area, also appearing soon after the initial occurrence of ME in a patient (Richardson, personal communication). The several other deaths mentioned were all due to cardiac disease. It is impossible to state how significant this is but in any other long-term follow-up the cardiac status of patients should be observed. It is perhaps more significant that six of the ten patients interviewed complained of cardiac fibrillation or dysrhythmias, all of which started with the disease and that, in some, these dysrhythmias persisted. In others, the dysrhythmias stopped, only to reappear 30 years later. This cardiac relationship to ME is also discussed in a more complete fashion by Leon-Sotomayor (1969). Behan and Behan (1988) have also referred to abnormal cardiac perfusion in patients with ME. They have biopsied these areas and found them to be abnormal.

Relapses

Relapses were noted by both Sigurdsson *et al.* (1950) and Gilliam (1938) as primary features that served to distinguish ME from typical poliomyelitis. This is a feature noted by almost all researchers who have published on epidemics of this disease. A curious feature of these ten patients is that, after the initial few years none mentioned recurrences of their disease. It is difficult to interpret this finding in light of the current thinking on relapses. However, so singular was the lack of recurrences, that I wonder if many reported breakdowns are not improperly interpreted. Some cases may represent quiescent disease that has simply become visible when the patient has gone beyond the physical limitations imposed by this disease. Other cases may represent reinfection.

For example, if a patient is very ill and seeks rest and quiet, after a short period that patient may look and feel well. Any physician's examination and history during that period might register a recovery. Yet, on returning to normal activity, the patient again appears to fall ill. In this manner, many instances of quiescent disease would be noted as recovery. It is very obvious to physicians that patients who have ME do recover and return to normal activity and then fall ill again after periods of several years of obvious good health. Is it possible that, in these cases, we are dealing with a reinfection rather than a reccurrence? In these ten Icelandic patients it would appear that the pattern is consistent with an initial severe viral injury, followed by a slow cyclical recuperation period. Some physicians may incorrectly consider return to some level of work activity as recovery from disease.

Mental and cognitive recovery

Many prepubertal patients appear to recover relatively quickly (one to three years) from their disease process. A small number of adults appear to follow a similar pattern. Ultimately all the patients stabilize at a level of recovery that is impossible to predict from the state of the patient's initial illness. The return of cognitive abilities, which appears to precede the return of physical abilities, seems to be the rule in Iceland, as it does elsewhere in clinical observations of many patients with ME (Hyde, in preparation).

Total recovery

In determining total recovery, one has to distinguish success in home and work life from complete physical, emotional and cognitive recovery. On clinical grounds, only two of the ten patients indicated a total physical and intellectual recovery. They were a five-year-old child and a gymnastics teacher. Both were also unique in that neither demonstrated a positive VP1. Due to the small sample size, it is impossible to obtain good prognostic features from these two cases.

SOCIOPSYCHOLOGICAL ASPECTS OF AKUREYRI DISEASE

None of the ten persons interviewed showed any obvious signs of hysteria or neuroticism. On the contrary, they were well adjusted and continued to lead successful lives. No suggestion of depression was noted in any of these patients at the time of the interview, although two said that they had had considerable reactive depression earlier in the disease. It is the authors' opinion that, had they been more carefully questioned during this recent survey, reactive depression early in the disease would have been noted as a more common feature, as it is in new patients seen by physicians today. Each of the ten individuals had reached or surpassed their socio-economic expectations. This was equally true whether the home or work life was considered. Marital or social relationships, rather than being placed in a situation of jeopardy, appear to have been strengthened. This strengthening of interpersonal relationships seems to be contrary to much of the experience in Britain and may represent greater psychosocial support systems in Iceland.

Two women who initially had been severely paralysed were transferred to long-term hospitalization, both to Denmark and later one to the Roosevelt Center in Georgia. Although their period of paralysis lasted for close to two years, in one case the father and in the other the fiancé accompanied the individual and gave considerable emotional support during a period full of uncertainty and great stress. It is of interest that, unlike typical paralytic poliomyelitis patients and despite the severity of the initial paralysis, both individuals recovered from all visual aspects of paralysis, although they continue to experience muscle weakness.

When problems did arise, it was because the doctor would not believe that the patient was really ill, but believed that the patient was suffering from an hysterical paralysis. One patient, E. G., stated that:

As far as I know I was the first to fall ill with Akureyri disease. It was the 20 October, and by the 21 October I was in severe pain, I had no fever, but I could not urinate and I was unable to move either of my legs. Then when the doctor came he would not believe that there was anything wrong with me.

Conversely, initially patients were frequently totally avoided by the general population, nurses and friends due to the universal fear that the illness was contagious.

This problem was not so evident in Akureyri, but when the patients were transferred to the infectious hospital in Reykjavik, such was the general fear of the population that some nurses were terrified of approaching the victims, or of entering their rooms. Since, in some instances patients were so weak that they were not able to raise their hands to eat, eating became a problem. In the few occurrences, these episodes were rapidly corrected, but they left frightening memories.

It is to be remarked that only one of the adults, the gymnastics teacher, returned to an active sports life within one year of illness, and, curiously, in both this case and that of the child, a low level of VP1 antigen was detected in the serum, indicating persisting enteroviral infection. The other eight patients demonstrated a complete spectrum that ranged from permanent paralysis to disabilities that would be considered minor or non-existent to a casual medical observer. Negligible as these disabilities might appear, the patients concerned have remained justly cautious of the limits of their physical abilities. One particularly successful patient who had fallen ill at the age of 18 and who after two years of severe muscular weakness returned to school and eventually became a major figure in Icelandic political and administrative life, stated:

This disease has changed my life. I have never since dared to attempt my physical limits for fear that they would fail me. After I was strong enough to return to school, even at dances I would go home early and in a way, this gave me an advantage over others since I knew I could count on my mental abilities as long as I did not push my physical abilities. Yet I have not met a man in Iceland who fell ill with Akureyri disease who has recovered as well as I have.

In 1988 this man, who stated that he had made a better recovery than all the others he had met, still had a positive Rhomberg test, nystagmus in upper outer quadrants and abnormal visual saccades. His small muscle control was such that he was still not able to write a long letter by hand without a marked deterioration of his cursive writing abilities. Yet he prided himself as being totally recovered. Part of his insistence of total recovery may be related to the fact that there was still a suspicion on the part of many Icelandic physicians that this disease was simply hysteria. It would be important for a person in a situation of major government trust to distance himself from any presumed 'neurotic' disease.

This denial of ME-type disease is not unique to Iceland. Ramsay (1988) noted that the nurses involved in the Royal Free Hospital epidemic were so upset by the claims of certain physicians that they were simply suffering from hysteria that they as a group have refused to respond either to physicians or the press, concerning the chronicity of their disease. This denial of disease is the opposite of what one would anticipate from an hysteric patient. Hysteria, it is assumed, exists as a public display to achieve an end. It makes no hysteric sense to keep one's symptoms secret.

CONCLUSION

Iceland is in an excellent position to study the long-term sequelae of ME. The population is small, approximately 242,000. The names of all the patients who originally fell ill with Akureyri disease are known. Those patients still alive are still resident in Iceland. The population in question are all on the Iceland medical computer. For those patients already deceased, it is an easy task to retrieve the cause of death. The autopsy rate of the country is high. Accordingly, Iceland affords a unique situation for a much needed comprehensive epidemiological study of ME.

Though the exact etiology of this particular epidemic may never be clearly demonstrated, a possible epidemic mechanism may be found in the fact that three of the ten patients interviewed had fallen ill with a similar but shorter disease episode in the year prior to the epidemic. Since the work of Yousef *et al.* (1988) indicates that one group of the viral causes of this disease can be recovered intact from the stools up to three years after the initial infection, the source of the epidemic may well have been carried over from the earlier episode.

The fact that eight of the ten patients examined, irrespective of their work and home successes, continued to have various forms of chronic disability is not surprising to someone who has worked with such patients. These figures are also consistent with the findings of Sigurdsson and Gudmundsson (1988) who noted that subjectively only 13% and objectively only 30% of 39 patients examined had completely recovered after six years. Sigurdsson and Gudmundsson did not define what they meant by nervousness, the most common complaint seen after six years. However, their descriptions of general fatigue, muscle pain, tenderness and weakness as well as various neurological complaints are similar to those noted 40 years later in this chapter.

The lack of any obvious ongoing psychological illness in these patients may be related to the considerable support given at all times by family, loved ones, their community and the state. There is undoubtedly at this stage, 40 years later, a degree of acceptance of their individual physical limitations that may have not been present immediately after the disease inception. The excellent and free medical services available in Iceland have certainly contributed to the Akureyri patients' integration as useful members of their society.

ACKNOWLEDGEMENTS

The authors would like to thank Drs Gunnar Fredriksson and Sigurdur Thoriacius and those members of the Icelandic medical community and their patients who assisted in this project.

REFERENCES

Arnold, D. L., Radda, R. K., Bore, P. J., Styles, P. and Taylor, D. J. (1984) Excessive intracellular acidosis of skeletal muscle on exercise in a patient with a post-viral exhaustion/fatigue syndrome. *Lancet*, i, 1367–1369.

Behan, P. O. and Behan, W. M. H. (1980) Epidemic myalgic encephalomyelitis. In *Clinical Neuroepidemiology*, p. 375. Atman Medical, London.

Behan, P. O. and Behan, W. (1988) Postviral fatigue syndrome. *CRC Critical Reviews in Neurobiology*.

Behan, P. O., Behan, W. M. H. and Bell, E. J. (1985) The postviral fatigue syndrome—an analysis of the findings in 50 cases. *Journal of Infection*, **10**, 211–222.

Gilliam, A. G. (1938) *Epidemiological Study of an Epidemic, Diagnosed as Poliomyelitis, Occurring Among the Personnel of The Los Angeles County General Hospital During the Summer of 1934*. Public Health Bulletin No. 240, United States Government Printing Office, Washington DC.

Hart, R. H. Correspondence. *New England Journal of Medicine*, **281**, 797.

Henderson, D. A. and Shelokov, A. (1959) Epidemic neuromyasthenia—clinical syndrome. *New England Journal of Medicine*, **260**, 757–764, 814–818.

Inoue, Y. K. (1971) Subacute myelo-optico-neuropathy. *Japanese Journal of Medical Science and Biology*, **24**, 195–216.

Jamal, G. A. and Hansen, S. (1985) Electrophysiological studies in the post-viral fatigue syndrome. *Journal of Neurology, Neurosurgery and Psychiatry*, **48**, 691–694.

Leon-Sotomayor, L. (1969) *Epidemic Diencephalomyelitis, a possible Cause of Neuropsychiatric, Cardiovascular and Endocrine Disorders*. Pageant Press International Corp., New York.

Marinacci, A. A. (1968) In *Applied Electromyography*, Leo and Febiger, Philadelphia.

Marinacci, A. A. and Van Hagen, K. O. (1965) The value of the electromyogram in the diagnosis of Iceland disease. *Bulletin of the Los Angeles Neurological Society*, **30**, 161–168.

Ramsay, A. M. (1988) *Minutes of Epidemic Myalgic Encephalomyelitis Study Group*, London.

Salahuddin, S. Z., Gallo, R. C. *et al.* (1986) Isolation of a new virus, HBLV, in patients with lymphoproliferative disorders. *Science*, **234**, 596–601.

Sigurdsson, B. and Gudmundsson, K. R. (1956) Clinical findings six years after outbreak of Akureyri disease. *Lancet*, **i**, 766–767.

Sigurdsson, B., Sigurjonsson, J., Sigurdsson, J. H. G., Thorkelsson, J. and Gudmundsson, K. R. (1950) A disease epidemic in Iceland simulating poliomyelitis. *American Journal of Hygiene*, **52**, 222–238.

Sigurdsson, B., Gudnadottir, M. and Peterson, G. (1958) Response to poliomyelitis vaccination. *Lancet*, **i**, 370–371.

Sigurjonssen, J. (1959) Poliomyelitis and the Akureyri disease. *Nordisk Medicine*, **61** (174), 1–10.

White, D. N. and Burtch, R. B. (1954) Iceland disease. A new infection simulating acute anterior poliomyelitis. *Neurology*, **4**, 506–516.

Wickman (1913) Acute poliomyelitis. *Journal of Nervous and Mental Disease*.

Yousef, G. E., Bell, E. J., Mann, G. F. *et al.* (1988) Chronic enterovirus infection in patients with post viral fatigue syndrome. *Lancet*, **i**, 146–150.

Part III

Clinical Assessment, Diagnosis and Approaches to Management

13

Presentation, Investigation and Diagnosis of PVFS (ME) in General Practice

Richard Stone

2 Garway Road, London, UK

You don't get a temperature with a nervous breakdown.

The above advice is from a GP who was an experienced doctor before World War II. He had many years of diagnosing without most of our laboratory techniques, and treating without penicillin and other modern drugs.

The GP of the 1980s and 1990s when faced with symptoms which could be due to myalgic encephalomyelitis (ME), is in the uncomfortable position of the pre-World War II doctor. She or he is faced with obvious illness, but without the tools we nowadays accept as standard. A thermometer in this situation can be the most helpful piece of equipment. The importance of taking the temperature can be shown by one example.

A woman of 29 came in asking for a tonic. The quickest reply in a busy surgery running half an hour late already is to prescribe a tonic and call the next patient. The doctor knows that all the scientific evidence shows that tonics are an expensive waste of time. However, prescribing this 'placebo' gives the patient what was asked for and allows the doctor to call the next patient quickly and make up, say, ten minutes. However, further questioning of this particular patient revealed a sexual problem. Her husband had told her to 'go to the doctor to get a tonic, or I'm leaving you'. Once again, the quick response is to give the number of the Marriage Guidance Council (= Relate), yet further questioning (we are now running three-quarters of an hour late) revealed a fairly sudden onset months previously of uncharacteristic tiredness, aches and pains of variable distribution, 'heaviness' all day, lack of concentration and, not surprisingly inability to face the effort of lovemaking. By now a GP who wishes to avoid loss of another doctor due to

Post-viral Fatigue Syndrome. Edited by R. Jenkins and J. Mowbray

nervous breakdown, or heart attack, will have found a way to organise something to be done which will end this consultation. However, it must bring the patient back, within a short enough time interval so that the patient is confident that the doctor is serious in trying to get to the bottom of the problem. It is actually quite easy and appropriate to order the necessary blood tests, the results of which will be available at a consultation in about a week. It is worth encouraging the patient to come in to the second consultation with her or his partner. The partner will be able to offer not just verification of the case history, but often extra insights and observations. The partners of ill people have good reason to be especially observant, often because of their frustration with not having 'the real you'. The natural desire to deny the illness may get in the way of noticing details. However, even the anger which results from that denial can produce flashes of clarity, e.g. 'it's always when you drink red wine' to which the ill person says 'but you never said that before'.

Above all, the patient must be asked to buy a thermometer 'and don't leave the chemist's shop until you have been shown how to read it'. The readings are pretty useless if done on a regular four-hourly basis as is usual for nurses to do in hospitals. The clinically logical thing to do is to 'take a full two-minute reading when you feel rotten, and again when you feel fairly all right. Then you can compare the readings to see if there is a pattern'. Women need to be informed (or reminded) that the temperature goes up in the second half of the menstrual cycle anyway.

If the temperature charts do show fevers, that is a proof of illness which is very helpful for the doctor. This is because the pursuit of the cause of a fever of unknown origin is a well-known clinical exercise for which doctors are well trained. For the patient it is a great reassurance to be able to see that there is a physical illness causing the vague symptoms.

Of course many people with symptoms suggestive of ME do not run fevers. However, it is alarming how many are told by their doctor that they are not ill, while the thermometer shows a physical feverish illness. The woman of 29 mentioned above took her positive temperature chart home to her parents for a rest. There she was seen by a GP who made a diagnosis of depression and referred her to a psychiatrist. It was only at the point where the psychiatrist recommended electroconvulsive therapy that she realised that 'this was no convalescence' and was certainly not an appropriate treatment for recurrent fever, and returned to her own flat, and her own GP.

INVESTIGATION

The preliminary laboratory tests to arrange, even in the absence of fevers, are FBC (full blood count), differential white count, ESR (Erythrocyte

Sedimentation Rate), Paul–Bunnell (for glandular fever), liver function tests and mid-stream specimen of urine (MSU). Other tests may be indicated by the history or examination, e.g. HIV test, or chest X-ray for TB. On the second visit a physical examination should include the heart, lungs, abdomen, glands, temperature, blood pressure and urinary sugar and albumen. It may be appropriate also to perform a basic neurological examination.

Two more specialised tests are recommended by Dr Charles Shepherd in his book *Living with ME—a Self-Help Guide* (Shepherd, 1989). These are (a) to exercise the patient to the point of fatigue, when it can sometimes be demonstrated that there is a definite muscle weakness, and (b) Dr Ramsay's test of exquisite points of tenderness in muscle—if found, these are also very suggestive of ME.

If the examination and the tests, as well as the temperature chart, are all normal, the doctor may dismiss the patient as fit and malingering. However, a sudden or even slow onset of rather vague symptoms in a previously fit active person is strongly suggestive of a physical cause. The onset may have been months or even some years previously, but the doctor must not be put off. Post-viral fatigue can persist for months after the viral fever has gone. The exhaustion, aches and depression of ME will similarly not show up on any tests.

Many patients do improve with one or two weeks resting in bed, off work and off alcohol. Those who remain ill warrant more specialist tests. These may require referral to a specialist in virology but the GP can at least take blood for paired sera for viral antibodies. Some GPs may have access to the viral protein 1 (VP1) test for enterovirus. The ME Association's booklet *Diagnostic and Clinical Guidelines for Doctors* (Myalgic Encephalomyelitis Association, 1989) can be very helpful at this stage.

PSYCHOLOGICAL ASPECTS

It is well worth explaining early on the diagnostic process to the patient and to her or his partner. It needs to be stressed that negative examination and tests could suggest either 'a physical illness for which doctors do not yet have a test, or a psychological response to some deep and severe stress'. It is all too easy in the recent enthusiasm for diagnosing post-viral fatigue and ME to ignore a psychological crisis or nervous breakdown. Given permission to look at physical and psychological causes of symptoms, patients may well come up themselves with an obvious psychological cause. Doctors must take up and deal with the psychological problem offered even when a physical cause is found. After all, we all know how emotional we can get when laid low with a fever or pain. The psychological problems that surface then are just as painful regardless of the physical illness going on.

In the same way, just because a psychological cause has been offered and accepted, the hunt for physical disease must not be called off. Apart from the fact that physical and psychological disease often coexist, for some distressed people it is a great comfort to have a physical diagnosis to hold on to.

DIAGNOSIS

The diagnosis is essentially based on the history, the current symptomatology and the exclusion of other illnesses which would account for the symptoms. ME must be remembered by GPs in the same way that in the old days we were taught that syphilis is the great mimic. Some patients have already made the diagnosis for themselves and professionals must not be put off because of this. 'Doctor, I think that I have ME. Please can I have a VP1 test.' This sort of apparently aggressive presentation should not be shrugged off, nor should it be yielded to without a full consideration of other possibilities.

The most common presentation is of a gradual or sudden change in activity level, and it is the change which is the cardinal sign. Somebody who was active and leading a normal life, and then became unable to continue it, must be considered as having acquired an illness, and the differential diagnosis is considered below. The classical presentation of ME is that the fatigue is overwhelming (far worse than is seen in patients who are simply depressed), and is accompanied by muscle pains, and paraesthesiae. However, the latter two symptoms are not always present and patients who have these symptoms do not always volunteer them, and it may be necessary to ask direct questions to elicit them. The muscle pains are characteristically variable in distribution, and are not focused on joints.

In the face of an obviously ill person in whom all tests and examination are negative, the possible diagnoses are:

(a) Post-viral fatigue.
(b) ME.
(c) Glandular fever syndrome (i.e. a persisting low-grade viral illness which is either glandular fever, cytomegalovirus, Epstein–Barr virus or other non-identifiable virus).
(d) Food allergy or intolerance.
(e) Psychological crisis.
(f) Mental illness, e.g. depression or phobia.

Medical science has little to offer in confirming the diagnosis and doctors may be tempted to dismiss the patient as either 'Not ill—go back to work' or else 'You are ill I suppose, but I cannot do anything about it.'

However, the opportunity should not be lost to reassure the patient that the normality of all the tests and examination in themselves show the patient and the doctor what illnesses the patient has *not* got, e.g. TB, cancer, AIDS, leukaemia. Doctors may take it for granted that none of these illnesses is present, but the patient or the patient's relatives may not have dared to ask about their worst fears. The fears will inevitably be exaggerated because the doctor, having excluded serious illness very early on, has not thought to spell out the exclusion of serious illness.

TREATMENT

Support

Whatever the cause, support of the patient by the doctor is in itself therapeutic.

Rest

Encouragement to 'listen to your body and do what it tells you' can give permission not to drive the body into a worse sick state. A short or even long afternoon sleep will break an otherwise long day, and such advice may need a letter from the doctor recommending it. Devising ways of conserving energy for only those activities which really matter needs a lot of discussion and support. The temptation 'to go back to tennis' is hard to resist.

Pain relief

When the pains are very severe, they do not respond to ordinary analgesics and from time to time doctors do have to resort to opiates. Obviously, these should be a last resort. Those patients who have to live with months of severe pain generally prefer to avoid chronic consumption of analgesics of any sort and they may benefit from alternative methods of pain relief.

No alcohol

For many people even a little alcohol brings on symptoms with a vengeance and it is worth encouraging even those who do not notice such a link to stop all alcohol for one year.

Food

Careful exclusion and re-inclusion diets can throw up a clear link with certain foods. This is a most satisfying cause of the illness to find, if it is

there. The book *Food Allergy and Intolerance* by Brostoff and Gamlin (1989) is
one of the best to sort this out.

Gammaglobulin

Particularly in the face of a raised VP1 test, triple doses of normal gammaglobulin can benefit as many as half of patients. All patients should keep a
daily log of their symptoms in order of their severity. Thus, for example, if
fatigue is the main symptom and generalized aches another, then the patient
could keep a score, e.g. 2 out of 10 or 8 out of 10 at the end of each day. If
scores are on the high side before gammaglobulin is given and markedly on
the low side for some weeks afterwards, then there is a strong likelihood
that it was the injection that caused the improvement. This benefit may last
for several months and occasionally even be permanent. If the improvement
is dramatically lost after weeks or months then it may be worth giving a
repeat injection. As the ABPI Data Sheet Compendium states, gammaglobulin 'is generally well tolerated without reactions', but it is worth checking with the data sheet that comes with the vials before giving an injection.
Further 'overdosage need not be expected to lead to more frequent or more
severe adverse reactions than the recommended dose'. The theory behind
giving high doses of gammaglobulin is that, in some patients with an ME-
like illness, the body may only produce 'partial antibodies' to a virus. The
result is that when viruses appear in the bloodstream there may be a low-
grade fever and/or the patient may feel ill. The body is able to neutralize
those viruses but is unable to eliminate the virus totally from the body and
therefore further viraemia (leakage of virus into the bloodstream) will cause
recurrence of the symptoms. If high doses of pooled normal antibodies from
the general population are given, the body will have a supply of complete
antibodies which will last until those are removed, as all antibodies are, in
two to three months (Mowbray, personal communication). The dose for
these patients may need to be two or even three times the normal maximum
recommended dose of pooled normal human gammaglobulin.

REFERENCES

Brostaff, J. and Gamlin, L. (1989) *Food Allergy and Intolerance*. Bloomsbury Publica-
    tions, London.
Myalgic Encephalomyelitis Association (1989) *Diagnostic and Clinical Guidelines for
    Doctors*. Myalgic Encephalomyelitis Association, Stanford Le-Hope, Essex.
Shepherd, C. (1989) *Living with ME—A Self-Help Guide*. Cedar, Heinemann Publica-
    tions, London.

14

Post-viral Fatigue Syndrome and the Cardiologist

R. G. Gold

Freeman Hospital, Newcastle-upon-Tyne, UK

The patient suffering from Post-viral fatigue syndrome (ME) is referred to a cardiologist almost always because of chest pain. A small number of patients who seek cardiological advice experience shortness of breath and/or palpitations as their main symptoms. The usual cause of the chest pain in these patients is chronic benign pericarditis. When we reviewed this condition in 1967 we suggested that 'viral pericarditis' was unlikely to be a direct result of a virus infection, as identical clinical features can be produced by widely differing mechanisms such as myocardial infarction (Dressler's syndrome), cardiac surgery (postcardiotomy syndrome), trauma and drug reactions. We felt then that the pericarditis was the final common pathway in an abnormal immunological response, and that the above 'causes' were triggering mechanisms for this response (Gold, 1967). In 'viral' pericarditis, as with ME, there is now abundant evidence that the disease process arises from an abnormal response to a virus infection, most commonly the Coxsackie B group (Muir *et al.*, 1989; Archard *et al.*, 1988; Easton and Eglin, 1988; Yousef *et al.*, 1987). The history of an antecedent virus infection is, however, often lacking in such patients, probably because of the chronic nature of the condition which may have been present for several years before a cardiological opinion is sought. At this stage, all the usual laboratory tests to provide evidence of previous or ongoing viral infection are negative. Although the presence of a pericardial friction rub provides strong clinical confirmatory evidence of the diagnosis, this is often absent or transient and the diagnosis frequently depends on a carefully taken history. Fortunately the pain of pericarditis has some highly characteristic features (see below) which suggest the diagnosis to the clinician who is aware of these.

Post-viral Fatigue Syndrome. Edited by R. Jenkins and J. Mowbray
© 1991 John Wiley & Sons Ltd.

All too often, however, the preconceived notion that the pain must be angina until proved otherwise leads to a label of 'atypical chest pain' being attached to the patient. To the experienced observer the pain of pericarditis is almost as typical of that condition as classical angina pectoris is of ischaemic heart disease. There are, however, several overlapping features between the two conditions and it is therefore not surprising that the patient often reaches the cardiologist with an erroneous clinical diagnosis of coronary artery disease having already been made. It is, of course, equally important that, because of an associated history of ME, the clinician does not jump to the conclusion that the chest pain is due to pericarditis, thereby missing coexistent coronary artery disease.

HISTORY

The patient may be of any age and of either sex but the condition is most common in the third and fourth decades. In chronic or recurrent pericarditis a history of an antecedent virus infection is often absent.

Chest pain is variable in character. It is sometimes severe, sharp and stabbing, or it may be dull and aching. It is unrelated to the act of exertion though the patient frequently feels the pain to be worse after a day of increased physical activity. Such a patient, when asked whether the pain is related to exertion, will often give a misleading affirmative response and the true relationship is only established by further questioning as to whether the pain occurs *during* exercise or *after* extra activity, perhaps several hours later. The pain may last for several hours or even days. It frequently occurs centrally but even in the same patient may recur on a different occasion in the right or left chest or the back. It is commonly aggravated by sudden movement, changes of posture, respiration or swallowing (McGuire *et al.*, 1954; Gold, 1967). It may radiate to the shoulder tip.

These features should help to distinguish the pain of pericarditis from that of ischaemic heart disease, but not infrequently pericarditic pain may radiate down the inside of one or both arms, thus making clinical differentiation difficult.

Although pyrexia may be present in acute pericarditis, this is seldom a feature of the chronic condition with which most ME patients will present.

The patient may complain of shortness of breath but this is, in our experience, rarely true dyspnoea. It is, rather, a subjective feeling of not being able to breath deeply enough, possibly a manifestation of fatigue of the voluntary muscles of respiration.

Palpitations are frequent, with sinus tachycardia being a common and at times troublesome symptom (Dressler, 1966). Other arrhythmias such as atrial fibrillation, supraventricular and ventricular premature beats and atrial flutter may occur (Soffer, 1960). Ventricular tachycardia seldom if ever occurs with pericarditis and its presence should suggest an associated myocarditis or dilated cardiomyopathy.

As with ME itself, severe listlessness and ready fatigue are very common symptoms but it must be emphasised that the other features of ME are frequently lacking in patients with pericarditis. The symptoms of ME and of pericarditis should thus not be regarded as part of a spectrum of symptoms from the one illness but rather as an expression of involvement of different and organs by a common abnormality of immunological response to a viral infection.

EXAMINATION FINDINGS

A pericardial friction rub is probably presesnt in most patients at some stage of the illness. However, it may be extremely transitory, disappearing within a matter of hours. Auscultation of the heart several times during the day in different postures may be necessary to detect it but even this may be unrewarding. The presence and behaviour of the pericardial rub is independent of the presence and intensity of pain. The effect of respiration is very variable and occasionally the patient's posture is critical, the rub being heard only, for example, when the patient bends forward or in a particular phase of inspiration or expiration (Bradley, 1964). The heart sounds are otherwise normal.

Manifestations of cardiac failure are universally absent in uncomplicated pericarditis and the presence of a third or fourth heart sound should suggest the presence of an underlying cardiomyopathy or myocarditis.

Pericardial effusion is seldom sufficient to be clinically detectable and the jugular venous pressure is therefore almost always normal. If it is markedly elevated, pericardial tamponade or constriction should be suspected though these again are rare complications of pericarditis.

INVESTIGATIONS

The chest x-ray is seldom abnormal in uncomplicated pericarditis. Radiological evidence of an associated pneumonitis may be present, but this is, in our experience, uncommon. Enlargement of the cardiac silhouette may be due to pericardial effusion or to a dilated cardiomyopathy. The presence of either of these conditions can be readily confirmed by echocardiography.

The electrocardiogram in chronic or recurrent pericarditis seldom shows the classical features (Porte and Pardee, 1929) of ST segment elevation with preservation of its upward concavity, and is usually normal or shows merely nonspecific T wave flattening or shallow inversion. Treadmill exercise electrocardiography is normal, showing at most mild exaggeration of any ST and T wave abnormalities present in the resting record, and is thus a useful diagnostic tool in excluding ischaemic heart disease as a cause of the chest pain. In a borderline case an exercise thallium scan of the heart should be carried out. Particularly in those patients who are thought to have been diagnosed erroneously as suffering from angina coronary artery disease, coronary angiography should be advised if, after the above investigations, the diagnosis remains in any doubt.

Echocardiography will often be completely normal, but should be carried out routinely as it may reveal some pericardial thickening or the presence of a subclinical amount of pericardial effusion. Furthermore, demonstration of normal ventricular dimensions and function is valuable reassurance that there is not an underlying myocarditis or dilated cardiomyopathy.

Laboratory investigations are almost always unhelpful. Their main role is to exclude other conditions which are associated with pericarditis. For example, a markedly elevated erythrocyte sedimentation rate may point to an underlying collagen disease responsible for the pericarditis. The various virological and immunological tests used as an aid to diagnosis of ME are discussed elsewhere. None of these, unfortunately, is of any specific value in diagnosing pericarditis of viral origin when ME is already present.

SUMMARY

The diagnosis of the cause of chest pain as a complication of ME rests almost entirely on careful clinical evaluation. The value of further investigation by the various methods discussed above is chiefly to exclude other conditions with a more sinister prognosis than chronic benign pericarditis. Although the latter may continue or recur for many years and, like ME, be a distressing and debilitating illness, the tendency is for the attacks to become less severe and less frequent with the passage of time and the ultimate prognosis is excellent. There is, alas, no way of predicting how long the condition will persist, and no reliably successful means of treating it.

Although we have found that some patients respond temporarily to immunoglobulin either by intramuscular injection (Al Kadiry et al., 1983) or by intravenous infusion, or to infusion of contact donor plasma (Gold, unpublished observations), the main role of the clinician is to provide symptomatic relief and sympathetic support, including a full explanation of the condition, guidance on how patients can adjust their lifestyles to cope with their illness and reassurance that their illness is not 'all in the mind' and that the ultimate outlook is favourable.

REFERENCES

Al Kadiry, W. A., Gold, R. G., Behan, P. O. and Mowbray, J. F. (1983) Analysis of antigens in the circulating immune complexes of patients with Coxsackie infections. *Progress in Brain Research*, **59**, 61–67.

Archard, L. C., Behan, P. O., Bowles, N. E., Bell, E. J. and Doyle, D. (1988) Postviral fatigue syndrome: persistence of enterovirus RNA in muscle and elevated creatine kinase. *Journal of the Royal Society of Medicine*, **81**, 326–329.

Bradley, E. C. (1964) Acute benign pericarditis. *American Heart Journal*, **67**, 121–132.

Dressler, W. (1966) Sinus tachycardia complicating and outlasting pericarditis. *American Heart Journal*, **72**, 422–423.

Easton, A. J. and Eglin, R. P. (1988) The detection of Coxsackievirus RNA in cardiac tissue by in situ hybridization. *Journal of General Virology*, **69**, 285–291.

Gold, R. G. (1967) Acute non-specific pericarditis. *Postgraduate Medical Journal*, **43**, 534–538.

McGuire, J., Kotte, J. H. and Helm, R. A. (1954) Clinical progress. Acute pericarditis. *Circulation*, **9**, 425–442.

Muir, P., Nicholson, F., Tilzey, A. J., Signy, M., English, T. A. H. and Banatvala, J. E. (1989) Chronic relapsing pericarditis and dilated cardiomyopathy: serological evidence of persistent enterovirus infection. *Lancet*, **1**, 804–807.

Porte, D. and Pardee, H. E. B. (1929) Occurrence of coronary T wave in rheumatic pericarditis. *American Heart Journal*, **4**, 584–590.

Soffer, A. (1960) Electrocardiographic abnormality in acute, convalescent and recurrent stages of idiopathic pericarditis. *American Heart Journal*, **60**, 729–738.

Yousef, G. E., Mann, G. F., Brown, I. N. and Mowbray, J. F. (1987) Clinical and research application of an enterovirus group-reactive monoclonal antibody. *Intervirology*, **28**, 199–205.

15

Chronic Post-viral Fatigue Syndrome: Presentation and Management in the Neurology Clinic

H. E. Webb and Linda M. Parsons

St Thomas' Hospital, London, UK

As practising neurologists, actively involved in research on virus-induced neurological conditions, it was natural for us to take an interest in this problem.

One of us (H.E.W.), having acted as general practitioner to the staff at St Thomas' Hospital since 1962, has over the years frequently encountered the symptom of abnormal fatigue in this particular population, following many different virus infections, including glandular fever, shingles, chicken-pox, influenza and enteroviruses. In 1967 amongst nursing and paramedical staff at St Thomas' there was an outbreak of a nonspecific viral-like illness similar to that described as Royal Free disease, with low-grade pyrexia, myalgia, paraesthesiae of extremities, headache, some photophobia and vague urinary symptoms. This lasted four to five days and was followed in a proportion of those affected by severe fatigue, persistence of muscle pain, sleep disturbances and depressed mood, which delayed a return to work. Personality studies carried out on 16 of those affected with this postinfection fatigue state showed no common personality pattern and no evidence that the condition was due to hysteria.

It is well accepted that a short period of nonspecific malaise may follow a viral infection but it is usually self-limiting. However, persistent disabling fatigue, often lasting months and sometimes years, is less common but a definite clinical entity. Well-known other associated features of this prolonged post-viral fatigue state include sore throat, myalgia, arthralgia, mood disturbance, poor memory and concentration and disorders of sleep pattern. Patients with these varying symptoms will usually present first to their general practitioner and then, because of the diversity of symptoms, may be

Post-viral Fatigue Syndrome. Edited by R. Jenkins and J. Mowbray
© 1991 John Wiley & Sons Ltd

referred to any medical sub-speciality, including general medicine, rheumatology and neurology. After several such referrals, associated usually with no abnormality of clinical findings or investigations and with no satisfactory explanation being offered, many patients feel that conventional medicine has failed them. They have then gone either 'doctor shopping' for help or have turned to alternative non-conventional treatments.

Over the years there have been sporadic referrals of patients with chronic fatigue states to the neurology department at this hospital but as interest in and awareness of this condition have increased so the numbers referred have grown. Recently we have been able to study a group of these patients who have been referred to the neurology clinic with a putative diagnosis of chronic post-viral fatigue. The majority have come to the clinic many months and, in some cases, years after their original illness (see Table 3). They provide a useful basis for describing our approach to the diagnosis and our management of this group of patients which we find has been of considerable benefit.

HISTORY

An accurate history taken from the patient is very important. Fifty-three patients were referred as having either 'myalgic encephalomyelitis' or post-viral fatigue. All except two had symptoms dating from a documented febrile illness which, with our present understanding, would be acceptable as viral in origin. This is an important point, as the *sine qua non* for a post-viral fatigue state is that the patient should actually have had an infection. Some patients who label themselves as 'ME' have not, on close questioning, ever had an illness, febrile or otherwise. It is useful to take a careful past history, particularly in relation to performance at school, jobs held, time off work each year due to sickness and, in women, how much time is missed due to problems at period times. In this way it is possible to identify people who have a low threshold for sickness and absence. They may also be genuinely suffering from post-viral fatigue but we find the prognosis in this group to be less good.

Post-viral fatigue can affect any age group, as illustrated by Table 1 which shows the age range and sex distribution of our 51 patients. This condition also crosses social divides, the occupations of our patients being shown in Table 2.

Whilst we have not carried out any formal personality studies, it is our strong impression that the majority of patients affected were normal people who were extremely confused regarding what had happened to them and were frustrated by their inability to get better. However, there were some in who a vulnerable personality could be identified, in that there was evidence

Table 1 Sex and age range of 51 patients having post-viral fatigue

	Number	Age range
Male	20	12–60
Female	31	17–55

Table 2 Occupations of 51 patients with post-viral fatigue

Doctor	3	Inspector	1
Nurse	5	Catering assistant	1
Solicitor	2	Secretary	2
Teacher	6	TV Producer	1
Scientist	1	Computer operator	1
Civil servant	3	Technician	2
Banker	2	Student	6
Company director	1	Housewife	3
Managerial	6	Unemployed	1
Social worker	4		

of a poor response to life events in the past, or a previous depressive episode or a cyclothymic mood tendency, or they had responded in a similar way to a previous viral infection (five of 51 patients).

Many patients have needed to take considerable time off work. In our series five had actually resigned from their jobs completely and four had over six months off sick. Some 16 patients managed time off, varying between odd days and some weeks and 14 had needed up to six months. In 11 of our patients the time between the original illness and being seen by us ranged between two and nine years and in 22 the time to referral was anything from eight months to two years (see Table 3). These figures indicate just how damaging this condition is to the quality of life and work output of the people affected and how important it is to reach a diagnosis and treat the patients appropriately as early as possible.

We have found it essential when first meeting the patient to indicate that their story as to how awful they felt would be believed in spite of all previous normal examinations and investigations. Many had been seen by 'unbelievers' in various specialities and needed careful sympathetic handling in order to build up rapport. Patients frequently stated that in the past they had

Table 3 Time between illness and first clinic visit

Under 1 year	25
1–2 years	15
> 2 years	11 (2–9 years)
Total	51

not been considered as having a genuine problem, which had caused considerable resentment.

The main complaints were usually intense lassitude, which was noted by all 51 of our patients. However, exertional fatigue was also prominent (reported in 33 patients). Poor concentration and poor memory were also common complaints (24 and nine patients respectively). Other symptoms which are often more associated with depressive illness were not volunteered, appearing only on direct questioning, but form a prominent part of the symptomatology of the syndrome. However, the patient may not relate them to the problem. It is our policy first to ask specifically about disturbance in sleep pattern (reported in 29 patients). This may take the form of early-morning waking, difficulty in getting off to sleep or indeed excessive sleepiness. Secondly, mood disturbance is also important. Although not as prominent as in more conventional depressive illness, it is nevertheless present in post-viral fatigue states with tearfulness and negative feelings. Suicidal intent is uncommon in our experience, but should be enquired about; suicides have been reported in relation to this condition. Feelings of paranoia and extreme worthlessness do not appear to be prominent. Thirdly, libido is often reduced (11 out of 52 patients admitted to this). This aspect is rarely volunteered by the patient and requires specific sympathetic enquiry.

Other somatic symptoms do occur. In our series of patients myalgia, headache, sore throats, weight loss and 'pins and needles' were mentioned by a minority of patients. These symptoms appear to be more prominent in the more acute stages of the illness as are fever, muscle twitching and lymphadenopathy. In our patients fatigue, lassitude, sleep disturbance and poor memory and concentration were the predominant complaints. In the case of 'pins and needles', enquiry should be made to exclude hyperventilation—often an accompaniment of an anxiety state. Where weight loss occurs, questions should be asked regarding eating patterns, and thyroid disease excluded.

It goes without saying that enquiry into other aspects of general health, together with medication, should be made. Family history may be relevant. We have had one patient whose father responded in a similar way following an attack of hepatitis A. There may also be a family history of depression (two of our 51 patients).

EXAMINATION

Full physical examination is essential. In post-viral fatigue, abnormal physical signs are conspicuously absent. A salutory tale is of the lady referred to as having post-viral fatigue who, on examination, had a spastic paraparesis from a spinal cord lesion. Special attention should be paid to muscle, particularly in those complaining of myalgia, to exclude the possibility of an active myositis. Recent work suggests that in patients who do not have viral myositis, muscle power is normal, there being altered perception of the effort required (Stokes *et al.*, 1988; Lloyd *et al.*, 1988).

INVESTIGATIONS

Many patients reach the neurological clinic having already been fully investigated. There is little point in repeating tests which have previously given normal results. However, it is often useful to ensure that some particular investigations have been done prior to starting medication (Table 4).

Most of the patients show little abnormality except for evidence of a past viral infection. In our series of patients we were satisfied that four had had herpes zoster, 12 glandular fever, four Coxsackie B infection, one hepatitis A and one cytomegalovirus. Twenty-nine had a flu-like illness, in which viral studies were not done at the right time or were not helpful.

MANAGEMENT

Our management of patients with post-viral fatigue is based on our belief that the condition forms part of the spectrum of a depressive illness, triggered by a viral infection. The rationale for this viewpoint is considered fully in Chapter 21. Suffice it to say at this point that the mainstay of our treatment is antidepressants together with careful sympathetic handling of the individual patient. As has been mentioned previously, the importance of rapport in the management of these patients cannot be overemphasised. Patients who reach our clinic after seeing several others are often deeply

Table 4   Investigations

Full blood count	Particularly in women for iron deficiency anaemia
Erythrocyte sedimentation rate	For collagen diseases, associated with myositis
Urea and electrolytes	
Serum calcium	Abnormalities may present as unexplained fatigue
Liver function tests	
Thyroid function tests	
Antinuclear factor	Particularly in women for collagen diseases
Creatine kinase	For active muscle disease
Viral antibody screen	If referred early enough and preferably with paired sera

suspicious of being labelled as depressive and this is carefully avoided. Careful explanation is needed in order to achieve compliance. The major emphasis of our explanation centres on our belief that viruses can alter enzyme systems and neurotransmitters in the brain, producing problems with energy, mood and drive without producing frank neurological abnormalities. We explain that we believe that the medication improves these biochemical changes in the brain and hence the symptoms.

We have found treatment with tricyclic antidepressants, chiefly amitriptyline or trimipramine, and monoamine oxidase inhibitors, mainly phenelzine, for periods ranging from three months to over a year extremely successful. Those who suffer sleep disturbance, particularly with early-morning wakening, are treated with tricyclics, which are always given at night. It is important not to start with too large a dose as some patients are extremely sensitive to this class of drug and even a small dose may produce excess drowsiness the next day, which they dislike and often causes them to stop taking medication. We allow our patients to adjust the dosage themselves so that they get a good night's sleep with minimal morning 'hang-over' but with a nightly dose limit of 150 mg. We find that the majority of patients, given this responsibility, handle their medication very sensibly. The average amount taken at night was 50 mg and none reached 150 mg. It is well known that tricyclic antidepressants have a lag phase of roughly 14 days before benefit is noticed. Because of this we have found it essential to explain to patients that although their sleep pattern might improve immediately on starting medication, their fatigue and other symptoms will not be affected for at least two to three weeks after starting treatment. Indeed, we point out that they might even feel more lethargic because of the sedative effect of these drugs initially. We emphasise that they must persevere for this length of time in order to find out whether the treatment will be helpful. In patients with excessive sleep, phenelzine has been the drug of choice, given in the dose of 30 mg in the morning and 15 mg at noon, again with strict instructions that they should persevere for at least three weeks for the same reasons. The appropriate food and drug restrictions are of course, explained together with warnings regarding postural hypotension. Patients with meticulous, obsessional personalities also seem to be suited better to phenelzine.

It is explained that the minimum length of time for medication will be three months and that they should not stop taking the tablets suddenly because they feel better. Once improvement has been maintained our policy is to reduce by one tablet every two to three weeks, the patient assessing how they feel following this reduction. It has sometimes been found necessary to increase the dosage again if symptoms return, until well-being is achieved and confidence maintained. Cautious reduction can then be recommended. Treatment has sometimes been continued for over a year, still with satisfactory withdrawal.

Of our 51 patients, 36 (72%) were greatly improved and returned to full-time work with an excellent quality of life, and 12 (23%) showed considerable improvement but as yet are not back to their pre-illness state. Unfortunately, two patients were not compliant, and one patient was loath to take treatment because she was pregnant.

Somatic symptoms such as headaches and myalgia were also greatly improved following treatment with antidepressants, suggesting that these too have a strong central component. Similar improvements have been documented in chronic pain syndrome following the use of antidepressants (Watson *et al.*, 1988).

In those patients who did not respond satisfactorily to one single drug, usually the tricyclic, phenelzine was added with obvious benefit. Apart from patients occasionally feeling worse during the initial period there have not been any significant problems from using these drugs together over the past 27 years.

Using this form of treatment together with sympathetic understanding, good rapport and gentle persuasion to build on any improvements, we have successfully treated this condition and feel that antidepressants should be considered the treatment of choice in the post-viral fatigue syndrome.

REFERENCES

Lloyd, A., Hales, J. and Grandevia, S. (1988) Muscle strength, endurance and recovery in the post infection fatigue syndrome. *Journal of Neurology, Neurosurgery and Psychiatry*, **51**, 1316–1322.

Stokes, M. J., Cooper, R. G. and Edwards, R. H. T. (1988) Normal strength and fatiguability in patients with effort syndrome. *British Medical Journal*, **297**, 1014–1017.

Watson, C. P. N., Evans, R. J., Watt, V. R. and Burkitt, N. (1988) Post hepetic neuralgia: 208 cases. *Pain*, **35**, 289–297.

16

Assessment and Diagnosis of ME in the Psychiatric Clinic

Rachel Jenkins

Institute of Psychiatry, London, UK

INTRODUCTION

Once one is familiar with the concept of post-viral fatigue syndrome, such patients are in practice not too difficult to differentiate from those with true psychiatric illness such as depressive illnesses, anxiety, hypochondriasis or hysteria. However, until practitioners are familiar with the concept, these patients present a puzzling diagostic and management dilemma. I well remember one patient, a man in his early 40s, whose psychiatrist had written in despair to the referring physician 'This man is extremely neurotic—I can do nothing for him'. This comment, of course, sums up the diagnostic fallacy. Neurosis is in general eminently treatable; depressive neurosis responds to antidepressants, supportive psychotherapy and appropriate management of social difficulties; anxiety neurosis responds to behaviour therapy and so do phobias and obsessional neurosis. Three years later, when I took over the man's care, neither the first psychiatrist nor myself considered the possibility that the primary diagnosis of neurosis was mistaken, and I continued to try psychological treatments with no benefits. However, about 18 months later, after I had become familiar with the concept of ME and read various descriptions of its history and presentation, I reviewed this man's case and there in the case notes found all the evidence which should have alerted me much earlier to the diagnosis of post-viral fatigue syndrome. In his first assessment interview, the patient had described severe fatigue and fluctuating physical and psychological symptoms following a severe viral infection. It was then possible to institute a more effective management programme.

Post-viral Fatigue Syndrome. Edited by R. Jenkins and J. Mowbray
© 1991 John Wiley & Sons Ltd

PSYCHOLOGICAL SYMPTOMS IN ME

In a depressive illness, *mood* tends to be more consistently low, whereas in ME, if depressed mood is present, it is labile and will characteristically include bursts of enthusiasm and cheerfulness. Rapid mood swings occur, closely related to physical energy and fatigue, and to the presence or absence of other physical symptoms, including fevers. The classical diurnal variation of mood in severe depressive illness, with the patient waking feeling suicidal, and then improving towards the evening, is not seen. The patient may start the day feeling reasonably well, but quickly become fatigued and low. Alternatively, the patient may waken feeling nauseated, aching, feverish and tired, but gradually improve towards midday and then fatigue again during the course of the afternoon. In general, the patient with ME will relate their depression to the frustration felt at not being able to do the active things they enjoy doing although they will maintain enjoyment of passive pursuits; whereas the depressed patient will have lost interest in doing all the things they used to enjoy, whether active or passive.

The *fatigue* in a depressive illness tends to be low grade and psychological in origin. The patient feels fatigued and will be unmotivated to exercise, but can do most activities if required and sustain them, including climbing a hillside, swimming for an hour, standing upright for two hours or carrying a heavy object, such as a bucket of water or a bag of shopping, without too much physical difficulty. The sufferer with ME, on the other hand, cannot do more than a fraction of these activities, and a very small amount of activity (e.g. climbing two or three flights of stairs) results in the person literally feeling as if they had just run a marathon. Patients with ME try to continue their previous levels of activity, and this results in severe relapses entailing days or weeks of bedrest. They subsequently learn, either unaided or with advice to restrict their physical and mental activity and to intersperse it with regular rest periods so that they can sustain some level of activity, albeit much reduced. Patients are often particularly exhausted at the end of the day, and tend to go to bed very early, and thus will report greatly restricted social and leisure lives.

Some patients say that they feel as if they have relatively normal amounts of energy at the start of exercise, but that the energy is quickly used up, leaving extreme fatigue in its wake. One patient, a middle-aged male civil engineer, with a two-year history of post-viral syndrome (which had necessitated him changing job to an administrative post), told me that he was sometimes still able to go to the gym and practise lifting weights for short periods of time, but that afterwards he felt 'as if the central motor isn't functioning properly'. Someone else (medically qualified) described the fatigue following activity as 'it's as if my body has suddenly used up all the available ATP'.

There are also subtle differences between the impairment of *concentration* in depression and that in ME. In depression, the impairment of concentration tends to parallel the depth of depression, whereas in ME, the impairment of concentration tends to be associated with the timing and severity of the fatigue. Mental fatiguability occurs in the same way as physical fatiguability, and a short period of mental concentration may leave the patient feeling physically drained. Likewise, physical activity may leave the patient unable to exert themselves mentally. In addition, *specific cognitive abnormalities* are present in ME, including difficulty in marshalling material, difficulty in finding the correct words in a sentence, and inappropriate syntax, which can cause amusement to family and friends. (These cognitive abnormalities are described in detail in Chapter 10.) Family may report that memory is affected, that speech is sometimes slurred, and that the patient appears more *clumsy* than usual. They tend to bump into doorways and furniture more frequently, may display old bruises, and may complain of a feeling of disequilibrium.

The *sleep pattern* is usually very disturbed. In the early acute phase of the illness, the patient may sleep for as little as one to two hours a night unaided. However, in the later phases of the illness hypersomnia is the norm, and the patient may regularly sleep for 12–14 hours a day. Patients often report that they dream very vividly during this period.

Irritability is often a prominent aspect of ME. Outbursts of irritability are common, and relatives may report that these are totally uncharacteristic of the patient. The patient may describe to the doctor how frustrated and angry they feel at their illness, and their inability to get better. In addition they may express hostility to the medical profession if they have received scant sympathy and understanding in the past.

Anxiety is also common, particularly in the early stages of ME. Patients with ME often report waves of severe psychic anxiety occurring for no reason, most often in the afternoons. In addition, patients who have had an alarming time at the hands of doctors, with extensive medical investigations, and no clear diagnosis, often become secondarily frightened and every new symptom serves only to terrify them further, until they acquire a continuous anxiety state, with the usual physical and psychological symptoms. Such a secondary anxiety state is treatable long before the ME itself resolves.

I have not in my clinic seen any worsening of pre-existing phobias or obsessive compulsive traits in ME. Some of the *physical symptoms* which patients may report should be an aid to diagnosis, although they may be wrongly attributed to primary psychological illness unless care is taken in eliciting them.

PHYSICAL SYMPTOMS IN ME

Palpitations in ME, usually described as a fluttering in the chest and some-times accompanied by pain over the left chest, are common, leading to anxiety over possible heart disease. Ectopic beats are also common. These phenomena may readily be distinguished from the regular rapid powerful heart beats of a panic attack. Occasionally the patient experiences angor animi. Paraesthesiae are also very common in ME, particularly in the early months, and tend to be continuous, unlike the paraesthesiae of overbreathing, which are essentially transient. Many patients complain of cold hands and feet. Most patients experience muscle twitches which can sometimes be observed, particularly in the muscles of the thigh. These are twitches or gross fasciculations of a group of muscle fibres, but are not the gross tremor seen in anxiety states. However, patients are often clumsy, and will report dropping things in the kitchen, bumping shoulders into doorposts, and hips against chairs and tables, and old bruises will be visible on examination.

Muscle pain is a common symptom, but the severity is variable, ranging from a few patients who are clearly in agony with muscle pains, particularly in shoulders and legs, to the majority of patients for whom the fatigue is a much more prominent symptom than the pain. The pains tend not to re-spond to simple analgesics, and in my view analgesic medication is best avoided in chronic pain because of the attendant risks of long-term consumption of analgesics.

Bowels are usually disturbed, with abdominal pains, and alternating constipation and diarrhoea is a common complaint. Bladder function is often disturbed with intermittent dysuria. The normal diurnal pattern of urinary production is often reversed, with concentration of urine in the day, and a diuresis at night, necessitating waking to void the bladder once or twice in the middle of the night. The menstrual cycle is usually disturbed in women, with missed periods, lengthened or shortened cycles, and heavy protracted bleeding all being reported.

THE HISTORIES

The histories presented by patients appearing in my outpatient clinic were all fairly similar, the principal features being previous good health and level of physical activity, some degree of 'overwork' for six months or more, followed by a severe viral infection from which a good recovery was not made. Instead the patient became progressively more fatigued over the ensuing weeks and months, irritable, with poor concentration and fluctuating depressive and anxiety symptoms, and displayed a number of characteristic physical symptoms, including mild fevers, aches and pains, lymphadenopathy, pain in the back of the neck, feelings of hot and cold sensation, dizziness, paraesthesia etc.

The family history and personal histories were generally unremarkable although there was a definite tendency for those patients with post-viral fatigue syndrome to have previously been in active, stressful occupations, but not necessarily professional ones. Although women are said to outnumber men, I saw roughly equal numbers of both sexes with this condition in my clinic.

SOURCE OF REFERRAL

Patients were referred to me from a variety of sources. Those with prominent psychological symptoms tended to reach me directly via the GP, those with prominent cardiac symptoms were referred to me by the local cardiologists, and those with prominent paraesthesiae tended to reach me via the neurologists.

I investigated these patients in the usual way, doing a physical examination, routine blood tests, including haemaglobin, Erythrocyte sedimentation rate, full blood count, and urea and electrolytes, liver function tests, and thyroid function tests. In addition, I would send blood to the immunopathology laboratory at St Mary's Hospital, Paddington for VP1 (see Chapter 3). The results of most investigations were essentially normal. The ESR was, interestingly, always extremely low, 0–2 mm/h. The VP1 test was only positive in a few of my patients, but all had damaged complement levels.

DIAGNOSIS AND MANAGEMENT

The diagnosis of post-viral fatigue syndrome is essentially a clinical diagnosis, based on the history of a viral illness from which complete recovery has not occurred, coupled with the onset and persistence of characteristic symptoms over a period of several months. Management is discussed in later chapters but, in essence, is adequate rest coupled with gentle, graded activity, always staying within one's limits and never overdoing it. Under this regime, the limits of physical activity gradually increase, whereas under a regime of pushing beyond the physical limits, severe relapses occur and physical limits decrease. This is the opposite of what happens in a depressed person who is otherwise physically well, where steady pushing beyond physical limits (within reasonable bounds) will extend those limits and increase physical fitness. It is of course very difficult to stay within one's limits, and careful planning is needed. A medical colleague, who had had the illness some years before, graphically described to me how he had gone for a walk until he was tired, only to discover that he was completely unable to walk back, and had to telephone his wife to rescue him. Anticipation is required, so that enough physical energy is left to complete the journey home.

Other features of good management include a healthy diet with plenty of fresh food supplemented by vitamins and appropriate minerals if there is evidence of deficiency. The mobilisation of social support from friends, family and colleagues is crucial; and antidepressants if the mood is consistently low, or if there is a suicidal risk. People with ME can often feel fleetingly suicidal when the pain and the malaise are severe and unremittent, and a few suicides are known to have occurred. The anxiolytic effect of antidepressants is also very helpful in the management of the acute anxiety sometimes experienced in acute post-viral fatigue syndrome. However, in my experience, people with this illness often do not tolerate antidepressants well, and social support may be the main weapon in the fight against secondary depression. Patients with post-viral fatigue syndrome are often very scared and in considerable pain, and, as a consequence, can be extremely demanding and difficult to care for. The psychiatrist in collaboration with the GP and their respective teams can do much to support the family as well as the patient. It may be necessary to arrange brief spells of respite care, so that the carer, whether spouse or parent, can have time to themselves.

17

The Presentation, Assessment, Investigation and Diagnosis of Patients with Post-viral Fatigue Syndrome in an Infectious Diseases Clinic

W. R. C. Weir

The Royal Free Hospital, London, UK

INTRODUCTION

Many patients with post-viral fatigue syndrome (PVFS) tend to be referred to an infectious disease physician because their symptoms are often suggestive of an infectious process, and the evidence in favour of this theory of causation is discussed elsewhere in this book. Nevertheless these symptoms can overlap with a large range of diagnostic alternatives, some of which may require an entirely different therapeutic approach. Furthermore, because the condition has a 'high media profile' and is consequently fashionable some patients tend to present with their own self-diagnosis of PVFS and may require to be otherwise convinced if they are found to have an alternative diagnosis. Such diagnostic alternatives include endocrine disorders such as hypothyroidism, chronic infections such as toxoplasmosis, Lyme disease and human immunodeficiency virus (HIV) infection, malignant disease, autoimmune disorders, metabolic syndromes such as sleep apnoea, and last, but not least, psychological disorder including depressive illness. A carefully taken history helps resolve some of these diagnostic problems and laboratory investigation is usually advisable when any definable alternative diagnosis is considered possible. In practice, this usually means a routine screen of various investigations, with additional ones such as HIV serology or thyroid function tests being required in the appropriate clinical context. Often the presence of a spouse, close friend or relative may be helpful during the process of history taking although the reliability of contributions from such a source has to be carefully assessed.

Post-viral Fatigue Syndrome. Edited by R. Jenkins and J. Mowbray
© 1991 John Wiley & Sons Ltd

PRESENTATION

History

In the great majority of patients an identifiable viral illness immediately precedes the development of PVFS (Behan *et al.*, 1985). This usually presents with upper respiratory symptoms and is usually attributed to 'influenza'; a subgroup of these will have infectious mononucleosis with serology indicative of acute Epstein–Barr infection (Hotchin *et al.*, 1989). A smaller number of patients have gastrointestinal upset with diarrhoea and vomiting as the predominant features, whilst vestibular neuronitis, rubella, Bornholm disease, chicken-pox and herpes zoster have all occasionally appeared in this context (Behan *et al.*, 1985; Behan and Behan, 1988). The author has also encountered two patients in whom vaccinations for typhoid fever and hepatitis B immediately preceded the development of PVFS. On closer questioning many patients will admit to having been simultaneously subject to some form of psychological or physical stress such as a divorce, bereavement or stressful period at work; a surgical operation or serious injury may also feature in this way. An interesting subgroup comprises top-class athletes in whom a punishing training schedule may coincide with this initial illness (Budgett, personal communication). In a small minority of patients there is no discernible combination of illness and stress at the beginning. Nevertheless, in each case a characteristic complex of symptoms ensues, the main features of which have been well documented by different authorities on the subject.

One of the most comprehensive accounts categorises these into 'major' and 'minor' diagnostic criteria (Holmes *et al.*, 1988), a modification of which follows.

Major criteria

(a) Persistent, or occasionally relapsing, lethargy unrelieved by sleep or daytime bedrest lasting for at least six months, with professional or social life or both being completely curtailed as a result.

(b) Exercise-induced muscle fatigue precipitated by trivially small exertion relative to the patient's previous exercise tolerance. Pain in the exercising muscles may also occur; this symptom may sometimes be immediate or delayed for a few hours and may persist for several days after comparatively mild exertion. As with (a) this symptom should have persisted for at least six months. Thus a previously accomplished athlete may liken the after-effects of climbing a single flight of stairs to those of running a marathon or a previously able-bodied housewife may find a normal day's housework beyond her physical capacity.

These two major symptomatic criteria must be present for the diagnosis to be made; the following 'minor' criteria lend further support to the diagnosis but if they occur in the absence of the major criteria then alternative diagnoses must be keenly sought.

Minor criteria

These can be subdivided into the following categories:

Autonomic. Bouts of inappropriate night or day-time sweating; Raynaud's phenomenon; postural hypotension; disturbances of bowel motility manifesting as recurrent diarrhoea or occasionally constipation (these symptoms are frequently indistinguishable from those of irritable bowel syndrome); recurrent or persistent nausea; epigastric bloating; photophobia; blurred vision due to disturbed accommodation hyperacusis; frequency of micturition; nocturia; small amounts of alcohol (up to one standard glass of wine) causing intoxication and/or severe hangover symptoms and/or a worsening of other PVFS symptoms.

Neuropsychiatric. Impairment of short-term memory; loss of powers of concentration; excessive irritability; nominal dysphasia; hypersomnia (i.e. a tendency to sleep for abnormally long periods relative to the patient's previous sleep routine); insomnia (commonly associated with depressive symptoms); acute hypersensitivity to trivial stimuli (such as the touch or weight of bedclothes); recurrent vertigo and/or tinnitus.

Immunological. Periodic episodes of low-grade fever (i.e. not exceeding an oral temperature of 38.6°C); sore throat which may be persistent or recurrent (i.e. present for at least one week per month); arthropathy of a fixed or migratory nature.

In the author's experience the presence of two 'qualifying' symptoms from two separate categories of the above is highly suggestive of the diagnosis and unless physical examination and/or laboratory investigation reveals alternative pathology the patient almost certainly has PVFS.

This list is by no means exhaustive; headache, for instance, is a common symptom in many patients but is not sufficiently discriminative because of its widespread occurrence in many other disorders. The curious intolerance to alcohol is highly specific in this context; its inclusion under autonomic symptoms is for want of a better category for it. It should also be emphasised that the symptoms of PVFS tend to vary capriciously from hour to hour and day to day (Ramsay, 1988); nevertheless it is absolutely characteristic that they tend to be exacerbated by physical or mental exertion and this association should always be sought whilst taking the history. Finally it must be emphasised that this should be taken using nonspecific generalised enquiry and that 'leading' questions, particularly those relating to the diagnostic criteria, must be kept to a minimum.

Physical Signs

Characteristic physical signs are seen in PVFS and in the right symptomatic context they contribute to the validity of the diagnosis. Nevertheless their absence does not exclude the condition, and they are as follows:

(a) Pharyngitis which is either persistent or recurrent (present for at least one week every month) with or without tonsillar enlargement. This is nearly always non-exudative and when present is usually accompanied by the low-grade fever mentioned under immunological symptoms.
(b) Tender enlargement of lymph nodes, particularly of the cervical group; these also may accompany the fever and they may decrease in size during the afebrile periods.
(c) Muscle tenderness with a particular predeliction for the neck and shoulder girdle and the major muscles of locomotion. Points of exquisite tenderness are occasionally found by palpating the affected muscles with the tip of a finger (Ramsay 1988).

ASSESSMENT, INVESTIGATION AND DIAGNOSIS

Clearly, many of the symptoms and signs described can be attributed to a number of other important diseases. Nevertheless the combination and context in which they present are very important in the making of what ultimately has to be a diagnosis of exclusion. The occasional 'leadswinger' may be encountererd in this context also and, as previously emphasised, generalised enquiry with minimal use of leading questions should help detect such patients. The major alternative diagnoses to be borne in mind before conferring the diagnosis of PVFS can be considered under the following headings:

Chronic infections

Toxoplasmosis, Lyme disease, HIV infection, chronic active hepatitis, schistosomiasis, brucellosis, occult sepsis, tuberculosis.

Endocrine disorders

Hypothyroidism, thyrotoxicosis, Addison's disease, Cushing's syndrome, diabetes mellitus, hyperparathyroidism.

Neuromuscular disorders

Myasthenia gravis, multiple sclerosis, mitochondrial myopathy.

Metabolic disorders

Sleep apnoea syndrome, chronic renal failure.

Malignant disease

Occult tumours such as undiagnosed lymphoma, retroperitoneal sarcomas; renal and liver tumours; frontal lobe tumours.

Autoimmune disease

Rheumatoid arthritis, systemic lupus erythematosus.

Haematological disorders

Leukaemias and anaemias of varying origin.

Miscellaneous

Heavy metal poisoning, chronic intoxications due to prolonged exposure to chemicals such as petrol, benzene, and methylene chloride; drug side effects such as those due to beta-blockers, and long-term benzodiazepine usage; chronic alcoholism; coeliac disease.

Psychiatric

Endogenous depression, anxiety neurosis.

Laboratory investigations

The laboratory is occasionally indispensable in the search for some diagnoses, and in the author's experience this applies particularly to the category of chronic infection. For example, toxoplasmosis occasionally causes prolonged debility and lymphadenopathy in otherwise normal individuals

(Christie, 1987) and the toxoplasma dye test is a good general screen for this. If this is strongly positive then a further test for the presence of a raised toxoplasma IgM antibody confirms the diagnosis in this symptomatic context. Lyme disease is of topical interest because of the relatively recent discovery of its causative agent, *Borrelia burgdorferi* (Benach *et al.*, 1983).

The characteristic early feature of erythema radiating outwards from the site of an infective tick bite—erythema chronicum migrans— may be elicited in the history but it is the later neurological and joint manifestations (Steere, 1989) which may overlap with some of the diagnostic criteria of PVFS.

Detection of IgM antibodies against *B. burgdorferi* is the standard means of diagnosing an active infection; it is especially important not to miss this diagnosis because the long-term sequelae in untreated cases can be crippling (Steere, 1989). HIV infection is also worth mentioning in this context. It can present with lymphadenopathy and generalised debility although in the UK it is still extremely unusual outside of the recognised 'high-risk' patient categories (Gill *et al.*, 1989). The current climate of opinion dictates that specific permission be requested from the patient before HIV serology is done and appropriate counselling be available in the event of a positive result.

Psychiatric illness

This aspect of PVFS is dealt with more fully elsewhere in this book but it is worthy of comment in this chapter also. The detection of those with genuine psychiatric illness can be a difficult task, not least because some patients, particularly those who present with their own self-diagnosis, are hostile to the proposal that their illness is possibly of a psychological nature. This often arises from an unnecessarily pejorative interpretation of the concept of psychiatric illness which may be as much the fault of the doctor as of the patient (David *et al.*, 1988).

The understandable secondary depression of genuine PVFS can often be very hard to distinguish from classical endogenous depressive illness, and sometimes a trial of antidepressant therapy is warranted in order to make this distinction. In the author's experience the patients with definite PVFS tend to suffer severe side effects with no beneficial therapeutic response, particularly with the tricyclic agents. It is often the case that the patient's own general practitioner may already have tried this approach and the absence of benefit associated with pronounced side effects lends support to the diagnosis of PVFS. Another condition which also deserves mention in the context of psychiatric illness is benzodiazepine dependence. This unpleasant condition can go undiagnosed because benzodiazepines have become such a part of the individual sufferer's way of life that their significance is overlooked.

CONCLUSION

In conclusion it is axiomatic to state that the history is by far the most important part of the diagnostic process and this applies particularly to the task of excluding the possible alternatives before settling on the diagnosis of PVFS. The physical examination should obviously be equally thorough with particular reference to the possibility of neuromuscular disease. Laboratory investigations are also important but 'blanket' screening should never be considered to be a substitute for a painstaking, clinically oriented approach in the accurate diagnosis of this distressing condition.

REFERENCES

Behan, P. O. and Behan, W. M. H. (1988) Postviral fatigue syndrome. *Critical Reviews in Neurobiology,* **4**(2): 157–178.
Behan, P. O., Behan, W. M. H. and Bell, E. J. (1985) The post-viral fatigue syndrome— an analysis of the findings in 50 cases. *Journal of Infection,* **10,** 211–222.
Benach, J. L., Bosler, E. M., Hanrahan, J. P., Coleman, H., Habicht, G. S., Bast, T. F., Cameron, D. J., Ziegler, J. L., Barbour, A. G., Burgdorfer, W., Edelman, R. and Kaslow, R. A. (1983) Spirochaetes isolated from the blood of two patients with Lyme Disease. *New England Journal of Medicine,* **308,** 740–742.
Christie, A. B. (1987) *Infectious Diseases: Epidemiology and Clinical Practice,* 4th edn. Churchill Livingstone, London.
David, A. S., Wessely, S. and Pelosi, A. J. (1988) Post-viral fatigue syndrome: time for a new approach. *British Medical Journal,* **296,** 696–699.
Gill, O. N., Adler, M. W. and Day, N. E. (1989) Monitoring the prevalence of HIV. *British Medical Journal,* **299,** 1295–1298.
Holmes, G. P., Kaplan, J. E., Gantz, N. M. *et al.* (1988) Chronic fatigue syndrome: A working case definition. *Annals of Internal Medicine,* **108,** 387–389.
Hotchin, N. A., Read, R., Smith, D. G. and Crawford, D. H. (1989) Active Epstein– Barr virus infection in post-viral fatigue syndrome. *Journal of Infection,* **18,** 143–150.
Ramsay, A. M. (1988) *Myalgic Encephalomyelitis and Post-Viral States. The Saga of Royal Free Disease,* 2nd edn. Gower Medical Publications, London.
Steere, A. C. (1989) Medical progress: Lyme disease. *New England Journal of Medicine,* **321,** 586–596.

18

Employment Aspects of Post-viral Fatigue Syndrome

Michael Peel

Occupational Health Unit, British Telecom International, London, UK

INTRODUCTION

Post-viral fatigue syndrome (PVFS) is a condition which predominantly affects young active adults. There is therefore a great likelihood that sufferers will be in employment. This adds an extra perspective to managing the case. The individual will almost certainly be off sick in the early stages of the disease. If the course is prolonged it may be necessary for the GP to discuss the situation with the employer, to advise on return to work, and to help to arrange rehabilitation. It may also be helpful to be able to reassure an individual on their job security.

If the patient does not recover fully, it may be necessary to discuss medical retirement with the employer. A doctor may also be asked for his or her opinion on the suitability of someone who has had PVFS in the past for new employment.

Most large companies and an increasing number of small ones have an occupational health service, either from occupational physicians or occupational health nurses. Occupational health is the study of the relationships between work and health, and between health and work (Edwards *et al.*, 1988), and this expertise is particularly relevant. If an occupational health unit exists, it is essential that its staff are involved at every stage, as they can perform the liaison role between the medical advisor and the employer.

BRITISH AIRWAYS STUDY

In the period September 1986 to July 1987, medical officers at British Airways identified 13 patients who were suffering from PVFS (Peel, 1988). They

Post-viral Fatigue Syndrome. Edited by R. Jenkins and J. Mowbray
© 1991 John Wiley & Sons Ltd

came from a total non-flying population of approximately 15 000, a rate comparing well with the highest reported one of 1 per 1000 per year.

The 13 cases comprised eight men and five women. The median age was 29 years, with a range of 20 to 57 (Figure 1).

The median time off sick was eight weeks. Duration of sickness absence is, however, an unreliable guide to severity. It is affected by a number of factors, particularly personality. In the case of PVFS, individuals, by their nature, frequently wanted to return to work as early as possible, even too early. This was compounded by the majority of them enjoying their work. Many of them also had domestic circumstances which meant they obtained the majority of their social support at work.

Six patients regressed at some time during their recovery, requiring either more time off sick, or a reduction in hours. The regression is particularly the case during and after further viral infections and following unavoidable or unrecognised pressures.

When I reviewed the group one year after the end of the study, all but two of the group had returned to normal duties. This represented up to two years after the onset of the disease. One sufferer had a multiple relapsing course, which meant that he was back to normal duties, but had several episodes each year which necessitated short absences. The other was still only able to work four hours per day intermittently, 20 months into the disease, and ultimately took medical retirement.

Their return to work went from four hours per day, to five hours, to six

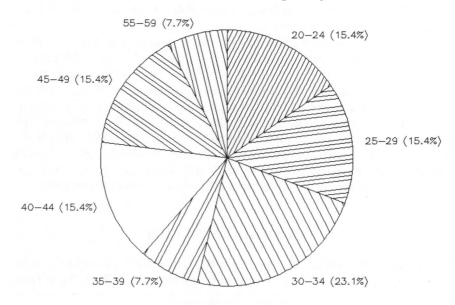

Figure 1   Ages of patients

hours, and then to normal duties. Although the pattern was very variable,the usual stay on any step was four to six weeks (Figure 2).

The 11 who were able to return to work took a median of 22 weeks to return to normal duties, with a range of seven to 66. One of them took a further two months to go on to shift work, and several others needed a similar period to go from normal to full duties. In a few cases I was able to follow the individuals up completely. This experience suggests to me that complete return to normal takes as long as 18 months to two years (Figure 3).

DIAGNOSIS

The key to the management in PVFS is making an accurate diagnosis. Rehabilitation is similar to that from many other diseases, but the time scale is longer. Rushing return to work will slow recovery, and may cause a relapse. Equally it would be damaging to treat individuals as though they had PVFS when their sole diagnosis was clinical depression.

Diagnosis is made mostly from the history. The literature is very clear that there are two groups of well-defined symptoms, the physical and psychological. The pathognomonic feature of the PVFS is excessive muscle

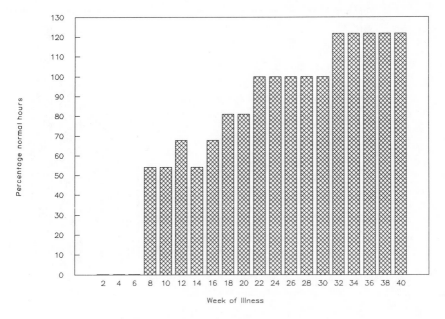

Figure 2 Typical recovery pattern

fatiguability, which recovers very slowly. Thus even the slightest exertion leaves a sufferer washed out, and this persists much longer than would normally be expected. This is so marked that one expert has suggested that ME should mean muscle fatigue on exercise. The other physical symptoms are an overall feeling of tiredness, generalised aches and pains, often muscle twitching, and sometimes paraesthesiae.

The psychological symptoms include poor concentration and memory, again out of proportion to the other symptoms. There may be associated clinical depression, which usually responds well to antidepressants. Even with the depression treated, the other symptoms persist, which tends to undermine the theory that these individuals are suffering purely from depression.

The consequences of this in employment are that all aspects of a job are affected. The physical tiredness affects the ability to travel in and out of work. It also has a significant effect on anyone who has a physical component to their job, even individuals who have to walk around large building complexes to get from meeting to meeting.

The psychological effects are also very damaging whatever the job. The ability to concentrate and remember may seem to be more important in clerical or managerial jobs, but skilled workers in manual jobs may need to use their minds just as much.

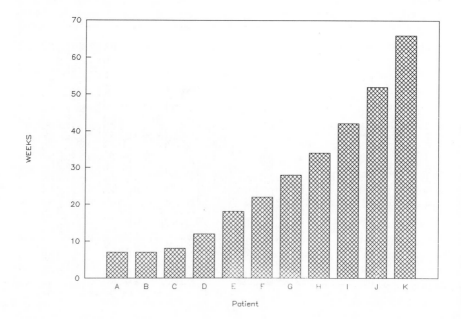

Figure 3   Length of recovery time to normal duties

UNDERSTANDING

Most sufferers recover much more easily if they understand the nature of the condition and its implications. There is considerable evidence now about the interrelationship between stress, exhaustion and impairment of the immune system (Anonymous, 1987). I therefore generally use the following model in explaining the condition.

My experience is that most of the sufferers are young, fit, and energetic. When they develop a minor illness, they continue working long hours, and taking regular exercise, long after their bodies tell them to stop. They therefore have no resources with which to fight the infection, with severe results.

The consequence of this is that by resting they allow the body to recover its natural resilience, so that they can slowly return to almost their previous level of activity. This does, however, take time, and cannot be rushed. Rushing simply causes the symptoms to get worse. Many sufferers complain of having good days and bad days. When it is explained to them that the bad days follow the good ones because they over-exerted the day before, the message gets home.

The rate of recovery is usually exponential, so that recovery is much slower in the later stages than early on. This, too, can be dispiriting if not explained. It is up to the doctor, therefore, to encourage a steady recovery, without going either too slow or too fast. It will seem like a long slog to the individual, but they can be encouraged to take a positive attitude by setting small short-term goals, and keeping their recovery in perspective.

RETURN TO WORK

Individuals are generally fit to return to work when they are reasonably mobile at home. Being able to walk without a load on the flat for about half an hour, and being able to carry a loaded tea tray, are useful guidelines. Being bored at home may also be useful, as this shows an improvement in concentration. I would advise someone to try regular reading at home to see if they can cope with more than watching television.

Many larger employers pay full pay for six months, then drop to half pay. Individuals working for smaller companies may notice this drop in income sooner. Often individuals ask to return to work at that point, but they should be discouraged. If they return to work too early, they will need to take further time off on half pay, and will lose more than if they stayed off until they were ready. Moreover, their sickness record will show several short absences rather than one long one, and this may also be misinterpreted.

If an occupational health service is available, then contact should be made prior to this point. The staff will understand the work pattern of the individual, and will know how to explain to managers why rehabilitation is necessary. If there is no occupational health cover, the GP can only make contact with the employer directly. This may be either the local manager or the personnel department, depending on the company. The individual should know who to approach.

It is important to explain that an individual will be better returning to work on reduced hours for two reasons. Firstly, the employer will get some work done rather than none in the early stages; secondly, the individual will return to full hours much sooner if they are allowed to return gradually. Having someone on prolonged reduced hours may seem like a nightmare to a manager, but if some idea of time scales is given, that will help. Even two years is a relatively short time over a career.

I would generally suggest that an individual returning to work after more than six months off should return on half time, generally between 18 and 24 hours per week. This is regardless of the cause of the absence. It is much better to do this by working up to four hours every day, split equally by the lunch break. This should allow travelling to avoid the rush hour.

The alternative is for the individual to return by working two or three longer days, e.g. Monday, Wednesday and Friday. This pattern has the disadvantage that the individual will be overtired after a work day, and will need the next day off to recover, thus producing a 'two steps forward and one step back' pattern. It is also better for the individual to return on a Thursday, so that they work their first two days and have a weekend off. The hours can then be increased on a monthly basis until the individual is working a normal day.

REHABILITATION

A significant number of these patients are in responsible jobs, or executive positions. For this reason, it is important to reduce not only the hours of work, but also its content. The combination of tiredness, poor memory, and difficulties with concentration means that work cannot be prolonged or open-ended. Once an individual is fit to return to work, the quality of work must be built up in parallel to the quantity.

Many individuals find meetings in particular to be too tiring to manage, because they have little control over duration, and may be asked to contribute to an unexpected extent. It is very difficult for a manager, particularly a junior one, to walk out of a meeting at half past three in the afternoon, and go home. Some senior managers seem to be more able to accept one of their staff members working short hours if they are not made too aware of it.

The rehabilitation programme obviously requires the co-operation of the line manager. Frequently, sufferers from PVFS are well respected in their team. Their managers are therefore very relieved to find that a trusted colleague is genuinely ill, rather than hysterical. They are usually then happy to co-operate with rehabilitation programmes. It helps very much to be able to quote figures such as those above in briefing managers. The more precise information they have on the restrictions required and the likely time course, the easier it is for them to plan departmental workload patterns. It is unhelpful to all concerned to give unrealistically short predictions. The manager will cease to trust the doctor, and the individual will become more depressed through having failed to meet targets.

RECOVERY

Recovery from PVFS is easy to define from an employer's point of view. The individuals can manage a normal day's work. That is not to say that they are fully recovered. They all need to preserve their energy for some time longer, usually by reducing domestic, family, and social commitments.

It is quite common in the early stages after return to work for patients to find that they are simply getting up, going to work, then collapsing into bed when they return home. It is important to reassure them that this is quite normal, and will pass. Only when they can do a full day's work without needing this should extended duties such as overtime be considered. This includes the sort of very long hours that certain 'macho' managers take as the norm, and which their staff think are expected. A normal day's work means exactly that, the contractual hours and no more. It is unlikely at this stage that they will produce anything useful in the extended hours, because the memory and concentration problems will recur with tiredness.

This does beg the question of the meaning of full recovery. The model of PVFS as I explain it to patients suggests that sufferers have been overdoing things. This means that it would be unrealistic to define recovery as the return to things exactly as they were before the illness. Moreover, these individuals will have experienced up to two years of relative immobility and its consequences, and even a 30 year old may not be able to return to previous full fitness after that time. That is not to say that I encourage individuals to overprotect themselves. They can still do all the things that they did before, just not all on the same day.

I would also not advise an individual to change jobs until they have been working normally for about a year. This is because of the prolonged nature of recovery, and the effect of extra stress on a recovering sufferer. A relapse at this stage would be disastrous for the individual and the new employer alike. After this time, I would consider the person to have recovered full capacity, and would see no objection to employing them.

MEDICAL RETIREMENT

The formal definition of medical (or ill-health) retirement varies from company to company, and pension scheme to pension scheme. Not all employers offer provision for medical retirement, but the vast majority of major companies do.

Generally the criteria require that an individual has a medical condition which prevents him or her performing their normal job, and that the condition is unlikely to recover in the foreseeable future. Sometimes it is necessary to declare that an individual is 'permanently unfit'. One difficulty with this is that a few patients may have moved to live a long way from work, so that they are either fit to travel to, or return from, work, but not both. This does not in principle constitute grounds for medical retirement, as the underlying problem is the journey, not the occupation.

Many companies add another criterion, which is that suitable alternative employment has been sought, but nothing suitable has been found. As well as being a way of losing an employee unnecessarily, it is possible that an individual who is medically retired when suitable employment is available could be found to have been unfairly dismissed.

The major problem with this is the unpredictable nature of PVFS. It is impossible to say in the early stages of the condition whether or not any particular individual will fully recover over a period of time, or have a relapsing course. It is therefore only when someone has been off sick for around nine months with no evidence of recovery that it would be fair to say that recovery is unlikely in the foreseeable future.

CONCLUSION

In this chapter I have discussed the results of a study performed at British Airways, and I have addressed the employment consequences of post-viral fatigue syndrome, with particular reference to the British Airways data. This includes sickness absence, rehabilitation, liaison with the employer, and medical retirement.

Post-viral fatigue syndrome is a condition which is gaining increasing recognition. If it is correctly diagnosed, then standard principles of rehabilitation hold good, but over an elongated time frame. It is up to the doctor to explain this to the sufferer and if necessary, the employer. If there is an occupational health department, this will make the liaison much simpler.

The key is in setting small, realistic targets, and encouraging the individual to work towards them. Once they have returned to work, this must become an agreed rehabilitation programme that the employer and employee both understand.

Now that the existence and diagnosis of PVFS are better understood, the employment consequences are becoming clearer. Adequate rest in the early stages is crucial to recovery, in terms of both sickness absence and steady rehabilitation. Understanding the condition and its effects is the key for employers and individuals. General practitioners are in a key position to help with this, and liaison with occupational health departments, where they exist, is invaluable.

Sufferers can recognise that recovery is usual in PVFS. They need to realise that they must put considerable effort into recovery, including holding themselves back when necessary. Two years may appear a long time for someone to be less than 100% effective, to the individual or their employer. In the context of a career or a lifetime, however, it should not be a significant period. The best thing that any doctor can do is to impart a sense of perspective. The key is to keep the sufferer motivated whilst they recover naturally.

REFERENCES

Anonymous (1987) Depression, stress, and immunity. *Lancet*, **i**, 1467–1468.

Edwards, F. C., McCallum, R. I. and Taylor, P. J. (1988) *Fitness for Work, the Medical Aspects*. Oxford University Press, Oxford.

Peel, M. R. (1988) Rehabilitation in postviral syndrome. *Journal of the Society of Occupational Medicine*, **38**, 44–45.

19

The Management of Post-viral Fatigue Syndrome in General Practice

David G. Smith

High Road, Horndon on the Hill, Essex, UK

INTRODUCTION—DISEASE DEFINITION

An effective disease management strategy requires a sound definition of the disease to be managed, so that accurate diagnosis can occur, and an understanding of the natural course of the clinical process. The boundaries of myalgic encephalomyelitis (ME) are not distinct and in the absence of any coherent move in Britain to develop criteria for the disease, the medical profession has generally had to fall back on the American working case definition of chronic fatigue syndrome (CFS) (Holmes *et al.*, 1988), although this is not synonymous with ME. This state of affairs has inevitably increased the confusion in the literature, as ME is only one subset of CFS. In my experience, the most identifiable clinical process within the umbrella of ME is acute onset post-viral fatigue syndrome (PVFS) (Smith, 1989a), which is defined as a 'new disease' process lasting for six months or more, seen in a previously fit and healthy person, who:

(a) Has a good premorbid personality and good psychiatric health.
(b) Experiences an acute onset illness, suggestive of a viral or 'flu-like' process, associated with general malaise and demonstrable pyrexia.
(c) As a result, suffers from undue perceived excessive muscular fatigue, in response to what would be a less than usual amount of physical activity for him or her.
(d) In whom this muscle fatigue has an extended period of recovery.

These symptoms are often associated with widespread polymyalgia after effort; muscle tenderness to palpation; loss of concentration; and short-term

Post-viral Fatigue Syndrome. Edited by R. Jenkins and J. Mowbray
© 1991 John Wiley & Sons Ltd

memory dysfunction. On clinical examination the patients demonstrate no focal or localising signs that could reasonably explain their symptomatology; routine haematological and biochemical screening show no significant abnormality. No other disease process can be discovered.

The features which distinguish acute onset PVFS from CFS are that acute onset PVFS, by definition, has a specific start, always associated with a presumed viral illness, and is subsequently associated usually with either the enteroviruses (Yousef et al., 1988) or with serological evidence of reactivation of Epstein–Barr virus (EBV) (Hotchin et al., 1989). A possibly different specific fatigue syndrome is found subsequent to a primary EBV infection (White, 1989; Smith, 1989). Acute onset PVFS sufferers exhibit levels of morbidity across the whole spectrum and not necessarily below 50% of premorbid activity. In my experience, unless there is an intercurrent infection, pyrexia is not observed after the initial infection. Despite frequent subjective fever and hot and cold sweats, the oral temperature tends to be either normal at 36.5°C or lower. There is a perceived subjective muscular fatigue but no absolute weakness can be demonstrated on formal testing. Sore throat, while common, tends to be a variable and fluctuating symptom. There is no specific test for PVFS which will support or refute the diagnosis.

SYMPTOMS OF ACUTE ONSET POST-VIRAL FATIGUE SYNDROME

The symptoms of acute onset PVFS fall into two groups: firstly, central nervous system symptoms (neurocognitive and neuropsychiatric), and secondly, peripheral functional symptoms which are suggestive of a centrally based autonomic nervous system dysregulation. It is vital to understand the nature and the origin of the fatigue and the associated symptoms if we are to manage the disease effectively.

There is increasing evidence that most of the peripheral symptoms are centrally generated, and, in my view, the most likely explanation is that the primary lesion of acute onset PVFS is potentially a fully reversible dysfunction of the hypothalamus (this hypothesis is discussed in Chapter 21).

It is necessary at this point to consider the work of Wagenmakers et al. (1988). These studies have been carried out on patients approximating to a Chronic Fatigue Syndrome, and various effort syndromes. Wagenmaker's introduction suggests that some of the patients studied had a virus infection at, or shortly before, the beginning of their symptoms. As a result of a subsequent discussion with the authors, I am in no doubt that many of the patients studied suffered PVFS, and that the assessment of their muscle power was wholly appropriate.

Using twitch occlusion, and a maximum force production (by programme stimulation electromyograms) before, during and in serial assessment, for several days after a specified exercise programme, there is no demonstrable peripheral skeletal muscular fatigue, and the muscles are physiologically normal, except where disease atrophy becomes apparent. This brings into serious question the effects of observed skeletal muscle abnormalities. Although single fibre EMG studies have demonstrated abnormal muscle fibre jitter in patients with ME (Jamal and Hansen, 1985), and enteroviral particles have been demonstrated in skeletal muscle samples (Archard *et al.*, 1988), the significance of these and other pathological findings for the genesis of the muscle fatigue remains unclear, and awaits further research. Some demonstrable muscle pathological findings are probably due to disease atrophy rather than anything else, and do not appear to play a significant part in the fatigue.

The cardiovascular symptoms of palpitations, cold hands and feet, and the sudden draining of facial colour, appear to be independent of any demonstrable cardiovascular disease, and are probably developed from central autonomic dysfunction. In addition, central hypothalamic dysfunction could explain the respiratory system symptoms of sensation of shortness of breath, and the hyperventilation which is sometimes seen (Dighton, 1980). Irritable bowel syndrome (IBS) is found in as many as 25% of patients (Smith, 1989b) and may be a result of autonomic dysfunction, as indeed has been suggested for IBS in general (Catnach and Farthing, 1989). Furthermore, autonomic nervous dysfunction could account for all the more minor problems: bladder frequency, menses upset, hot and cold sweats and perspiration. Centrally originated autonomic problembs may account for temperature dysregulation and intolerance, sleep disturbance and a sudden feeling of increasing strength, observed by some patients after eating sweet foods, which can on occasion lead to excessive weight gain.

Thus a hypothalamic dysfunction could account for most of the symptoms seen peripherally. However, there remain a few peripheral symptoms for which a central explanation is more difficult. These are the widespread myalgia and polyarthralgia, intermittent sore throat, and tender cervical lymph glands. The vast majority of central nervous system symptoms could also be explained by a hypothalamic dysregulation. These include emotional liability, psychiatric symptoms of depression, anxiety and panic attacks, loss of concentration, short-term memory and cognitive dysfunction, and sleep disturbance, particularly initiating sleep and increased sleep restlessness, seen so often in the acute stages of acute onset PVFS.

Clinical experience shows that the majority of PVFS patients spontaneously remit, and that the condition is fully reversible. Thus there is no clinical evidence of any permanent tissue damage to the central nervous system. However, there are a small number of acute onset PVFS patients who do not improve and it is possible that they have developed some kind of permanent central nervous system abnormality.

NATURAL HISTORY OF PVFS

I have seen approximately two thousand cases of acute onset PVFS and have taken the opportunity to chart each clinical course. Whilst the severity and duration of the illness is variable, nonetheless a general pattern can be observed, and Figure 1 represents the clinical course of a typical case of unmanaged acute PVFS. The horizontal axis represents the duration of illness, typically here seen extending into two years with full recovery. After a period of six months, a diagnosis of acute onset PVFS can reasonably be made. (Hopefully, in the future, earlier recognition will be possible.) The vertical axis represents the subjective reflection of the sum total of all the symptoms which influence the patient's functioning. Most patients express marked polysymptomatology, including that of being ill, without being able to specify precise symptoms. The bottom of the vertical axis marked '0% ill' represents the condition of an international athlete. Therefore most people would be '5% ill'. The top of the vertical axis '100% ill' represents a patient needing hospitalisation 75% cent ill might represent having to spend the majority of the time

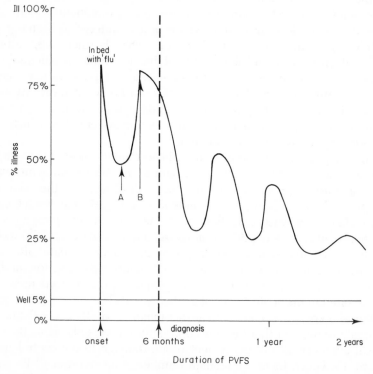

Figure 1   Clinical course of a typical case of *unmanaged* acute onset post-viral fatigue syndrome

in bed or resting in a chair, as the result of the disorder. 50% ill might represent a level of function which allowed the patient to be able to carry on with his or her job or look after house and family, but with only 50% efficiency, needing help, or having to take time off because of the illness. 25% ill might mean being able to cope with the house and occupation and most aspects of life, but losing social capabilities, i.e. having to go to bed early, resting at weekends, and/or not being able to participate in sport or leisure activities.

In this typical example, on the day of onset the patient went to bed with a 'flu-like' illness. Point A represents the crucial phase of partial recovery which may come variously after a few days, weeks or even months. Having lost the acute 'flu-like' symptoms but not having fully recovered, the patient might return to his or her occupation prematurely, thus exacerbating the symptoms, and causing a relapse at point B.

In the acute phase, during the first six months, the symptoms are at their most florid. They show marked degrees of fluctuation in both severity and variability, and there appears to be no particular cause for either remission or exacerbation with the sole exception that any physical effort produces generalised deterioration.

As the illness progresses, there is more stability in the rate of change. The severity of the symptoms diminishes and exacerbations become more predictable.

The patient finds that increasing physical and/or mental activity exacerbates both the peripheral and central symptoms, seemingly in proportion with the amount of exertion. In general, all of the symptoms are improved by mental and physical rest; and the patient, like one of Pavlov's dogs, avoids overactivities in both of these areas in order to prevent a generalised increase in his or her symptoms. Patients notice that not only do they suffer for their activity immediately, but also their recovery period can be extended to several days, or even a week, if the activity has been particularly strenuous. The more vigorous the activity, the longer the period of recovery. During the recovery period, any further activity undertaken, either mental or physical, has a cumulative effect, so that an exponential deterioration pattern can be observed, leading to periods of illness that appear to 'poleaxe' the sufferer. Recovery from these episodes can be protracted, and if patients continue to push themselves to exhaustion, not only is the recovery period from each episode slower and longer, but also the whole illness process can be substantially extended, and the degree of eventual morbidity can be increased. At this stage, persistent overactivity can lead to permanent ill-health and perpetual morbidity. Usually the general clinical pattern demonstrates, albeit slowly, a trend towards recovery. The periods of exacerbation diminish in length and severity as the condition improves. As the severity of symptoms declines, activity is increased.

Apart from mental and physical activity, there are other factors that influence the process of recovery to full health. However, more usually, the sufferers make a fairly rapid recovery from these episodes, returning to the previous level of activity. Operations, general anaesthetics and trauma (e.g. road traffic accidents) appear to have the same deleterious effect as intercurrent infections. Vaccinations with tetanus, typhoid and cholera have also been observed to produce severe exacerbations from which recovery can be exceedingly slow—such vaccinations should therefore be avoided unless medically essential. Many patients also experience chemical (e.g. petrol fumes, alcoholic beverages, artificial preservatives and colourings in foods) and food intolerance. Avoidance of these factors, while ensuring that the diet remains balanced, may improve some of the symptoms such as depressions, sleep disturbance, myalgia and IBS.

PROGNOSIS OF PVFS

The vast majority of the population would recover from an acute viral infection in a period of approximately one week, and return to normal health. Recovery over a slightly more extended time period, such as up to eight weeks, occurs in a minority of the population. If recovery has not occurred by six months then the criteria for acute onset PVFS are met. This occurs in a tiny fraction of the population recovering from acute viral infections. Of those with acute onset PVFS at six months, about half will recover completely within two years of onset. By five years, a further quarter will have recovered, albeit with varying levels of residual morbidity. Even after the illness has lasted five years, there is still a general tendency to improvement in most sufferers, but morbidity can be high. Table 1 represents a computerised average of some 1500 personal graphs, taking the symptom severities at six months, 12 months, 24 months etc. and averaging the scores.

It is my opinion, having followed the case histories of patients over a decade, that medical mismanagement frequently contributes to permanent ill-health. For example, I have seen a number of patients who, after receiving thorough investigations from their GPs and consultants, have been told not only that the tests are negative, but also that there is nothing wrong with them, and that they are simply psychologically disturbed, this being variously attributed to hysterical conversion, depression, anxiety or some other neurotic illness. The mistaken logic inherent in such an approach has been discussed elsewhere in this book (Chapters 1 and 5). Such patients are often older than average, and have poor relationships with their spouses and families who, having had the opportunity to hear the GP's and consultant's views, often feel that the ill member is simply 'putting it on'. By the time this situation has lasted for a year or two, such patients certainly do tend to have an increased percentage of psychiatric symptoms and problems.

Table 1 Time to recovery in 1500 patients with acute onset ME and a duration of illness greater than six months

Time to recovery	No. of patients	Percentage
6–12 months	60	4
1–2 years	150	10
2–4 years	555	37
> 4 years	500	33
> 4 years (still > 25–50% disability)	180	12
> 4 years (still > 50% disability)	60	4

Those patients with acute onset PVFS who recover within two years tend to be younger, in the age range 16 to 40. They are mainly female (80%) with good family support and, even more importantly, good medical support. They are told that they have some kind of post-viral syndrome and even though their illness is not specifically managed they are encouraged to believe that they will get better in the 'near future' although often the estimates of recovery times are over-optimistic. If they do recover in a year or two then all is well. However, if the anticipated recovery is not forthcoming by two years, the support from family and doctor may begin to waver and doubt as to the accuracy of the diagnosis creeps in. Relatives, colleagues, and doctors may comment ' isn't it time you were better?', and everyone starts to wonder whether the illness was primarily a psychiatric illness after all. In my experience it is likely that those who end up with severe unremittant morbidity do so because of poor medical management in the past. The severe psychiatric symptomatology and evidence of muscle disuse atrophy have both been acquired during the course of the illness and were not present at the onset, and have become a self-fulfilling prophecy by the doctors concerned. (Skeletal muscle biopsies done in this group tend to show type 1 fibre atrophy and unfit skeletal muscle; and some even have interstitial fibrosis.) The condition of these patients can become apparently irrecoverable. In order to avoid this unfortunate situation, the patient's condition must be accurately identified much earlier in the course of the illness. Doctor and relatives need to communicate their understanding of the nature of the illness to the patient so that the patient knows they understand he or she is ill, and he or she is not then constantly having to prove that the illness is 'real'.

Acceptance and appropriate management of the frequent psychological symptoms is vital, but is not at all the same thing as telling the patient that the whole illness is psychological, psychiatric or all in the mind. The patient who is experiencing recurrent lymphadenopathy, sore throats, very severe myalgia etc. will know the doctor is wrong, and will cease to have any faith in their judgement.

MANAGEMENT OF ADULTS

Explanation

After careful diagnosis, the next consultation should be one of counselling and sympathetic explanation, not only to the patient, but also to their spouse and/or relatives, of what is known about acute onset PVFS. This usually produces immediate relief, as patients discover, perhaps for the first time, somebody in the medical profession who acknowledges their symptoms and has an understanding of the condition. Patients are frequently relieved to find that they are not suffering from something more serious that medicine had missed, such as tumours or some other malignant process. They need to know that they have an active viral infection from which they will eventually recover, and that recovery can be assisted by appropriate management.

Identification of exacerbating factors

The patient should be asked to keep a daily diary over the next few weeks, recording the severity of their symptoms, their activities and any factors which seem to influence the condition. At the next consultation, this can be plotted graphically with the patient, identifying obvious exacerbating and ameliorating factors. This process should help the patient to understand that *they* are in control of their own disease process and that a positive approach is an essential aid to recovery.

How much activity?

Good management is dependent upon using the information in the subjective daily diary, plotted as a graph if this is helpful, to give careful advice about how much activity should be undertaken, both from a physical and mental point of view, in order to prevent exacerbation and facilitate full recovery. How much activity is advisable depends upon the morbidity level of each patient. More general activity can be advised in those who are less afflicted. Detailed statements are required of how much activity patients are currently undertaking and managing without making themselves worse. Whereas even with quite severe exercise a normal person will recover within a few hours (less than a day), the PVFS patient able to perform the same amount of work may not recover for several days, or even a week.

In order to understand the rational of pacing 'power output' in a modified activity programme, one needs to look at the alteration in recovery after physical work that occurs in patients suffering acute onset PVFS.

Figure 2 shows a comparison of recovery times in normal individuals and sufferers of acute onset PVFS. Normals, fatigued after maximal exercise, recover in a few hours. The acute onset PVFS patient does not recover from maximal exercise in a day. Hence the fatigue of the subsequent days' exercise is cumulative.

Thus a continued high activity level can produce an exacerbation. The patient then feels that further exercise is impossible and this would probably result in their return to total rest and even bed from which the recovery process can be very slow. These features can be seen clearly when talking to patients who do not manage their problem well, where a story of 'ups and downs' of fluctuation with good days, bad days, good weeks or bad weeks is all too common.

Similar graphs can be produced using a vertical axis of mental activity or 'stress' instead of muscle fatigue. Excessive or undue mental activity produces increasing fatigue, both mental and physical. With enough mental stress and strain, physical exacerbations can be seen to be produced in a similar fashion to excess physical activity. There is a close relationship between overproduction of power and excessive mental stress and strain.

With this kind of understanding of the effects of excessive mental and physical activity and the generation of relapses, one can develop disease management programmes to aid the stabilisation of the disorder and its subsequent improvement.

A gradual recovery programme is essential, as is the advice that too much rest is as bad, if not worse, than too much activity. Prolonged periods of rest are to be avoided as they lead to a perpetuation of the very symptoms being complained of.

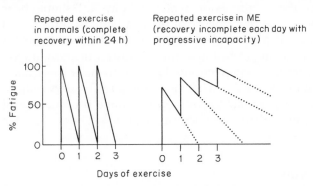

Figure 2 Comparison of recovery times in normal individuals and sufferers of acute onset post-viral fatigue syndrome

The improving patient will notice that the recovery time shortens and the degree of recovery increases. It becomes possible to suggest an increase in exercise. The degree of increment should be small. Again the activity should be regularised and paced, and using such small incremental steps the disease is found to gradually improve and recovery is usual.

Each patient needs an individual programme of daily activity, splitting the day up into smaller periods of rest and activity, both mental and physical. The ratio of mental and physical depends upon the severity of the symptoms and the relative preponderance of mental and physical symptoms which can vary quite markedly from patient to patient. It is better to divide such activity into smaller portions throughout the day. For instance, two quarter-hour walks, one at either end of the day, may be more rewarding and less fatiguing than one half-hour walk. The same kind of rationing should be applied to mental study, which should be based upon an assessment of the degree of concentration and memory, seen in the patient's capacity for reading a book or paper.

This baseline programme of mental and physical activity should be repeated every day at the same level for a couple of weeks or so. There should be no uncontrolled outbursts of strenuous activity. The regime is, of necessity, one of rather monotonous regularity. When reviewing the clinical responses at the end of this period, it is likely that the marked fluctuation in the illness will have disappeared or at least lessened, because of the controlled pattern of activity which secures the necessary time lag to smooth the passage of recovery.

At the end of this introductory time, the patient should be seen to be as well or better than they were before. If the patient is worse, then the programme of activity should be reduced, and if the patient's condition remains the same, the programme should be continued for another similar period of time, at the same level of activity. If the patient has improved and feels better, the activity (both mental and physical) should be increased by a small amount at the expense of the rest periods in the day. This part of the treatment is a good place to regularise the time of getting up in the morning and going to bed at night. This is particularly important for the sufferer in employment, who should revert to his or her usual waking time in preparation for the day when he or she is ready to try returning to work. Adoption of a graduated activity programme prevents the likelihood of deleterious exacerbations which can lead to a substantial extension of the whole illness.

Return to work

The same graduated approach should be used in the return to work, school or college. It will be necessary to discuss the need for a transitional phase with the occupational physician, welfare officer or line manager as appropriate. A gradual return, starting with one or two half-days a week, is advised, building up slowly (see Chapter 18). In some cases, it may be a good idea to bring work home for a part of the day.

Where the illness is a long one, patients can sometimes be pressured to return to work or school far too soon by 'threats' of job loss, or retirement on medical grounds. These pressures in themselves can trigger anxiety, depression and mental stress, and actively exacerbate the disease process. Hence alleviation of these pressures, where possible, is very important.

Exacerbations

Exacerbations are commonly caused by intercurrent infections, such as a new cold or 'flu'. As these infections exhibit the same symptoms as those already experienced, it can be difficult to differentiate the new from the old. It is important to note that when a fever can be demonstrated by a thermometer, it is not usually due to exacerbation, but to a new infection. When this occurs, the activity programme should be cut back, and recovery to the previous level of functioning may take a little longer than would be normal in an otherwise healthy person. The same approach should be adopted if the sufferer has to have a general anaesthetic and surgery, as these procedures can also cause a temporary setback.

Use of antidepressants

As we believe that the fatigue is of central origin, and as psychological symptoms are frequently present, it is appropriate to discuss the use of antidepressants (see Chapter 2). Patients are often reluctant to use these medications as they are inclilned to feel that, once again, the medical advisor is suggesting that they are simply depressed. But, with encouragement, it can be understood that disturbed sleep patterns, which are so frequent, can be rectified with sedative antidepressants. A good rewarding sleep maximises rest, both mental and physical, and optimises the patient's energies for the day. The other neuropsychiatric symptoms that are frequently present in this disorder, symptoms like depression, agitation, mood swings and emotional lability, can also be alleviated by the use of antidepressants. The quadricyclic antidepressants are usually preferred: maprotiline hydrochloride (Ludiomil) and trazodone hydrochloride (Molipaxin). More recently the 5-HT reuptake agonists have been found to be particularly beneficial: fluoxetine hydrochloride (Prozac) and fluvoxamine maleate (Faverin).

Because there is a strong likelihood that patients may have chemical sensitivities that were not present before the onset of their illness, it is sensible for the doctor to introduce drugs at very low doses, and to increase the dosage slowly. Intolerance to one antidepressant should not prohibit the trial of others. However, I believe that the use of minor tranquilisers has no place in the drug treatment of acute onset PVFS. Reassurance that anti-depressants are non-addictive, non-habituating and easily withdrawn should be given.

Diet

Most patients find they benefit from the avoidance of alcohol. Many patients also develop food intolerance, and avoidance of the offending food can be helpful. However, it is vital to ensure that the patient takes a balanced diet, and exclusion diets should only be undertaken with the knowledge and advice of the medical advisor.

Other remedies

A modified activity programme and the use of antidepressants are the main-stays of recovery. However, there are many other therapies which may also be beneficial, but they do require to be proven safe and effective.

Referral to a psychiatrist

In a few patients the psychiatric symptoms become very severe. In these circumstances it is advocated that the disease is best managed by a psychia-trist. Patients may be extremely reluctantly, especially if they have already had an unsympathetic encounter. However, the medical advisor with a good knowledge of PVFS should encourage them, pointing out the benefits of a positive and sympathetic approach from an expert with experience in prescribing pscyhotropic medication. It is obviously helpful if the GP al-ready has a good working relationships with the psychiatrist in order to facilitate this type of referral and to ensure adequate communication.

WHEN WILL RECOVERY OCCUR?

Figure 3 shows the subjective recovery graph of a patient whose illness might be identified after one year at point A. The axes are the same as for Figure 1.

   The patient has been suffering from a fluctuating disease, with exacerba-tions and remissions, but over this period has made an improvement of some 25% in functional terms. Using the management guide suggested earlier, one might expect improvement along the lines B, C or D, making the

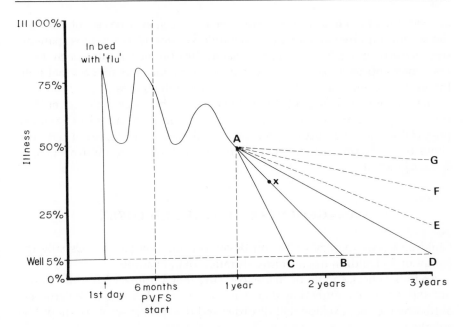

Figure 3 Subjective recovery graph of a patient suffering from acute onset post-viral fatigue syndrome, whose illness might be identified one year after the symptoms emerge at point A

recovery time two years two months, one year seven months or three years respectively.

At point A the outcome is uncertain, except that eventually the patient is likely to improve. When the patient is reviewed at two and four months into a management programme, they might indicate a rate of improvement, which, if it is plotted on the graph, may be at point X. From this starting point it should then be possible to extrapolate in the direction of the fit line, striking point B and giving a forecasted recovery date of approximately two and a quarter years.

Inevitably this forecast tends to be rather optimistic, as there are almost bound to be a few 'setback' occasions. For instance, a superimposed viral infection can delay the whole recovery period.

If the patient returns after the management programme instigation, and suggests a greater rate of improvement, then the forecast may improve to point C (one and a half years); equally, slower improvement may unfortunately indicate point D (a three-year recovery period). Once the second year of illness has been reached, the recovery appears not to be linear, and the impetus is lost and tails off, leaving some degree of morbidity, here suggested by levels E, F and G.

From my observations, I am sceptical that if the illness has extended beyond two and a half to three years, recovery can ever be complete. From the several hundred cases that I have followed for 12 years, most patients seem to recover to a level of approximately 10% but never quite reach the fit line. They appear to have residual minor complaints and suggest that their fitness and strength are not the same as prior to the illness.

The capability of being able to tell the patient when they will recover is, of course, of great importance. The rate of recovery in acute onset PVFS is fairly predictable. No other disease process has quite the same degree of certainty about the slow progression towards recovery, in that the improvement is always gradual.

MANAGEMENT OF AFFECTED CHILDREN

Children under the age of 16 can develop acute onset PVFS. Usually the condition in children has a shorter duration than in adults.

An initial check should be made to ensure that a primary EBV infection is not the cause, remembering that a negative Paul–Bunnell or heterophile antibody does not exclude that disorder and the specific serology should be sought.

In the event that a primary EBV has been excluded, the problem of diagnosing acute onset PVFS in children is fraught with difficulty. As the child's activities and attitudes are largely controlled by their parents and doctors it is far more difficult to assess their condition and then ensure the correct management of their illness. Here a multidisciplinary approach is essential, and a careful well-balanced interface is needed by parents, who usually need to be guided about the psychological consequences of their children's illness. I have noticed a very high incidence of behaviour problems and psychological disturbance in children with this condition. This is frequently caused when polarised attitudes are taken by parents and/or doctors.

The basic principles of recovery, using antidepressants and modified activity programmes, apply equally to children as to adults. There is the complication of trying to continue their education: where possible, home tutors should be used more frequently than they are at present.

Occasionally it is possible to observe a family in whom all the members are struck down by the same virus at the same time, with two members or more developing acute onset PVFS. If, on the other hand, two members appear to develop acute onset PVFS or another type of fatigue syndrome at differing times, it is more likely that one, if not both, are psychologically based. The chances of two members of a family independently developing this type of illness are remote.

REFERENCES

Archard, L. C., Behan, P. O., Bell, E. J. *et al.* (1988) Virus aetiology of the postviral fatigue syndrome. Myalgic encephalomyelitis: Persistence of enterovirus RNA in muscle and its correlation with elevated creatine kinase values. *Journal of the Royal Society of Medicine,* **81,** 326–329.

Arnold, D. L., Bore, P. J., Rada, G. K. *et al.* (1984) Excessive intracellular acidosis of skeletal muscle on exercise in a patient with a post-viral exhaustion/fatigue syndrome. A31P Nuclear magnetic resonance study. *Lancet,* **i,** 1367–1369.

Behan, P. O., Behan, W. M. H. and Bell, E. J. (1985) The post viral fatigue syndrome— an analysis of the findings in 50 cases. *Journal of Infection,* **10,** 211–222.

Catnach, S. M. and Farthing, M. J. G. (1989) Irritable bowel or irritable body? *Postgraduate Update,* 1 December, 993–997.

Dietrichson, P., Coakley, J., Smith, P. E. M. *et al.* (1987) Conchotome and needle percutaneous biopsy of skeletal muscle. *Journal of Neurology, Neurosurgery and Psychiatry,* **50,** 1461–1467.

Dighton (1980) *General Practitioner* 25 January.

Holmes, G. P., Kaplan, J. E., Gantz, N. M. *et al.* (1988) Chronic fatigue syndrome: A working case definition. *Annals of Internal Medicine,* **108,** 387–389.

Hotchin, N. A., Read, R., Smith, D. G. *et al.* (1989) Active Epstein–Barr virus infection in post viral fatigue syndrome. *Journal of Infection,* **18,** 143–150.

Jamal, G. A. and Hansen, S. (1985) Electrophysiological studies in the post viral fatigue syndrome. *Journal of Neurology, Neurosurgery and Psychiatry,* **48,** 691–694.

Manou, P., Matthews, D. and Lane, T. (1988) The mental health of patients with a chief complaint of chronic fatigue. A prospective evaluation and follow-up. *Archives of Internal Medicine,* **148,** 2013–2017.

Smith, D. G. (1989a) Myalgic encephalomyelitis. *Royal College of General Practitioners Handbook,* pp. 247–250, London, Royal College of General Practitioners.

Smith, D. G. (1989b) *Understanding ME.* Robinson Publications, London.

Wagenmakers, A. J. M., Coakley, J. H., Edwards, R. H. T. and May (1988) Post viral fatigue syndrome. *Egonomics,* **31,** 1519–1527.

Yousef, G. E., Bell, E. J., Mann, G. F. *et al.* (1988) Chronic enterovirus infection in patients with post-viral fatigue syndromes. *Lancet,* **i,** 146–150.

20

Management of Symptoms of Myalgic Encephalomyelitis in Hospital Practice

Peter Merry

Burnley General Hospital, Burnley, UK

Myalgic encephalomyelitis (ME) suffers from being a symptom complex with, until Professor Mowbray's work, little laboratory evidence to support it. I believe that after almost a century of spectacular advances in diagnostic techniques, we as doctors are ill-suited to coping with a condition which does not fit our neat pigeon-holes. We are in danger, like Procrustes, of tailoring conditions to fit our present views just as he cut travellers' feet off or stretched them on the rack to make them fit his bed.

It is interesting to consider what some of the great physicians of the last century like Freidreich and Charcot would have made of ME; one feels that at least they would have been a good deal more flexible in their approach.

As always in any form of treatment, diagnosis is of paramount importance. While a typical history of symptoms following a viral infection may be suggestive of the condition, a differential diagnosis must include a number of conditions which may give similar pictures. Such a list would include anaemia, exhaustion from stress at work or in the home, and an early inflammatory polyarthritis. It must also include tuberculosis, as this is more common than it was, and multiple myeloma, which may present with bone pain, giving a similar clinical picture.

Every patient who has not been investigated should have a chest X-ray, examination of haemaglobin, sedimentation rate and white blood count, a biochemistry profile and, if there is a degree of suspicion, tests for the rheumatoid factor. Numerous other investigations are often carried out but a feature of the disease is that they are within normal limits.

Professor Mowbray's work on the virus particle 1 (VP1) test has been an enormous boon for sufferers from ME; even where it has proved negative,

Post-viral Fatigue Syndrome. Edited by R. Jenkins and J. Mowbray
© 1991 John Wiley & Sons Ltd

the knowledge that there is an accurate scientific test involved in the investigation of the disease has been a great morale booster after the disbelief and
hostility that many patients have encountered.

The VP1 test has been developed recently by Professor Mowbray and
detects enterovirus antigen in the serum. In it a labelled monoclonal antibody to VP1 is employed which detects the virus particle which is present in
the coating of all enteroviruses. As there are 75 enteroviruses, this cuts down
enormously the time needed for testing.

There are two reasons for the occurrence of negative results in the VP1
test. It is thought that about a third of cases of ME are caused not by an
enterovirus but by the Epstein–Barr virus, which would not be detected by
the test. A more interesting problem which is being investigated at present is
how long the VP1 test remains positive and whether in a disease with such
wide variations it remains uniformly positive all the time.

When a diagnosis has been made it is vital to discuss the clinical picture
with the patient and go with them into every detail of their life to provide all
the help we can. In a condition that varies so widely and so quickly from
complete exhaustion to virtual normality from day to day, the patient must
be in control of their own treatment.

FATIGUE

ME is characterised by severe fatigue, both physical and mental. This is an
abnormal exhaustion which is well beyond anything that happens in normal
life and is difficult to explain to those who have not experienced it. It can reduce
a fit, very strong man whose job was working on the roofs as a slater to a
condition where it is impossible for him to rise from his bed to open the door.

This fatigue can be mental also, and memory and concentration may be
profoundly affected. Simple facts like well-known telephone numbers and
addresses may be lost.

In normal fatigue, after rest there is a tendency when recovery has occurred for the same task to be performed more easily. This does not occur in
ME and after very moderate exercise the recovery period may stretch into
days or weeks.

TREATMENT

Rest

Although there have been a number of counter-claims, rest is the only treatment which seems to help all patients and to hasten the occurrence of a

remission. This may vary from complete bedrest in severe cases, with the patient too exhausted to move, to needing 20 minutes rest at lunchtime.

While this is easy to write, the effects are wide-ranging and must be discussed fully. A stiff upper lip and a resolve to beat the illness by drive and determination are not a useful means of treatment and usually result in a severe exacerbation. The patient must operate within their own limits, which may mean a period or a whole day off when the condition is active. It is very important that employers and families should be prepared for these variations, as if they know that they are going to occur, it is much easier to cope with them.

If one has a car it is very useful to take 30 minutes off at lunchtime, when the patient can retire to a quiet car park for a rest or, if possible, a sleep. In work it is important to have colleagues who can cover for the patient. It is at such times that a VP1 test is particularly important as, if positive, it is very useful confirmatory evidence.

What applies to a patient's working life is even more important in social life and this may be the hardest of all to arrange satisfactorily. Any late night must be carefully judged and followed by increased rest in the following days. It is particularly in this managing of working and social life that every person with ME is an individual and takes a different path from any other; and, despite all the help and support that doctors can provide, the patient's own management of their lives is of paramount importance. This is, of course, not uncommon in medicine and it is quite wrong to think of ME as being a disease apart. In rheumatoid arthritis, despite the new generation of drugs available, rest is still a most important part of treatment, both total bedrest and rest in splints. This is also a disease which varies from day to day and where the fine tuning of the programme must be left to the patient.

Pain

Apart from the abnormal exhaustion which characterises ME, one of the most distressing symptoms is pain. In an exacerbation this is widespread through the body, sometimes seeming to concentrate on a previous weak spot, causing, for instance, severe intractable low back pain. In 60% of patients with ME, aching pain in the muscles, bones and the joints is a prominent symptom. Patients complain of a burning muscle discomfort similar in some ways to the pain after very severe muscle exercise but occurring after only minimal effort.

It is interesting to wonder if this pain is in anyway related to interference with the production of muscle energy by aerobic and especially anaerobic processes in the muscle and some experimental work is being carried out to investigate this.

This muscle pain is generally global in distribution and affects all muscles but tender spots may occur in varying areas, the chest, heels and Achilles tendons being often affected.

Although ME has a tendency to improve over a period and does not leave anatomical sequelae it may be a long illness and therefore any drug regimes which are considered must be carefully checked for side effects.

The patient is once again the only person who can decide whether an analgesic medication is necessary but I feel that many people deny themselves the considerable benefits of relief of pain partly from natural inclination and partly from the hostility which their condition has aroused. Relief of pain, particularly at night when it often disturbs sleep is very important.

For those who have a genuine antipathy to tablets, I would recommend a strategy used by the first rheumatologist I worked under, who was as skilled in the workings of human nature as in those of rheumatic disease. Remedies were less extensive at that time and large doses of aspirin were an important part of treatment. If a patient was upset at taking the aspirin, the rheumatologist used to say that he had a small amount of tablets prepared from distilled extract of Willow Bark that he could let them have. Perhaps because this sounded more natural and wholesome, very few patients refused and he then used to give them the aspirin and explain how this had been developed from the original gypsy remedy, and give a short talk on salicin.

As ME may be long continued with a variable course, any medication must be carefully screened for possible side effects.

Painkillers or analgesics

Paracetamol in a dose of two tablets up to four times a day may be very helpful when pain is severe. Like all medication it should be taken regularly over a period and if possible under a doctor's direction, although it and numerous proprietary brands are available over the counter.

This method of taking controlled medication over a period is important, as most analgesics and most drugs generally are only effective when a therapeutic blood level is reached, and taking them irregularly and haphazardly will not produce a satisfactory result.

While paracetamol is normally very safe, and it must be remembered that it can cause liver damage with prolonged use and overdosage. This is particularly likely to occur if there has been previous liver damage due to alcohol.

Aspirin is a very useful analgesic but even in the enteric coated form can cause indigestion and gastrointestinal irritation with slight asymptomatic blood loss. With any medication which is taken over a long period, regular blood tests to test haemoglobin levels and to warn of blood dyscrazias should be taken.

Anti-inflammatory drugs

Just as in the treatment of an inflammatory polyarthritis, anti-inflammatory drugs can be very helpful in controlling the aching, burning pain which combines with severe exhaustion to reduce resistance in ME. As with painkillers, it is important to use the simpler remedies if possible.

Ibuprofen sold as Brufen and Ebufac does not need a prescription and can give a good deal of relief. The bedtime dose is particularly important as it will help to give a better night. Side effects are rare but dyspepsia, rash and thrombocytopenia may occur. Non-steroidal anti-inflammatory drugs appear to have one property in particular that should be mentioned. There seems to be a considerable variation in the effect which various drugs in similar doses have on different people. This means that, with the help of their doctor, it is well worth the patient 'shopping around' to find an anti-inflammatory drug which suits them personally.

I have found in a number of cases with severe muscle pain and stiffness that a small dose of indomethacin 25 mg three times a day or 50 mg three times a day may be very helpful. This is a powerful drug and can cause severe side effects. It must be prescribed by a doctor. It should be taken with food and can cause indigestion, headache and dizziness. In prolonged therapy, ophthalmic and blood examinations are necessary.

If indigestion causes severe problems, indomethacin can be taken rectally in the form of suppositories of 100 mg. These have the useful property that they take about eight hours to be absorbed so that if one is taken with food or milk at night, it is exerting its maximum effect in the early morning on first waking when many people experience their most severe symptoms.

In a condition with symptoms as varied as ME, numerous other remedies have been used in some cases to improve the condition but in most cases to ameliorate symptoms. Trials of gammaglobulin have so far been inconclusive although they are a hopeful avenue of research. So far, the use of specific antiviral remedies has been disappointing although this may be because we do not know the condition sufficiently well to make the best use of the agents involved.

Loss of sleep

Loss of sleep, and particularly the sleep which, although it appears to be deep, does not refresh, is common in ME. It seems likely that this phenomenon occurs because relaxation is never complete. As they have been prescribed a great deal we must consider sleeping tablets and antidepressants.

Sleeping tablets and antidepressants

Although they are so exhausted, patients with ME often have great difficulty in sleeping. Although sleeping tablets can reduce this period of wakefulness, my experience is that most patients feel a great deal worse after taking them.

Sleeping is at least partly a matter of habit and altering one's life a little can provide a much more satisfactory solution than sleeping tablets. So long as one can rest comfortably during the night, loss of sleep, except for a very long period, is not as harmful as people think and a good book and a carefully shaded light can work wonders.

One of the tragedies of ME is that so many of the symptoms can so easily be ascribed to vague psychiatric illness without the doctor concerned bothing to investigate either condition properly.

My feeling is that the symptoms of ME are usually made worse by antidepressants and I do not generally recommend them. However, if there are signs of overt clinical depression with physical signs of early-morning waking, loss of weight and constipation, antidepressants may be very useful. It is worth considering that with the hostility and antagonism which is raised in some quarters by the diagnosis of ME it is surprising that depression is not more common.

Medications, however bland, always carry some danger of side effects. Particularly in a condition which may be long-lasting, other methods of treatment may be effective and may carry far fewer dangers.

General considerations of treatment

A quiet discussion with the patient about what we know and assume about the diagnosis can be very helpful. One should always emphasise two points about ME. The first is that there is no evidence of anatomical crippling occurring with the condition, however long it lasts. This is in marked contrast to such diseases as rheumatoid arthritis and mutliple sclerosis, where anatomical changes are the rule.

The second hopeful feature is that there is a tendency in most cases for the condition to improve. Although a number of celebrated cases have lasted many years, in my practice, especially with young, otherwise well, patients, the majority have improved a great deal within two to three years. While this is still a long time, it is a great deal better than the indefinite sentence to which some patients feel they have been condemned.

Relaxation

Symptoms of anxiety and tension are common in ME and it is likely that while some of this may be engendered by external events, some is inherent and is caused by the effect of the disease on the central nervous system. Relaxation techniques can help this a great deal.

Relaxation classes run by an experienced psychologist or occupational therapist are very useful and will include discussion of troublesome symptoms and may be supplemented by a relaxation tape which the patient can use at home. One of the advantages of a relaxation tape is that the patient can use it whenever they feel the need.

In some cases, Yoga or meditation may suit the patient better than other forms of relaxation and these can form valuable adjuncts to treatment.

As a general rule in any form of treatment, cost is well worth considering. Althogh prognosis for long-term cure in ME in most cases is good, it is often a long-lasting illness. This can make the cost of any treatment outside the National Health Service a formidable burden and means that possible benefits must be weighed carefully against cost. Few things are more likely to increase the stress and anxiety of this condition than financial worries.

While exhaustion and muscle pain are perhaps the most common symptoms in ME, this is a wide-ranging illness and there are a number of other symptoms that can give great distress. Careful psychometric tests of the Wechslar type, although so far small in number, suggest that there is in many cases a marked effect on the central nervous system.

This would be a logical consequence, as a number of viral infections like poliomyelitis have shown a predilection for nervous tissue. Symptoms may be particularly upsetting because they are linked in people's minds and perhaps in the mind of the patient or doctor with psychiatric disturbances.

Slowed thinking and mental exhaustion

This occurs in 60–70% of patients with ME and often defects in short-term memory and visuospatial appreciation can be demonstrated. It can be particualrly worrying to a patient who has previously had a keen and active brain and whose job perhaps depends on these qualities.

A major step in dealing with these symptoms is to recognise them as a natural extension of the disease process and to be able to discuss them both with the doctor and with other sufferers. It is here that the ME Association can be of great help. Few things are worse than the feeling that one is alone, and chatting with other people who have experienced similar symptoms can help a great deal. From a practical point of view, once the symptoms have been recognised a great deal can be done.

Keeping a diary of one's life is extremely useful. It helps to record the progress of a very variable disease and it can always be referred to when short-term memory defects have blurred decisions and courses of action which have been previously taken.

Various memory techniques can also be very useful. Most people can remember a great deal more if they are provided with a series of cues. The memory techniques can provide these. The simplest cue is a list written in a diary, for instance of jobs that need doing. It is, however, possible with a little practice to link the jobs together in one's mind so that one job suggests another. This is a very old technique and is called catenation, from *catena*, a chain.

A very important factor in dealing with this slowness of memory and of thought is to recognise it and to make provision for it. Where possible patients should leave themselves longer for tasks than would normally be necessary and gear their work and domestic life to a slower pace. Colleagues, friends and family can be of great help at this time and a full and frank discussion is always valuable.

Emotional lability

Emotional lability is a common outcome of diffuse brain damage as those who deal with severe head injuries are well aware. It has been noted in a number of previous episodes of ME, for instance in the outbreak in Los Angeles. It can vary from minor irritation to outbursts of rage that are so vivid it has been suggested that they might represent epileptic equivalents. This emotional lability is particularly difficult for family and colleagues to accept.

Once again the most important step is to acknowledge that these mood changes are occurring so that steps can be taken to reduce the damage that they cause. Medication has little part to play as even large doses of tranquilising drugs do not appear to affect this symptom even when undesirable side effects like drowsiness and even disorientation occur.

A frank discussion with the people most likely to be involved is very useful. If a patient's family and colleagues are warned of the chance of lability of mood, steps can often be taken. While it is impossible to remove all sources of irritation from life, slight changes of routine and programme can often help to give a smoother course.

Dizziness and vertigo

This occurs in up to 70% of patients with ME. It seems to be more common early in the illness and can cause severe problems, particularly when it is sufficiently severe to interfere with walking. This is one of the symptoms that can be improved by drugs, although it must always be remembered that all patients differ and those with ME have a particularly wide variation. Stemetil and Avomine can often help with particularly severe attacks although they may cause drowsiness which makes driving or controlling machinery unwise. They can also act with alcohol to produce an enhanced depressant effect on the central nervous system. A less dangerous but annoying side effect is that they cause a dry mouth.

In a number of cases dizziness and vertigo is a passing symptom, but if it persists that there are dangers in prolonged regimes of medication. In these cases exercises of the Cooksey–Cawthorne type can be useful where retraining of the vestibular apparatus is carried out by a course of exercises where balance is maintained by eye fixation when the head is turned from side to side at first slowly and then with increasing speed. This appears to be helpful in some cases but as yet only a small number of cases have been treated in this way.

At first dizziness may be brought on by sudden movements of the head, and a deliberate policy of only making such movements slowly and carefully can help a great deal. When considering such movements one must remember that they can occur as part of an established procedure. For instance, when backing a car even quite simply out of a garage, the sudden rotation of the head can bring on a severe attack of vertigo.

If the occurrence of dizziness and vertigo passes off as it does in most cases, no further action is needed, but if it is persistent there are various mirror systems which can be fitted to a car which reduce the amount of head movement which is necessary. Sometimes when an attack of vertigo is severe a period of lying down is the only measure that brings relief.

Tinnitus or hyperacusis

This may cause a great deal of distress. In non-medical language, tinnitus is a ringing or buzzing in the ears. This can be very irritating especially as it tends to be more noticeable in conditions of quiet when the patient is trying to rest.

Often this symptom tends to improve or perhaps the patient merely becomes accustomed to it. If it continues it can present a major problem. In this case, there is some work which is being developed by some audiology clinics, which may be helpful, in which a pure tone of a different frequency is fed into the ears.

Hyperacusis is abnormal loudness of sounds and can occur in a number of conditions in which there is damage to the central nervous system. After a severe head injury, it can sometimes be a major cause of difficulty in returning to work where there is considerable engine noise in the workplace. The increase in volume of sounds also seems to carry with it an unpleasant piercing quality which does not occur in normal circumstances even when noises are loud.

Blurring of vision

This and difficulty in focusing are common problems in ME and this may be accompanied by intolerance of bright lights so that it is uncomfortable to go out, for instance in bright sunlight. It seems possible that both these symptoms are mediated through functional damage to the muscles of the eyes which are no longer working normally.

Although blurring of vision is inconvenient, it does not seem, on careful questioning, to be associated with misjudgement of distance and thus to present major hazards, for instances when driving. It should, however, be borne in mind if tasks requiring keen visual acuity are to be attempted. To cope with bright light there are a number of lightly tinted spectacles available which are a major help and do not make the patient conspicuous, as dark sunglasses do.

Headache and eye pains

These are extremely common in ME and may indeed be the first symptom following a viral illness. A differential diagnosis is always difficult and can be extensive.

Paranasal sinuses should always be checked, as infection or vacuum effects can often cause a similar headache. A simple analgesic may be helpful but spending an hour or two in bed, if this is possible, is often the most effective remedy.

In elderly patients with headache, and eye pain in patients with muscle stiffness and malaise similar to ME, a diagnosis of polymyalgia rheumatica with temporal arteritis should be considered. Here a sedimentation rate will be very much raised and a trial of steroids will produce an almost magical clinical improvement. This is in marked contradistinction to ME, which appears to be made worse by steroids, as one would expect in a condition associated with a live virus.

Thoracic symptoms

In company with symptoms which suggest damage to the nervous system, those which suggest an effect on the heart are a great source of anxiety. Two symptoms are particularly worrying.

Chest pain

This can be severe but is usually superficial in type and is altered by positioning of the left shoulder and arm and of the chest wall. There is often a tender spot over the sternoclavicular joint. Although the benefits may be only temporary, injecting the tender spot with 1% lignocaine may be useful. If the tenderness is diffuse, as it usually is, rather than pinpoint, a fan of several injections through the same entry puncture seems to be most useful. Round the joint itself it is best to inject deeply with the needle as near the periosteum as possible.

Palpitations

These are associated in many people's minds with heart trouble, and indeed in ME they may indicate a primary or secondary effect on cardiac muscle. They often seem to occur early in the course of the disease and may be associated with breathlessness. Reassurance can be offered that as yet there is no evidence of persistent pathological lesions being caused by this condition despite the alarming symptoms.

Occasionally, palpitation becomes a major problem and seems to intrude into every part of a patient's life. In these cases a small dose of a beta-blocker under careful medical control can be helpful.

Diarrhoea and a feeling of blocking

Less worrying than cardiological symptoms but causing a great deal of alarm and discomfort are gastrointestinal problems.

A high proportion of patients with ME develop intermittent diarrhoea and rather nonspecific stomach upsets with symptoms suggestive of an irritable colon with distension and discomfort. Constipation may occur intermittently and is helped by a moderately high fibre diet. In these days of central heating it is easy for patients to become slightly dehydrated and a pint of water taken just before going to bed will often promote a regular bowel habit.

Dysuria and frequency

These can be prominent symptoms; although a urine specimen for culture and sensitivity should be taken, it is normally found to be sterile and therefore it would not be appropriate to treat the condition with antibiotics. Fluid intake should be increased and the old-fashioned remedy of Mist Pot Cit 10 ml three times a day may be very helpful in reducing the irritability of the bladder.

Coldness of the extremities and extreme sensitivity to external temperature change

This may present as cold hands but it is much more common for feet to feel cold although this is not always obvious to an observer. It is possible that this is due to delays in adaptation of the circulation and there is certainly a tendency for all patients with active ME to look extremely pale. Treatment, however, is disappointing. Warm woollen socks and gloves do not seem to help a great deal and even electrically heated gloves were not effective in the few patients that have tried them, unlike the result in Raynaud's phenomenon, in whichi they are moderately successful.

Persistent sore throats

These appear in some cases to be the precipitating cause and may last for a considerable time. Throat swabs show only commensal organisms and the condition appears to be virus-mediated. Cervical lymph nodes, in my experience, are not usually enlarged.

Although there are a large number of medicated pastilles that can be used to help the condition it is doubtful if any of them do more than keep the mucous membranes of the oropharynx moist and this can be done just as efficiently by a simple boiled sweet.

Resumption of activities

Despite its often protracted course there is a tendency for all cases of ME to improve but care is needed in the adjustment of the programme when the patient begins to feel better. It is vital to avoid over-exertion and becoming exhausted as this will cause a severe recurrence of symptoms.

When planning a resumption of activities always err on the side of caution and make your plans as fluid as possible, as recurrences are common.

When cautiously increasing the amount of exercise taken, remember that walking, especially on moors and rough country, is severe exercise and would not be appropriate especially in the early stages of recovery. Gentle swimming is excellent exercise as the majority of the weight is taken by the water. One problem, however, can be the effect of the cold on the vascular instability that we have previously mentioned. Hydrotherapy pools with their much higher temperatures are ideal but are in short supply.

Many young male patients are desperate to return to weight-lifting gyms when they begin to feel better after such a debilitating illness. It is very important for this to be done very carefully. The form of exercises must be considered as well as their intensity and duration. Isometric exercises, where muscle contractions are achieved without movement, seem to produce much better results in the improvements of power without causing a return of the severe exhaustion.

Just as with exercise, a patient who is feeling better should only alter his social life slowly. Extravagant resumptions of activity should be avoided. It should be remembered that most patients with ME find that even a small amount of alcohol makes them feel a great deal worse.

Immunisations should be avoided if possible as there is a tendency for them to make the condition worse.

ALTERNATIVE TREATMENTS

I have not so far mentioned a large number of the treatments that have been advocated for ME. This is because I have not had a sufficient number of patients on those treatments myself to judge whether they have been of benefit nor have I been able to find adequate controlled trials to support their value. In all conditions where curative remedies are not available, a vast fund of anecdotal evidence grows up. It is very important to consider this dispassionately, as otherwise a great deal of disappointment and expense may be incurred.

It is well to remember also that judging the efficacy of treatment is particularly difficult in a condition with a very varied course. For instance, when I had only recently begun a career in rehabilitation, I had a patient with severe multiple sclerosis. He was a most intelligent man who single-handed had built up a large business. He was being treated at considerable expense with baths of homogenised seaweed.

I will list some of the more common treatments because in a disease with as wide a variation as ME it would be as unscientific to insist that none of them will work without trial as that they will be instantly successful.

Mineral and vitamin supplements

Trace elements like zinc and magnesium have been found by some workers to be low in ME. These substances are not routinely tested for in most biochemistry profiles, which may be why this finding is not more common. Zinc has been shown previously to have a marked effect on the healing of ulcers, while magnesium can affect muscle contraction. If these elements are significantly low, a short trial of a supplement would be appropriate.

The place of vitamins in ordinary life has always been controversial. Most of the experimental work has been done on grave states of deprivation like scurvy and beri beri, and vitamin needs in ordinary life have been much less clearly defined. There is, for instance, little hard evidence on the vitamin needs of a physically very energetic life like that of a professional footballer. It may well be that some vitamin needs are increased in such circumstances.

Equally, in a disease like ME, it is possible that vitamin needs are increased although there is as yet no hard evidence for this. It is reasonable to take a small vitamin supplement so long as moderation is practised. In a disease with so wide an individual variation it seems likely that benefit will only occur with a percentage of patients.

The vitamin which in the winter may be in greatest danger of being taken in sub-optimal levels, if not deficiency levels, is vitamin C. This is usually a matter of an ill-advised diet, which is all too easy in these days of fast food, rather than a really unsatisfactory diet.

Allergy

Many patients feel that food and chemical allergies contribute to their feeling of ill-health in ME. There is as yet little hard evidence available on this subject and it is a vast study with many ramifications. A full assessment of a patient's allergic state may be very expensive and confer only limited benefit. A useful start is using the invaluable diary to practise an exclusion diet to see if removal of any particular articles of food and drink appears to have a beneficial effect.

Hypoglycaemia

This can cause many of the symptoms that are common in ME, e.g. muscle weakness, fatigue and nervousness. In some cases the low blood glucose has been proved biochemically. The normal reaction is to take sweets or glucose tablets but these can cause a severe rebound hypoglycaemia. A slight increase of long-lasting carbohydrate in normal meals and preventing long intervals between meals will give better results.

Candida

Candida albicans is felt by some authorities to be involved in the causation of ME. This is an attractive theory because candidiasis is associated with a number of debilitating conditions like diabetes mellitus, and it also tends to occur where antibiotics have been intensively used. This occurs in many patients, especially early on before a diagnosis has been made.

If *Candida* does contribute to the long-term symptoms of ME, there are at least effective anti-yeast remedies like nystatin that can be used together with a low sugar and carbohydrate diet with restricted yeast.

The major difficulty with these patients is that *Candida* infection is most likely to occur when there has been a major breakdown of the immune system, where an infection with *Candida* can become a life-threatening emergency.

Acupuncture

Acupuncture is believed to work best in conditions in which there is disturbance of function but not anatomy. This would seem in our present state of knowledge to apply to ME and it has been widely used to alleviate symptoms. It has a very ancient lineage and although the mechanism by which it produces its effect is by no means entirely worked out, it has an impressive list of practical problems, like anaesthesia during operation, to which it has been applied. I would, however, counsel very earnestly about choice of an acupuncturist. Just as one would rightly hesitate to have an operation carried out by a surgeon who only did one or two a year, it is important to choose a well-trained and experienced practitioner of acupuncture, as poor results result otherwise.

CONCLUSION

This chapter has, I fear, contained a good deal of gloom and doom; may I close with a message of hope. First, there is a great deal of research being done on ME, as illustrated by Professor Mowbray's magnificent work with the VP1 estimation.

Secondly, and equally important, the climate of medical opinion, although as you know this is as slow to move as the bowels of the earth, seems to be shifting gradually towards regarding ME as an organic disease and less as a figment of the imagination. This will help a great deal in providing a broad base for research.

The active support of the ME Association is of great benefit and means that information is always readily available.

Things are a great deal better than they were at the time of the Royal Free epidemic and I think that we can look to the future with confidence.

REFERENCES

Achison, E. D. (1959) The clinical syndrome variously called benign myalgic encephalomyelitis, Iceland disease and epidemic neuromyasthenia. *American Journal of Medicine*, **26**, 569–595.

British National Formulary (1988) No. 16.

Dowsett (1988) Human enteroviral infections. *Journal of Hospital Infection*, **11**, 103–115.

Franklin, M. and Sullivan, J. (1989) *The New Mystery Fatigue Epidemic ME*. Century Hutchinson, London.

Gray, J. A. (1983) Some long term sequelae of Coxsackie B virus infection. *Journal of the Royal College of General Practitioners*, **34**, 3–6.

Jamal, G. A. and Hansen, S. (1985) Electrophysiological studies in the post-viral fatigue syndrome. *Journal of Neurology, Neurosurgery and Psychiatry*, **48**, 691–694.

Ramsay, A. M. (1986) *Post Viral Fatigue Syndrome. The Saga of the Royal Free Disease*. Gower Medical, London.

Smith, D. G. *Understanding ME*. Robinson Publishing, London.

21

Treatment of the Post-viral Fatigue Syndrome—Rationale for the Use of Antidepressants

H. E. Webb and Linda M. Parsons

St Thomas' Hospital, London, UK

As clinicians we are firmly of the opinion that depression itself is an organic disorder associated with neuroendocrine and neurotransmitter disturbances in the central nervous system (CNS). Depression may follow many different types of insult—head injury, stress, virus infections and bereavement—and may also be inherent in an individual through genetic determinants.

It cannot have escaped attention that many of the features of the post-viral fatigue syndrome (PVFS) bear a similarity to those found in depressive disorders where there is often somatisation. We believe that post-viral fatigue constitutes one end of the spectrum of a depressive illness, the main complaints being overwhelming fatigue and loss of drive, together with poor concentration and memory, loss of libido and sleep disturbance. Somatic symptoms also occur, e.g. myalgia, headache, sore throat, weight loss and 'pins and needles'. This picture is in contradistinction to the other end of the spectrum of depression where the features are more characteristic of 'classical' depressive illness with obvious mood disturbance, feelings of paranoia and worthlessness, nihilism and suicidal intentions. It is the lack of these latter more clear-cut symptoms which may have provided the stumbling block in the diagnosis in this group of patients and hence their rational treatment, a formal diagnosis of depressive illness being rejected by both patient and doctor, or not even considered in the first place.

Why then should a viral infection be associated with an illness which appears to be associated particularly with fatigue? We suggest that there could be a reasonable explanation for this and for the success of antidepressant medication.

As fatigue is such a prominent complaint amongst this group of patients,

Post-viral Fatigue Syndrome. Edited by R. Jenkins and J. Mowbray
© 1991 John Wiley & Sons Ltd

interest has been directed towards its origin. The occurrence of myalgia in some patients and an association with viruses which are known to be myotropic, for example Coxsackie B, would suggest that peripheral muscle involvement may be responsible for continuation of the myalgia and partly for the fatigue. In those patients who have no evidence of a myositis, studies have failed to detect any differences in muscle function between patients with chronic fatigue and controls (Stokes et al., 1988; Lloyd et al., 1988). These authors have suggested a central rather than peripheral mechanism for the fatigue, relating it to the perception of the effort required rather than any true muscle disease, and we would agree with this. Support for this view is provided by Wessely and Powell (1989). They compared patients who had unexplained chronic fatigue with a group with peripheral fatiguing neuromuscular disorders and a further group with depressive illness. They found that 72% of those with chronic fatigue had evidence of a psychiatric illness, mainly depression. Although there was no difference in subjective complaints of physical fatigue between the three groups, mental fatigue and fatiguability were equally common in chronic fatigue and the depressed patients but only occurred in those neuromuscular patients who also had a psychiatric illness. Overall the chronic fatigue patients more closely resembled the affective than the neuromuscular patients. The symptoms displayed by the chronic fatigue group did not enable the clinician to discriminate between chronic fatigue states and an affective disorder. The conclusion drawn was that the fatigue was of central origin.

Patients with post-viral fatigue have usually had a febrile illness which, with our present understanding, would be described as viral. No one virus has been shown to be exclusively involved. The fatigue which can follow glandular fever (Epstein–Barr virus) is well recognised. However, enteroviruses have received more attention recently. Yousef et al. (1988) have proposed that detection of the enterovirus antigen virus particle 1 (VP1) in serum is a sensitive method of investigation for these patients. They found VP1 in 51% of a group of patients with chronic post-viral fatigue. The number of patients positive for VP1 antigen was greater when IgM complexes were detectable than when they were not. These data suggest that persisting infection with enteroviruses may occur in some patients. However, Halpin and Wessely (1989) have pointed out that although there appears to be a relationship between VP1 and chronic fatigue syndrome, there was a lower frequency of positives in their study (30%) compared to that of Yousef. Also 12% of controls (randomly chosen inpatients from a general neurological ward with no history of fatigue) were positive, suggesting that the association may not be as helpful as previously proposed. It is well recognised that many people have Coxsackie infections with transient myalgia and no further sequelae. Those who develop prolonged post-viral disturbances may have a genetic susceptibility to react to a virus in this particular way. Many patients with post-viral fatigue have no evidence of prior enterovirus infection and the syndrome has been described following proven infections with other viruses.

It is accepted that many common viruses reach the CNS during the course of an infection, for example Epstein–Barr virus (Gautier-Smith, 1965), measles virus (Pampiglioni, 1964; Dubois-Dalcq, 1979), measles vaccine viruses (Pampiglioni *et al.*, 1971; Morgan and Rapp, 1977), herpes zoster, herpes simplex, mumps, many enteroviruses (Wood and Anderson, 1988) and many arboviruses. Viruses replicate well in brain tissue and many have been shown to have the capacity to persist in the nervous system for long periods of time, replication not necessarily producing overt neurological illness. Certain viruses have been shown to infect particular cell types within the CNS or subpopulations of neurones specific to particular regions of the brain (Johnson, 1980). Experimental studies using herpes simplex virus in the mouse have shown localisation of viral antigen predominantly to large neurones in the hippocampus, temporal cortex and limbic system, in particular cingulate cortex, septum and amygdala. In the pons and brain stem, antigen has been localised to the locus coeruleus, substantia nigra and dorsal raphe nucleus, primarily in large multipolar neurones (Cross *et al.*, 1984; Neeley *et al.*, 1985).

It is recognised that the hypothalamus and limbic system are important in the control of energy, drive, mood and libido. The locus coeruleus and raphe nuclei in the brain stem are thought to be important in the control of sleep. Experimentally, localisation of virus has been demonstrated in these areas. Hence changes occurring in or having a secondary effect on these particular areas may be important following viral infection and, in view of the known functions of these areas, would support a central origin for the fatigue and associated symptomatology seen.

What is it then about a viral infection of specific areas of the CNS which may produce a depressive disorder with a particular emphasis on fatigue?

There is increasing evidence showing that viruses can affect enzyme systems and neurotransmitters. In the experimental studies referred to previously it was shown using herpes simplex virus that a two- to three-fold increase in dopamine and serotonin metabolism, measured in the form of homovanillic acid and 5-hydroxyindolacetic acid respectively, was found in cortex, striatum, diencephalon and brain stem (Neeley *et al.*, 1985). Further work using an avirulent strain of Semliki Forest virus, an alpha virus, in the mouse, has shown selective changes in neurotransmitters, e.g. glutamic acid decarboxylase and homovanillic acid, some of which persist after infectious virus can no longer be detected (Barrett *et al.*, 1986). Other workers using Semliki Forest virus have shown the majority of focal lesions produced in mouse brain following this infection to be located in the midbrain, brain stem and cerebellum (Suckling *et al.*, 1977).

Suckling *et al.* (1976) have also shown that following an inapparent viral encephalitis in the mouse the levels of several lysomal glycosidases were elevated. Not all parts of the brain were affected equally, cerebellum, midbrain and spinal cord showing the most severe changes. Levels remained elevated at least 28 days after infection, infectious virus being undetectable after day 11. This effect has also been shown for other arboviruses (Suckling *et al.*, 1978).

It is apparent, therefore, that viruses may affect cellular metabolism in a subtle way which alters the specialised function of the cell without causing cell death. Oldstone (1989) has shown this effect using lymphocytic choriomeningitis virus (LCMV) in thyroid epithelial cells and in the islets of Langerhans with resulting impaired thyroxine, triodothyronine and insulin production respectively, but no change in cellular morphology. Klavinskis and Oldstone (1989) have also shown that LCMV infection in mouse CNS is associated with a growth hormone deficiency syndrome and that the decrease in growth hormone and its messenger RNA (mRNA) in these infected mice is related to a decrease in the initiation of transcription of the gene. Lipkin *et al.* (1988) have shown that LCMV infection in mice is accompanied by a decrease in brain levels of somatostatin mRNA, there being no change in mRNA for cholecystokinin and no morphological evidence of injury to the cell. There is, therefore, evidence of changes in differentiated, 'luxury' function of specific cells following a viral infection whilst cellular 'housekeeping' function remains unchanged.

Present evidence, therefore, suggests that many viruses reach the CNS and that virus may be localised to specific areas of brain associated with mood, drive and sleep pattern. There is also evidence that viruses can affect neurotransmitters and enzyme systems without causing cell death.

Although there is no general consensus as to the cause of depressive illness, it is accepted that neurotransmitters and the hypothalamic–pituitary–adrenal axis are important (Gold *et al.*, 1988). The first major hypothesis of affective disorder grew from the observation that depressive symptoms developed in 15% of patients being treated with reserpine for hypertension, reserpine being an amine-depleting agent. Subsequently monoamine oxidase inhibitors were found to be effective as antidepressant agents. Their mode of action was thought to be interference with the enzymic degradation of biogenic amines. Similarly, tricyclic antidepressants were found to block the synaptic reuptake of amines into presynaptic neurones. These observations gave rise to the original catecholamine hypothesis of depressive illness which suggested that it arose from a deficit in noradrenaline at critical effector sites in the CNS (Schildkraut, 1965; Bunney and Davis, 1965; Schildkraut, 1978). Further studies have shown that patients with major depressive illness have hypercortisolism, which is thought to derive from increased secretion of corticotrophin releasing hormone (Gold *et al.*, 1984, 1986). Subsequent studies have shown other neurotransmitter systems to be altered in depression and there appears to be a functional relationship between the locus coeruleus and corticotrophin releasing hormone, noradrenergic systems, gamma-aminobutyric acid, and cholinergic systems. Serotonin may also be involved. The interested reader is referred to Gold *et al.* (1988) for a full review. It is clear that there are many interactions amongst neurotransmitters and neurohormonal systems, and it is likely that many more still await discovery. The final explanation is likely to be complex. Regrettably, neuroendocrine and neurotransmitter studies in post-viral fatigue patients are lacking.

However, we feel that on the evidence available at present, it is reasonable to propose that many different viruses enter the CNS without producing overt acute neurological illness. Instead, neurochemical changes are induced, giving a pattern of symptoms with the emphasis on fatigue, the predominant symptom of the post-viral syndrome, rather than those of a more classical depressive illness. From our experience (see Chapter 15), antidepressants, both tricyclic and monoamine oxidase inhibitors, are highly successful in treating post-viral fatigue states. Because of the good response of this group to antidepressants, some light may be shed on the underlying cause of fatigue states and depressive illness in general, or at least directions may be suggested for further studies.

A final important point is how this information is conveyed to the patient. It is essential to overcome the stigma and rejection which some patients feel, particularly if they have been labelled as 'depressed'. We have found it useful to take time to discuss with the patient, in simple terms, the rationale for our treatment with tricyclics or monamine oxidase inhibitors. We explain that we believe their overwhelming fatigue to be due to the infection that they have had, that viruses can upset vital 'chemicals' in the brain which are responsible for controlling energy, drive, mood, memory, concentration and libido and indeed are often associated with control of pain. We do not make any reference to depression as such, except to say that the tablets prescribed are those used incidentally in the treatment of depression and that they will improve these abnormalities and make them feel much better. We emphasise, as stated previously, that the tablets must be taken for at least three weeks in order for there to be any benefit and will need to be continued for a minimum of three months. When the treatment is expressed in these terms, the patients appear to understand, accept treatment without problems, and persevere, particularly over the first three weeks when drowsiness may be a problem. It is then crucial that when the patients feel they have improved they do not stop the tablets abruptly but reduce them gradually, one at a time, at two to three week intervals. The pleasure they get from recovery, which may have eluded them for some considerable time, is very rewarding to the clinicians looking after them.

REFERENCES

Barrett, A. D. T., Cross, A. J., Crow, T. J., Johnson, J. A., Guest, A. R. and Dimmock, N. J. (1986) Subclinical infections in mice resulting from the modulation of a lethal dose of Semliki Forest virus with defective interfering viruses: neurochemical abnormalities in the central nervous system. *Journal of General Virology*, **67**, 1727–1732.

Bunney, W. E. Jr and Davis, J. M. (1965) Norephinephrine in depressive reactions; a review. *Archives of General Psychiatry*, **13**, 483–494.

Cross, A. J., Crow, T. J., Johnson, J. A., Neely, S. P. and Taylor, G. R. (1984) Effects of experimental herpes simplex virus encephalitis on monamine systems in mouse brain. *Journal of Physiology*, **350**, 30P.

Dubois-Dalcq, M. (1979) Pathology of measles virus infection of the nervous system: comparison with multiple sclerosis. *International Review of Experimental Pathology*, **19**, 101–135.

Gautier-Smith, P. C. (1965) Neurological complications of glandular fever (infectious mononucleosis). *Brain*, **88**, 323–334.

Gold, P. W., Chrousos, G., Kellner, C., Post, R., Roy, A., Avgerinos, P., Schulte, H., Oldfield, E. and Loriaux, D. L. (1984) Psychiatric implications of basic and clinical studies with corticotrophin-releasing factor. *American Journal of Psychiatry*, **141** (5), 619–627.

Gold, P. W., Loriaux, D. L. Roy, A., Kling, M. A., Calabrese, J. R., Kellner, C. H., Nieman, L. K., Post, R. M., Pickar, D., Gallucci, W., Avgerinos, P., Paul, S., Oldfield, E. H., Cutler, G. B. and Chrousos, G. P. (1986) Responses to corticotrophin releasing hormone in the hypercortisolism of depression and Cushing's disease: pathophysiologic and diagnostic implications. *New England Journal of Medicine*, **314**, 1329–1335.

Gold, P. W., Goodwin, F. K. and Chrousos, G. P. (1988) Clinical and biochemical manifestations of depression. Relation to the neurobiology of stress. *New England Journal of Medicine*, **319** (6), 348–353; **391** (7), 413–420.

Halpin, D. and Wessely, S. (1989) VP-1 antigen in chronic post viral fatigue syndrome. *Lancet*, **i**, 1028–1029.

Johnson, R. T. (1980) Selective vulnerability of neural cells to viral infections. *Brain*, **103**, 447–472.

Klavinskis, L. S. and Oldstone, M. B. A. (1989) LCMV selectively alters differentiation but not 'housekeeping' functions; block in expression of GH gene is at the level of transcriptional initiation. *Virology*, **168** (2), 232–235.

Lipkin, W. I., Battenberg, E. L. F., Bloom, F. E. and Oldstone, M. B. A. (1988) Viral infection of neurons can depress neurotransmitter mRNA levels without histologic injury. *Brain Research*, **451**, 333–339.

Lloyd, A., Hales, J. and Grandevia, S. (1988) Muscle strength, endurance and recovery in the post infection fatigue syndrome. *Journal of Neurology, Neurosurgery and Psychiatry*, **51**, 1316–1322.

Morgan, E. M. and Rapp, F. (1977) Measles virus and its associated diseases. *Bacteriological Reviews*, **41** (3), 636–666.

Neely, S. P., Cross, A. J., Crow, T. J., Johnson, J. A. and Taylor, G. R. (1985) Herpes simplex virus encephalitis. Neuro-anatomical and neuro-chemical selectivity. *Journal of the Neurological Sciences*, **71**, 325–337.

Oldstone, M. B. A. (1989) Viral alteration of cell function. *Scientific American*, August, 34–40.

Pampiglioni, G. (1964) Prodromal phase of measles, some neurophysiological studies. *British Medical Journal*, **ii**, 1296–1300.

Pampiglioni, G., Griffiths, A. H. and Bramwell, E. C. (1971) Transient cerebral changes after vaccination against measles. *Lancet*, **ii**, 5–8.

Schildkraut, J. J. (1965) The catecholamine hypothesis of affective disorders; a review of supporting evidence. *American Journal of Psychiatry*, **122**, 509–522.

Schildkraut, J. J. (1978) Current status of the catecholamine hypothesis of affective disorders. In M. A. Lipton, A. DiMascio and K. F. Killam (eds) *Psychopharmacology: a Generation of Progress*, pp. 1223–1234. Raven Press, New York.

Stokes, M. J., Cooper, R. G. and Edwards, R. H. T. (1988) Normal strength and fatiguability in patients with effort syndrome. *British Medical Journal*, **297**, 1014–1017.

Suckling, A. J., Webb, H. E., Chew-Lim, M. and Oaten, S. W. (1976) Effect of an inapparent viral encephalitis on the levels of lysosomal glycosidases in mouse brain. *Journal of the Neurological Sciences*, **29**, 109–116.

Suckling, A. J., Jagelman, S. and Webb, H. E. (1977) Brain lysosomal glycosidase activity in immuno-suppressed mice infected with avirulent Semliki Forest virus. *Infection and Immunity*, **15** (2), 386–391.

Suckling, A. J., Jagelman, S. and Webb, H. E. (1978) A comparison of brain lysosomal enzyme activities in four experimental togavirus encephalitides. *Journal of the Neurological Sciences*, **35**, 355–364.

Wessely, S. and Powell, R. (1989) Fatigue syndromes. A comparison of chronic 'postviral' fatigue with neuromuscular and affective disorders. *Journal of Neurology, Neurosurgery and Psychiatry*, **52**, 940.

Wood, M. and Anderson, M. (1988) Enterovirus infections. In *Neurological Infections*, pp. 145–152. WB Saunders, London.

Yousef, G. E., Bell, E. J. Mann, G. F., Murugesan, V., Smith, D. G., MacCartney, R. A. and Mowbray, J. F. (1988) Chronic enterovirus infection in patients with post viral fatigue syndrome. *Lancet*, **i**, 146–150.

22

The Cognitive Behavioural Management of the Post-viral Fatigue Syndrome

Simon Wessely*, Sue Butler†, Trudie Chalder†
and Anthony David*

*Institute of Psychiatry, London, UK
†National Hospital for Nervous Diseases, London, UK

INTRODUCTION

In the following chapter we shall discuss the pragmatic management of patients with the post-viral fatigue syndrome. Before embarking on such a task, however, it is necessary both to define the group of patients we are attempting to treat, and describe the rationale behind such an approach. This is particularly important as our approach differs in certain respects (although often in name rather than form) from that practised by other contributors to this volume.

Post-viral fatigue syndrome (PVFS) is a broad church that means different things to different people. It is even called different things. However, for the remainder of this contribution we will follow the convention adopted in this book and retain the label 'post-viral fatigue syndrome'. We will use the term as a clinical, as opposed to aetiological, description of a syndrome characterised by the following:

(a) Severe physical and mental fatigue induced by physical or mental effort.
(b) Myalgia, both at rest and on exertion.
(c) An absence of abnormalities on conventional medical investigations.
(d) Duration of at least six months.

Additional features include a variety of somatic symptoms, such as breathlessness, paraesthesiae, headache and dizziness. Furthermore, many, but not all, report an initial association with a 'viral'-type illness.

We are excluding from further discussion the rare patients with evidence

Post-viral Fatigue Syndrome. Edited by R. Jenkins and J. Mowbray
© 1991 John Wiley & Sons Ltd

of end organ damage which results from chronic viral infection. These include those with chronic active Epstein–Barr virus (EBV) infection, in which there is gross elevation of a variety of EBV antibodies and multisystem damage, with a high mortality from lymphoproliferative cancers (Jones et al., 1988). We also exclude those with clinical cardiomyopathy secondary to enteroviral infection (Muir et al., 1989). In practice most doctors can distinguish such patients from those who are the subject of the rest of this chapter.

A NEW MODEL OF PVFS

In order to explain our treatment approach, it is necessary to introduce our model of PVFS. Understanding this model is not only of theoretical importance, but also forms part of treatment, for, as we shall be constantly repeating, patients will only co-operate with such a programme if they understand the rationale behind it. We do not claim that the model is comprehensive, but instead suggest that it is heuristically useful and may explain many of the otherwise confusing elements of PVFS.

The model we have developed to explain the clinical predicament encountered by many of our patients is essentially a dynamic one, involving a combination of infective, physical, behavioural and psychological factors. It does not preclude the influence of infective agents and/or immune dysfunction, but places these within a psychosocial framework. We have divided it into six sections.

Virus

Starting the discussion with a virus is not arbitrary, since that is how most of our patients describe their illness as commencing. In our series of 50 subjects this was reported by over 75%. Such factors as the frequency of infections in the community, and the effect of 'search after meaning', suggest that this figure is an overestimate of the true association, but a viral-like infection remains the starting point of many clinical illnesses. The influence of prior psychological and general health on susceptibility to infection and their sequelae remains a complex area in need of further study.

Others have already described the immunological and serological consequences of viral infection. What about the behavioural consequences? No one can be in any doubt that during an acute viral infection the symptoms of pain, myalgia, fatigue etc. force most people to rest. Not only is this inevitable, but it may also be adaptive, since there is evidence of short-term subtle abnormalities in skeletal muscle (Astrom et al., 1976), cardiac muscle (Montague et al., 1988) and neuromuscular transmission (Friman et al., 1977) during acute viral infection, although the relevance is unclear (Friman *et al.*, 1985). Lerner (1988) has cautioned against the extremes of exercise during acute viral infections, although again this does not seem to apply to all viral infections (Repsher and Freebern, 1969). The immediate behavioural consequence of this is rest. However, this is the acute situation, not the post-viral syndrome. By the time the patient has been ill for sufficient time to warrant specialist referral, the situation has changed.

It must first be conceded that some people doubt that any change has occurred, other than the passage of time, and that 'PVFS' is simply a continuing infection. The evidence for such active persistence is reviewed in other chapters, but probably does not apply to the majority of patients with the clinical syndrome (Swartz, 1988; Straus, 1988; Wessely and Thomas, 1990).

What alternatives are there? Pasteur is reported to have said 'la germe c'est ne rien; c'est la terre qui est toute' (Laudenslager, 1987). There is increasing evidence in favour of his intuition, which implies a shift of attention away from the properties of the precipitating organism, to consider models which do not need ongoing viral infection to explain recurrent symptoms (Straus, 1988). We will concentrate on physiological, cognitive and behavioural changes occurring in the host.

Myalgias and mood

Myalgia is characteristic of PVFS, and, together with fatigue, is a major cause of the severe functional disability found in patients. It is a nonspecific symptom with a variety of causes (Edwards, 1986). One type is a muscle pain that is 'commonly experienced some few hours after exercise, and reaches peak intensity, which may be severe, about 24–48 hours later' (Editorial, 1987). This is one version of the muscle pain frequently described in PVFS (Ramsay, 1986; Smith, 1989), but in this instance is a description of the pain experienced by those taking unaccustomed exercise. The reason for such pain is eccentric contractions occurring in untrained muscles. Eccentric muscle contractions (when the active muscle lengthens whilst doing work) are potentially damaging to the muscle fibre, and may produce delayed muscle pain (Evans *et al.*, 1986; Editorial, 1987; Newham, 1988).

What is the relevance of such myalgias? We, along with others, have noticed how athletes are over-represented among those with PVFS. One explanation is the immunosuppressant effects of overexercise, and the other is the rapid physical deconditioning that occurs in the 'superfit' after even a brief period of forced inactivity. A further piece of the PVFS jigsaw is the anecdotal evidence that many chronic sufferers initially adopted too vigorous an approach to physical exertion during the immediate post-infective convalescence, perhaps again reflecting the possible over-representation of physically fit people in the final disease state. Assuming that recovery from viral illness follows a normal distribution from the rapid to the prolonged, the combination of this prolonged, albeit non-pathological, recovery with early vigorous exercise may cause unexpected severe delayed myalgia, and set in motion the rest of the cognitive behavioural cycle we describe later. However, neither too early activity, nor physical deconditioning, is a complete explanation of the myalgia/fatigue experienced in PVFS, since it cannot explain the evidence for central disorder (Lloyd *et al.*, 1988; Stokes *et al.*, 1988; Wessely and Powell, 1989). It is probable that delayed recovery coinciding with a liability to mood disorder is the most likely beginning to PVFS.

This introduces a second cause of pathological myalgia: affective disorder. Regardless of whether mood disorder is seen as the primary cause of symptoms, a secondary reaction to disability, or the result of a joint predisposition or pathology, a vast literature confirms it as a potent cause of fatigue and myalgia, including muscle pain both at rest and after exertion (Wessely and Powell, 1989). The mechanisms underlying fatigue and myalgia are obscure, although some authors have speculated on the role of hypothalamic dysfunction in both PVFS and mood disorder, and others on the direct effect of viral agents on mood disorder (see Chapter 21) and on sleep and myalgia (Modolofsky, 1989). Again, the direction of causality is by no means obvious, but even if explanations are tentative, the importance of central factors in fatigue and myalgia is widely accepted.

In published series of PVFS, operationally defined affective disorder is common, occurring in between a half to two-thirds of cases (Taerk *et al.*, 1987; Gold *et al.*, 1990; Manu *et al.*, 1989a; Kruesi *et al.*, 1989; Wessely and Powell, 1989; Millon *et al.*, 1989; Hickie *et al.*, 1990). These prevalences are higher than occur in other medical conditions without central nervous system involvement, and suggest that at least some of the observed mood disorder is not so-called 'reactive' depression, that is a 'psychological' reaction to illness.

The importance of these observations goes beyond the association between depression and fatigue/myalgia. The relationship between depression and PVFS is complex. Helplessness is a symptom of depression, and contributes to the expectation that fatigue and pain will follow exertion. Alternatively, myalgia and fatigue fulfil the description of stimuli that are associated with the genesis of depression in the 'learned helplessness' model (Abramson *et al.*, 1978), being potent, uncontrollable and aversive. In practice it is probable that both explanations are relevant to PVFS, forming the first of many self-perpetuating cycles that contribute to the clinical picture.

Attributions

Not only fatigue and myalgia, but also many other symptoms of PVFS, overlap with those found in affective disorder, including palpitations, breathlessness, sensations of altered temperature, paraesthesiae, dizziness, headache etc. These symptoms are also common during an acute infective illness. The confusion between the symptoms of acute viral infection, mood disorder and chronic fatigue syndromes was highlighted by Imboden (1972), who, when discussing the syndrome once attributed to 'chronic brucellosis' (Imboden *et al.*, 1959), wrote that 'vaguely described symptoms such as fatigue, apathy, weakness, restlessness, feeling "blue", various aches and pains, anorexia and insomnia' occurred in both 'chronic brucellosis' and affective disorder. He continued 'such complaints are also extremely common in the aftermath of any acute, febrile, debilitating illness' and finally 'in patients who become . . . depressed, these symptoms become severe and persistent and, when this occurs, they are apt to be regarded as evidence that the original illness itself is persisting'.

The consequence of such overlap may be that the patient (and doctor) blames all ills on continuing viral infection, unaware of other competing influences. The word 'blame' is used deliberately, as issues of guilt, blame and responsibility affect both patients with PVFS and doctors making the diagnosis.

Blaming symptoms on a viral infection conveys certain advantages, irrespective of its validity. It is simple, frequent, and easily accepted. Attributing ill-health to external causes is the 'norm' (Pill and Stott, 1982), whilst those who attribute somatically based symptoms to internal, psychological causes may be unnecessarily disturbed by them (Watts, 1982). It is also beneficial to self-esteem by protecting the individual from guilt and blame. 'The germ has its own volition and cannot be controlled by the host. The victim of a germ infection is therefore blameless. The cardinal attribute of germs is external . . . There is no malevolence or 'maleficium' involved' (Helman, 1978).

The situation becomes more complex and less clear-cut in a chronic condition. Continuing to attribute symptoms to an external cause continues to maintain self-esteem, and avoids guilt and self-blame (Powell *et al.*, 1990). However, there is a price to pay (Table 1). The simple explanation may be misleading, and if uncritically accepted may ensure that potentially treatable mood disorder is missed, with disastrous consequences. Equally important is the loss of self-efficacy. The patient feels in the grip of something which he or she is powerless to influence, be it a chronic virus or chronic allergy (see Folkman, 1984, for a more detailed discussion). External attributions increase helplessness, and may also increase the severity of fatigue, as has been demonstrated in anxiety (Hoehn-Saric and Mcleod, 1985). Levi-Straus (1963) alludes to this problem when describing the role of symbolism in explanatory systems: 'The sick woman . . . does not accept the incoherent and arbitrary pains which are an alien element in her system'. The healer's role is to give a symbolic model that permits the patient to understand, and thus get well. 'But no such thing happens to our sick when the causes of

Table 1 Possible consequences of attributing symptoms to an external agent

Advantages	Disadvantages
1. Simple to understand	1. Simple explanation may be misleading
2. No self-blame or guilt	2. May obscure symptoms of depression
3. No stigma	3. No control over symptoms
	4. No treatment
	5. Decline in self-efficacy

their diseases have been explained to them in terms of secretions, germs or viruses' (Levi-Straus, 1963). In terms of treatment the patient has no sense of 'what action to take beyond following the doctor's orders for medication' (Kirmayer, 1988).

These issues are raised because orthodox medicine has hitherto been unable to offer an explanatory model for PVFS. Into this vacuum have come a variety of 'alternative' theories—many taking preliminary or dubious laboratory theories and embellishing upon them. The demoralised patient naturally finds comfort in these 'explanatory systems', and may be reluctant to consider comparatively mundane mechanisms such as those raised in this contribution.

Cognitions

Modern cognitive theories emphasise the way our conscious thoughts (cognitions) mediate between our experiences and our actions. Through the seminal work of Beck (1976), it is also clear that cognitive errors are important in the development and maintenance of both anxiety and depression. What we think about symptoms and illness plays an important role in determining the eventual outcome of disease.

Returning to the initial precipitating illness, we have already discussed the role of prolonged recovery and early exercise in causing persistent myalgia and thus avoidance. There are cognitive consequences as well. Most people who present to the doctor with an acute viral-type infection are told they will 'soon get over it'. This is true in the majority of cases. However, some people will take far longer than others, without this implying a disease process. These people will experience a gradual increase in concern about recovery (not to mention loss of confidence in the doctor), especially if they are not prepared for the possibility of a prolonged convalescence. Advice about recovery which turned out to be faulty plays a similar role in perceived 'loss of control' in chronic pain (Philips, 1989).

We have encountered in patients with PVFS frequent examples of misguided assumptions analogous to those described by Beck. For example, behind many illness-provoked cognitions is the thought that 'I am suffering from an ongoing disease process in which activity exacerbates the illness'. In cognitive theory this is labelled a 'dysfunctional assumption', since it is a cause of disability (note that dysfunctional is not synonymous with inaccuracy). In consequence patients experience a variety of automatic thoughts (ideas that come rapidly and habitually in a specific circumstance), all of them negative, such as 'If I do more I'll cause myself serious harm', or 'I attempted to do more but feel exhausted, so I must have caused myself more muscle damage'. The former is an example of 'fearing the worst', usually called 'catastrophising' by cognitive therapists, the latter of misinterpretation, and their importance is that both may have a deleterious effect on mood, and emphasise avoidance of activity.

Discounting alternative explanations is common in PVFS, especially if sufferers are not aware of other explanations for their symptoms. Expectation is also important—based on previous experience, patients may think 'I am going to find this impossible' before attempting any activity. This will lead to either an upsurge in symptoms on attempting any activity, or feeling too dispirited to even commence. All this will be reinforced by the advice currently available to patients from the self-help literature.

A further cognitive factor in PVFS is that many patients, in an understandable effort to control and reduce symptoms by varying activity levels, become hypervigilant and oversensitised to physical sensations. Our knowledge of attention and awareness suggests that such symptom focusing may serve to further exacerbate unpleasant sensations. For example, increasing the attention paid to one's heart rate may lead to the detection of non-pathological ectopic beats which in turn gives rise to anxiety, and hence more palpitations.

We therefore propose that cognitive factors (in this case beliefs about health and illness) play an important part in perpetuating disability. These so-called 'dysfunctional beliefs' act as mediators of dysfunction, as has again been observed in chronic pain—the belief that pain invariably implies disability is a better prediction of the severity of impairment than subjective measurements of the severity of pain (Riley *et al.*, 1988). These dysfunctional attitudes concerning the interaction between rest, exercise and health also affect treatment outcome (Riley *et al.*, 1988).

Behavioural response

Dysfunctional cognitions are not sufficient to account for prolonged disability; their importance is linked to the development of maladaptive behavioural patterns. Simple operant conditioning shows that it is natural to avoid situations associated with distress. However, as the duration of illness lengthens, the reasons for this distress change, and avoidant behaviour no longer serves such a useful purpose.

Acute pain is a signal to the organism of danger, of tissue damage, but chronic pain fulfils no such role, and has no such readily identifiable physiological cause (Weisenberg, 1987). Instead, chronicity is influenced by the choice of coping strategies, and in particular avoidance of situations previously associated with symptoms.

'Avoiding situations plays an active part in reducing the sufferer's sense of control . . . and increasing his or her expectation that exposure will increase pain. These cognitive changes encourage further withdrawal from normal activities and a growing intolerance of stimulation.' (Philips, 1987)

Overall, chronic pain leads to major changes in lifestyle, activity and behaviour that are *independent* of the original stimulus (Weisenberg, 1987; Philips, 1987; Keefe and Gil, 1986).

We have extended this parallel to fatigue syndromes. The patient experiences genuine symptoms, learns that carrying on makes them worse, attributes them to a continuation of the initial viral infection, assumes also that symptoms are a warning of damage, and ceases the activity. This may have been adaptive, but is no longer so. Avoidance leads to decreased tolerance, both physiological and psychological. At each successive re-exposure to activity, decreased tolerance means symptoms occur at progressively lower levels of exertion, thus further convincing the patient of the accuracy of their explanation. Demoralisation, fear and depression soon compound the problem. Finally a vicious circle of pain, misery, avoidance and inactivity is established, in which the patient feels trapped and powerless to influence. Just as fatigue leads to inactivity, so does inactivity both cause and perpetuate fatigue.

The link between physical activity and well-being has been studied extensively. Hughes *et al.* (1984) found a correlation between fatigue and physical inactivity independent of physical health and fitness, whilst Stephens (1988) concluded that the positive correlation between physical activity, better mental health and lower levels of anxiety and depression (and hence fatigue) occurred independently of physical health status. In an eight-year follow-up study of nearly 2000 healthy adults it was shown that lack of activity was independently associated with a two-fold increase in the risk of depressive illness (Farmer *et al.*, 1988). Looking at coping strategies, Montgomery (1983) studied fatigue in a student population. He found significant differences in the response to the question 'when tired, what do you typically do?'. For tired subjects the sensations of fatigue serve as a stimulus to reduce their level of activity, acting as a cue to slow down or stop, whilst non-tired subjects tend to ignore similar sensations. Finally, in pain patients' rest is a potent reinforcer of both symptoms and disability (Keefe and Gil, 1986). Inactivity can, and does, cause fatigue. Nevertheless, with the occasional exception (Edwards, 1986; Dobkin, 1989), patients with PVFS are usually told from a variety of sources that lack of activity is invariably and permanently a consequence of fatigue. Such advice may be both inaccurate and counterproductive, and may serve to perpetuate the very disability that it is intended to minimise.

So far we have discussed avoidance and its role in PVFS. However, other behaviours that fall short of complete avoidance may also contribute. For example, many patients modify their activity to prevent exacerbation of symptoms. One example is one of our patients who chose to descend stair-cases on his bottom, rather than in the normal fashion. Others may take precautions, such as keeping a wheelchair handy even when not necessary, further limiting activity.

Modern behavioural medicine also emphasises the role of reinforcers in perpetuating disability. The behaviour of family and friends may inadver-tently reinforce the sick role, and mitigate against improvements when ap-propriate. Other family members may take on responsibilities previously carried out by the patient, or, out of their own concern, may prevent the patient from initiating recovery themselves. Social pressures, in particular the fear of being seen as psychologically ill, may contribute towards continu-ing illness affirmation.

It cannot be overemphasised that such behavioural responses are both understandable, and inadvertent. Yunus, talking about the same processes in fibromyalgia (a disorder also characterised by fatigue, muscle pain and affective changes and which overlaps with PVFS, and may be the same condition (Goldenberg, 1988; Goldman, 1988)), has pointed out a key issue: 'Operant behaviour is not the same as malingering, and any hint that the patient is consciously avoiding duties should be avoided'. Objective studies provide no evidence that the PVFS sufferer uses illness as a way of avoiding responsibilities (Beal, 1989), or attains any overall gain from ill-health. Any suggestion that the explanations advanced in this chapter seek to blame the patient for his or her predicament are without foundation.

Fear and uncertainty

Fear plays an important part in PVFS. First, we, and others, have found that clinical anxiety and phobias are common among patients. Second, fear of illness is an important part of PVFS, although this is not the exaggerated fear of illness found in hypochondriasis. This has been confirmed by Robbins *et al.* (1990), who compared fibromyalgia patients with rheumatoid arthritis controls. They found no differences in fear of illness and illness worry be-tween the two groups, the opposite of what would be predicted in hypoc-hondriasis. Nevertheless, worry about illness did play a role in the fibromyalgia patients, and correlated highly with overall functional disability. The authors suggest that 'feelings of vulnerability and apprehension about having an illness of unknown origin may contribute to sufferers' activity limitations, inability to sustain a work effort and varied somatic distress'. This is in accordance with our own observations, that it is the lack of both guidance about, and information on, the nature of PVFS, and of the origins of symptoms repeatedly experienced, that contribute to fear and hence disability. A further factor is ambiguity concerning the patient's medical status. Jerome Frank wrote that

Patients suffering from unfamiliar diseases tend to develop emotional reactions which impede recovery, such as anxiety, resentment and confusion. To keep disability at a minimum, therapeutic efforts must be directed not only to overcoming the pathogenic agent but to maintaining the patient's confidence in the physician, and encouraging his expectation of return to useful activity. (Frank, 1946)

Most important of all, fears of symptoms provokes and fuels avoidance behaviour (Lethem *et al.*, 1983; Philips, 1987; Weisenberg, 1987). As the patient's expectation that symptoms will follow activity increases, so do the precautions taken to avoid such symptoms. If these prove unsuccessful, fear increases. Stimuli that are anticipated, but unpredictable and uncontrollable, are particularly likely to lead to the final stage, when fear becomes fixed by the development of phobic anxiety. Avoidance of situations, including work, social activity, and travel, may result in the development of a phobic response on re-exposure. This is signalled by anxiety which in turn exacerbates fatigue (Folgering and Snik, 1988), a further vicious circle.

Conclusions

We are proposing that for many patients an initial infective trigger, with its associated myalgia and inactivity, begins a cycle in which both attributional and cognitive factors trigger avoidant behaviour. Avoidant behaviour itself sustains symptoms, as does any associated mood disorder, of whatever cause. The results explain much of the prolonged disability we associate with PVFS. The model can be summarised as follows. Figure 1 is the conventional view of the origin of symptoms in PVFS, and is the one that most patients are familiar with. Figure 2 shows that an initial virus may actually cause several different responses, any one of which may trigger the cycle described in Figure 3.

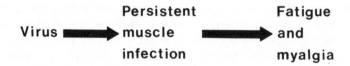

Figure 1   Conventional view of the origin of symptoms in PVFS

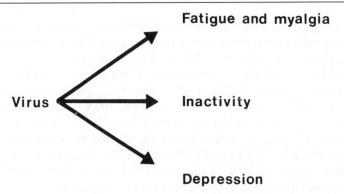

Figure 2   Initial virus may cause several different responses

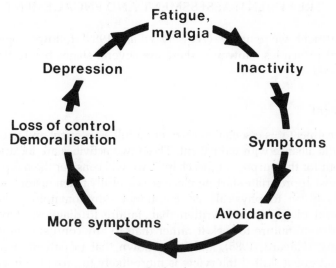

Figure 3   Cycle of responses

CURRENT TREATMENTS

At present there are no established treatments for PVFS. Other chapters have discussed the role of antiviral drugs, as well as agents acting on the immune system. No beuefit and considerable danger has been obtained from the former (Straus *et al.*, 1988). Trials of the latter are in progress, but to expect them to produce a complete solution to the problem is optimistic.

Instead, most patients receive very little in the way of help. If fortunate they may have a sympathetic medical adviser, and the fact that any professional takes them and their illness seriously is of inestimable therapeutic value. As regards practical advice, the mainstay of treatment remains rest, and to wait either for remission or a medical cure. This has been appropriately described as 'therapeutic nihilism' (Bayliss, 1988).

The situation is clearly unsatisfactory. What little we know about the natural history of these conditions (Wheeler et al., 1950; Valdini et al., 1987; Nelson et al., 1987; Kroenke et al., 1988; Wessely, 1990a) shows that untreated they can be severe and persistent. In the largest current series of sporadic cases 'Most of the cases seen do not improve, give up their work and become permanent invalids' (Behan and Behan, 1988). No satisfactory explanations have been advanced for this alarming tendency to chronicity. The rehabilitation package outlined below is an attempt to overcome it.

TREATMENT: ASSESSMENT AND ENGAGEMENT

The treatment we employ (Wessely et al., 1989) follows cognitive behavioural principles. However, there are several stages before that can be commenced.

Assessment

Before treatment it is essential to carry out a full assessment and to construct a therapeutic alliance with the patient. These two activities are inextricably entwined, but for the purpose of this chapter we will consider them separately.

The most appropriate starting place is a carefully taken history, with equal emphasis given to physical and emotional symptomatology. Discussing lassitude, a physician has written that 'failure to diagnose depression is usually due to failure to seek it rather than to any confusion in diagnostic symptoms' (Havard, 1985), and it is known that in patients with severe, chronic fatigue a skilled interview is more likely to provide information of use to the physician than further sophisticated investigations (Manu et al., 1989a; Kroenke et al., 1988; Valdini et al., 1989).

Certain areas are, however, of specific importance. It is essential to learn exactly what the patient thinks is the problem (which may or may not correspond to what he or she has been told). Next, one must build up a picture of the extent of functional impairment. This may be extreme, and is often equal to, or in excess of, that found in chronic medical patients (Kroenke et al., 1988). Finally, the nature, extent and reasons for all behavioural avoidances must be enquired into. It is not untypical to find a patient who is relatively free of symptoms, but on enquiry this is because they are leading an astonishingly restricted life. Many patients have rationalised such disability as 'living within limits' and have accepted extreme restrictions on functioning. One method is to go through a typical day hour by hour.

The final part of assessment, which merges into treatment, is obtaining a day-to-day record of symptoms and behaviour. We ask the patient to keep a diary of activity, including the minutiae of their response to symptoms. We pay particular attention to any variation in symptoms, and to the associations, both positive and negative, of such change. At every stage the patient is asked to list their corresponding cognitions.

Engagement and offer of treatment

At present the approach we favour is usually provided by professionals whose training and background is in mental health—psychologists, behaviour therapists, cognitive therapists and psychiatrists, the exceptions being general practitioners. There is no doubt that many PVFS patients are hostile to such an approach (Sharpe, 1990; Wessely, 1990b), seeing it as a denigration of their illness, and, no matter how politely phrased, a way of saying 'it is all in the mind'. No treatment can proceed before this hurdle is overcome.

One of the many paradoxes of dealing with PVFS is that the 'all in the mind' view is indeed held by many physicians, and may be the reason for referral in the first place. Many doctors, especially those in hospital practice, continue to see those illnesses which they are unfamiliar with, unable to treat, or even unable to find a pathological process for, as 'psychiatric'. They may adopt a punitive attitude towards the patient they have been unable to help. Kirmayer (1988) has pointed out 'if the norms for illness behaviour are contravened or pathophysiological explanations evaded, the patient may be blamed for diagnostic or treatment failures'. Many doctors are also intimidated by patients who have 'researched' their own illness and/or made their own diagnosis. The consequence is, all too often, a psychiatric referral. The patient may have appreciated these motives, and probably shares the common assumptions. It is an understatement to say this is not a propitious beginning to any therapy. Even if the patient does accept the referral, it may be with the sole intention of demonstrating that they are not mad after all.

We find that such attitudes must be tackled directly and openly. The initial interview is thus an explanation of our aim, which is to seek pragmatic ways of improving disability. We also permit the patient to admit to any previous, often unsatisfactory, medical encounters. This does not involve joining in criticising colleagues, but rather allowing the patient to discuss their feelings and experiences with the medical profession. A breakdown in the doctor–patient relationship seems to be part of the experience of ME (David *et al.*, 1988; Millon *et al.*, 1989; Jenkins, 1989; Wessely, 1990b). Our intention is therefore to enable the patient to discuss their own frustrations, and to observe how dealing with a difficult and intractable illness causes similar feelings in the doctor. The intention is also to confront the hidden (or sometimes not so hidden) message and assumptions behind the initial referral. We also openly discuss (and reject) allegations, spoken or un-spoken, of hysteria, malingering etc.

Over 50 years ago a consultant physician at the Mayo Clinic noted the same phenomenon. In an article entitled 'What to do with the patient who feels tired, weak and toxic' (Alvarez, 1935), he wrote 'The average doctor may feel the patient is neurotic, and will be disgusted with them. Often he sends them away with as little ceremony as possible . . . yet these poor people suffer the tortures of the damned.' Nothing has changed.

Treatment offer

The next stage is the offer of treatment. This may not be straightforward, and considerable difficulties may be encountered before a satisfactory treat-ment alliance can be formed. Many will remain wary of any treatment that is called 'psychological'. Before making an offer of treatment it is hence necess-ary to spend time discussing many of the principles outlined above. 'It is absolutely critical that the patient's goals and explanations be consistent with that of the treatment program, or the intervention will be doomed to failure' (Follick *et al.*, 1983).

A related problem is that of unreal expectations. Some patients have been told that the only prospect lies in a medical breakthrough, exemplified by the quote 'The hope is that one day a breakthrough will come, and that some substance will be isolated which has the power to zap the ME virus' (Hodgkinson, 1988). Such expectations are not only unrealistic, but also may obstruct real improvements, even if they fall short of 'cure'. A physical analo-gy is very helpful here. One physician discussing the management of these conditions advocated a pragmatic approach, writing that 'a surgeon can deal with a fracture without making inquiry into the details of the automobile accident during which it occurred' (Allan, 1945). We continue the analogy of being involved in an accident, and that pursuing the car to read the number plate will bring no benefit, as a way of emphasising the importance of the here and now, and that further investigations will serve little purpose. We also acknowledge that although patients usually wish to know why this has hap-pened to them ('Why me?'), definitive answers cannot always be given.

Treatment of mood disorder

Considerable research suggests that before embarking on any cognitive or behavioural approach it is necessary to treat any associated severe mood disorder. Not only is this a major cause of non-compliance and treatment failure, but also the illness needs treatment on its merits. Suicide remains the only recognised cause of death in ME.

The treatment of affective disorder is beyond the scope of this chapter.

Nevertheless, there is a wealth of evidence of the efficacy of tricyclic anti-depressants in the treatment of fatigue states associated with affective disorder. No formal trials of antidepressants exist in PVFS (see Chapter 21). Clinical evidence from the USA (Jones and Miller, 1987; Manu *et al.*, 1989b) suggests that 70% of these patients improve on low doses of tricyclics, but this may be an overestimate (Salit, 1985). Tricyclic antidepressants have also been used in placebo-controlled trials in fibromyalgia, and have significantly reduced muscle pain, insomnia and fatigue (Carrette *et al.*, 1985; Goldenberg *et al.*, 1986), and may have a direct effect on sleep disorder.

Criteria for treatment

Before treatment can commence, several criteria must thus be fulfilled:

(a) Patient and therapist agree on goals of treatment, that are both definable to the therapist and important to the patient.
(b) The patient understands the model of treatment, and is prepared to test out the suggestions, even if not agreeing with them.
(c) Mood disorder, if severe, is being treated appropriately.
(d) No further investigations will be performed without discussion with the therapist. It is assumed that reasonable measures will have been taken to exclude other treatable conditions.

TREATMENT: THERAPY

Introduction

The theoretical basis of cognitive behaviour therapy in PVFS does not depend, as many think, on the disorder having a psychological origin. This must be stressed, since most patients would find such a starting point unacceptable (Kruesi *et al.*, 1989; Matthews *et al.*, 1989; Sharpe, 1990; Wessely and Powell, 1989). The precise pathogenesis of the disorder is in fact irrelevant to the success or otherwise of cognitive therapy. Salkovskis, describing the role of cognitive behavioural therapy in somatic problems, has written

Patients commonly believe that their problems have a physical cause or manifestation; this perception may be accurate, exaggerated or completely inaccurate. However, when patients have a distorted or unrealistic belief that their bodily functioning is, or is going to be, impaired in harmful ways, this belief is a source of difficulty or anxiety (Salkovskis, 1989)

Thus the accuracy or otherwise of illness attributions is irrelevant; what is important is the extent to which they are behaviourally limiting. Evidence of an 'organic' basis is also not a contraindication, since treatment depends upon the differentiation between precipitating factors and maintaining factors. The maintaining factors, as outlined above, could be called secondary disabilities, but in persistent illness may have become the principal clinical problem.

Watts (1982) sums up thus:

The aim in working with disease conviction should not be to move the patient from a belief in organic aetiology to belief in a psychological one. This would not only be an unrealistic aim, it would usually represent one distortion of reality with another . . . The aim should be to encourage patients to see the full range of aetiological factors that apply. Patients will initially have a crude dichotomy of aetiologies, believing they must either have genuine symptoms with an organic aetiology or that they have psychological symptoms that are simply 'all in the mind' (Watts, 1982)

Regrettably it is our experience that other health professionals and the media seem equally likely to adopt such false dichotomies (David et al., 1988).

Methods

The principles and techniques of cognitive behaviour therapy are well known, and ably described in several books (Beck et al., 1979; Hawton et al., 1989). Therapy consists of working with the patient to identify maladaptive thinking patterns, and explaining how such thoughts may affect how they feel, and thus how they act. Some examples have already been described. Others include 'muscle pain means the virus is continuing to damage me', or 'viruses can't be treated, I'll never get better', a further example of catastrophic thinking. Having identified such thoughts, usually by self-monitoring, the therapist encourages the patient to generate alternative explanations. Thus a patient who began by saying 'I feel tired when I walk upstairs—I must still have ME', later came up with an alternative explanation: 'I may still have ME, but I may be feeling tired because I haven't done anything for a long time and am depressed'.

Therapy usually involves more education and explanation than is found during more conventional cognitive therapy, since many PVFS patients have a great deal of information about the condition, perhaps reflecting their frequent medical background. For example, therapy in PVFS may involve a discussion of both cardiac and muscle physiology. Patients need a valid explanation of how symptoms may have arisen, which must balance both the physical and psychological. A valid physiological explanation is particularly valuable, since 'it is difficult for the patient to reconcile [the absence of such an explanation] that this does not indicate, at least on the surface, that their pain was not real' (Follick et al., 1983). It is often necessary to share with the patient recent evidence of normal dynamic muscle function during and after activity (Stokes et al., 1988; Lloyd et al., 1988; Riley et al., 1990; Gibson et al., 1990).

Other somatic symptoms, such as breathlessness and palpitations, can be approached in the same way as in conventional anxiety management techniques. Some have argued that all the symptoms of ME can be explained by hyperventilation (Rosen *et al.*, 1990). However, such a unitary explanation of a complex phenomenon seems as inaccurate as any other attempt to invoke a single 'cause', especially as there is no direct link between subjective fatigue and objective biochemical data in hyperventilation (Folgering and Snik, 1988), or even normal individuals (Vollestad and Sejersted, 1988). Nevertheless, many patients are significantly troubled by hyperventilation-related symptoms, and will respond to conventional management, once again following basic cognitive behavioural principles (see Clark *et al.*, 1985; Salkovskis, 1988).

From beliefs, attention shifts to behaviours, although in practice no such sharp distinction can be made. The therapist explains how cognitions, which include misinterpretations of symptoms, lead to behavioural avoidance. Such avoidance is initially successful, since it is associated with immediate relief of symptoms. However, on re-exposure to activity these symptoms return, but even more intensely. Treatment is thus aimed at reducing avoidant behaviour, and reintroducing the previously abandoned activities.

The method we chose is to first establish predictable patterns of activity, and then to work towards a graded increase in that activity, based on the particular pattern of impairment encountered in each individual patient. This has been reported in some quarters as an exercise programme, which it is not. Instead, it involves joint agreement of behavioural targets between patient and therapist which are then practised between appointments. It is not the prescription of set amounts of exercise, but is based upon re-exposure to avoided behaviours. Targets may involve virtually no exercise at all—such as going to the toilet unaided, or spending five minutes every hour out of bed. The important point is to choose an activity which the patient feels is attainable. It must simply be something the patient has stopped and wishes to resume—its physiological/ergonomic consequences are immaterial. At no stage do we endorse intensive exercise retraining. Some authors have found that PVFS patients can tolerate such activity (Manu, personal communication; Stokes *et al.*, 1988), and others have not (Montague *et al.*, 1989). Either situation is irrelevant to our management.

Having reached agreement, the patient is asked to perform this activity regularly with the aim of ensuring consistency. He or she agrees to undertake the activity even when symptomatic, and not to abandon it if symptoms develop. It is crucial that the patient is warned that an initial rise in symptoms can be expected—but is told that he will become habituated to these symptoms. The patient agrees to carry out this minimal activity regularly, and not to miss out on a 'bad day'. Thus the patient is being asked to undertake the activity in response to an agreed timetable, and not the absence of symptoms.

So long as activity has been set at a low enough level, the patient avoids the severe discomforts associated with overexertion. He or she then has an opportunity to test out the hypotheses discussed, and to determine whether or not habituation to a fixed amount of activity does take place over time. This usually takes a few days, but we have managed patients for up to two or three weeks before habituation occurs. Regular contact, often by telephone, is important, and also prevents the frequent strategy of doing too much too early, followed by a total cessation of activity during the inevitable reoccurrence of symptoms, thus perpetuating the physiological and psychological limbo. Only when habituation to the principal symptom, usually fatigue, has taken place is a new target set. Adaptation occurs not just to fatigue, but also to a variety of other symptoms, including muscle pain, dizziness, paraesthesiae, sensitivity to noise and light etc., although such somatic symptoms seem to take longest for the patient to become habituated to them, and often do not disappear altogether.

It is essential to avoid too strenuous activity at first, since that will cause the delayed severe muscle pain that we wish to avoid.

Many patients are so discouraged by the experience of muscle soreness after the initial session that they never make another attempt . . . the only factor that seems to prevent soreness is previous exposure to a similar exercise task; even if the initial exercise exposure is of low intensity, severe soreness will not result (Editorial, 1987)

Return to activity takes place in planned stages. Like so much else, this is not new. Hough (1902) showed that in the untrained muscle the fibres are damaged by exercise, causing late soreness, but that this 'tearing' does not apply in the trained muscle. This has been noted in fibromyalgia, where if patients resist activity because of pain intensification, experts advise commencing with flexibility programmes before more aerobic exercise (Bennett, 1986). Once again, however, avoiding such soreness is not the goal of treatment—but provoking it would undoubtedly have a deleterious effect on morale and confidence.

Exactly the same applies to rest. It is not banned in any way, but is also made predictable, to be taken at set times and for set durations, rather than in response to symptoms. The amount of rest is decided by patient and therapist according to the subjective need—it is then made consistent and regular.

Measurement is also an important part of therapy. This is done by both patient and therapist, and includes both general measures, such as the current degree of handicap, or any changes in mood or other symptoms, and specific measures, including previously identified key problems and also the goals of therapy. Equally important is the involvement of a co-therapist, usually, but not always, the spouse, who is encouraged to come to sessions, and to help with monitoring etc. We also find that it is as important for the spouse to understand the treatment rationale as the patient (Yunus, 1988).

The key to this approach is to abolish the handicapping stimulus-driven cycle of PVFS, in which symptoms are always a signal to rest, and to replace sensitisation by tolerance. Instead, patients, having reassured themselves of their own safety, are encouraged to gradually cease using symptoms as a warning to stop, but to carry on to the agreed target. By careful setting of the target this can happen without the risk of causing new symptoms by overexertion. In the context of neurasthenia, an illness with many parallels to PVFS (Wessely, 1990b), Waterman (1909) wrote that the aim of treatment was to enable 'the knowledge that experience has shown that certain sensations have resulted from certain activities must be replaced by a conviction that these efforts may be made without harm, (Waterman, 1909).

BENEFITS

What are the benefits of this approach? First, and most important of all, is the return of self-efficacy—the idea that it is the patient, and not the virus or ME, that is in control. This has obvious effects on mood and morale, which in turn lessens symptoms. Insisting on consistency, and that behaviour is predetermined rather than symptom-driven, also decreases the need for constant symptomatic vigilance which can be extremely disabling. A similar approach is now the conventional wisdom for fibromyalgia: 'Successful management is facilitated by a caring and understanding doctor who gently but firmly guides the patient to assume responsibility for her own well being' (Yunus, 1989).

It must, of course, be conceded that such an approach is not specific for the problems of PVFS. Increasing the perception of control of symptoms has been shown to aid recovery from a number of conditions, including strokes and fractures (Partridge and Johnson, 1989). A further example is that of cardiac rehabilitation, where the benefits of 'exercise training' in preventing excessive morbidity after physical insult is due more to increased confidence rather than physical retraining (Mayou, 1981).

As an additional benefit, useful physiological changes can be expected. After all, rest, with its inevitable deleterious effects on cardiac, respiratory and muscle physiology, is hardly the treatment of choice for a chronic fatiguing condition (Edwards, 1986). It also appears that activity restores the deficits in muscle mitochondrial enzyme function (Wagenmakers *et al.*, 1988), and perhaps can increase muscle protein synthesis (see Chapter 7) and alter immune function (Bannister, 1988). Shepherd, a general practitioner and sufferer, has written that 'Prolonged bed rest . . . should be advised with great care in the long term cases, who may then become trapped in a vicious circle of immobility and weakness, and become almost bedridden (Shepherd, 1987). The physicians skilled in treating neurasthenia came to the same conclusion: 'Disuse is as hurtful as misuse' (Taylor, 1907).

What is the practical evidence? We will present some of our own results later, but controlled evidence comes once again from the treatment of chronic pain (Keefe and Gil, 1986; Weisenberg, 1987) and fibromyalgia. In the latter, controlled trials show that increased activity is beneficial on over-all symptom scores, sleep and pain (Bennett, 1986; McCain, 1986). The de-scription given by Yunus (1988) of standard therapy for fibromyalgia has obvious analogies to that adopted by us: 'start gently, avoid strenuous ex-ercises that will aggravate pain, stop before the pain is increased, and gradu-ally increase the limits of pain tolerance'.

Most experience, including our own, is in selected, chronic populations in whom spontaneous recovery is not expected (Behan and Behan, 1988; Smith, 1989; Shepherd, 1989). Peel (1988), an occupational physician, retorted a less selected, and more acute, sample of PVFS patients. The description he gives, of a gradual, steady, slow rehabilitation, attending to both 'quality and quantity' of work, is both sensible and consistent with our approach. He reports that the median period of sickness absence was 'painfully slow'— although the quoted figure of eight weeks seems more optimistic.

CONTRAINDICATIONS

There are very few absolute contraindications to the programme as outlined above. One is acute denervation, which does not occur in PVFS. Loss of more than 90% of muscle strength is a reason for caution, as research in neuromuscular disorders has shown a benefit of increased exercise in most patients, except those whose initial muscle strength was below 10% of nor-mal (Milner-Brown and Miller, 1988). However, the actual amounts of ac-tivity that are involved in our approach are small. Finally, it would be unwise to embark on therapy in the presence of untreated cardiac disorder. Again, this has not been a problem in practice.

RESULTS

Treatment setting

Most patients can participate in the programme outlined above on an out-patient basis. However, the therapist must be prepared to allocate consider-able time to each patient. The initial interview usually lasts up to two hours, followed by a further assessment of similar length. Treatment then involves regular (usually fortnightly) contact, lasting between a half to one hour. In our series the mean number of sessions has been eight, but with a range of two to 30.

We have also treated six severely disabled patients, who were either partially or completely confined to a bed or wheelchair. All had firm diagnoses of ME and had been told to expect little other than a lifetime of permanent invalidism. Given the severity of their disability, all were managed on an inpatient ward, the longest admission lasting eight weeks. Obviously, this involves skilled nursing and a highly motivated team, not often available for adult patients. Facilities for rehabilitation of the chronic sick remain woefully inadequate.

Successes

This chapter has described our standard clinical practice, which we believe represents the best approach currently available. We have used these techniques to treat a series of patients at the National Hospital for Nervous Diseases, and are able to report the preliminary results. Full details will be presented in the customary manner later (Butler *et al.*, 1991). We emphasise that we have not conducted a randomised, controlled trial, but a pilot study, the necessary preliminary to a more formal assessment.

We offered the management outlined above to 50 patients seen at the National Hospital for the assessment of severe fatigue; the sample thus consisted of nearly all the patients referred for a neurological (and not a psychiatric) assessment. Full details of the sample have been reported elsewhere (Wessely and Powell, 1989), but it will be noted that the patients resembled samples reported elsewhere as being typical of PVFS. Nearly all the patients felt they were suffering from PVFS, and half were members of the 'ME' Association. Like most of the samples reported in the literature, they had long durations of illness (mean 4.8 years), and severe disability. Illness had undoubtedly ruined the lives of many of them.

Thirty-two accepted treatment. At the end of therapy all completed a variety of self-rating scales. Ratings of global outcome are given in Table 2.

Table 2 'How do you feel compared to before treatment?'

	Completed	Drop-out
Much better	16	0
Better	6	1
About the same	4	2
Worse	0	0
Much worse	1	2
Total	27	5

Very significant improvements were noted in fatigue (both physical and mental), myalgia, number of somatic symptoms, psychological symptoms, and overall health. Perhaps the most important improvements of all took place in the levels of disability. This was self-assessed using four visual analogue scales of functional impairment, in which the maximum rating, indicating a complete inability to do the activity in question, was eight (the minimum being zero).

Follow-up has now taken place to three months post-treatment. Of the eight patients who finished symptom-free, seven still are. One has re-experienced some symptoms, but remains able to work. Ten finished the trial with symptoms still present, albeit considerably improved. Of these, four have continued the improvement, one of whom is now symptom-free. Three more are stable, whilst two have experienced a gradual worsening of affective symptoms, but with the improvement in functional disability being maintained. In conclusion, at three months follow-up the 18 who improved during the treatment all remain far better than before.

Failures

What about failures? These can be divided into three groups: first, those who refused to participate (these will be considered in the next section); second, those who dropped out; and third, those who did not do well. We include both of the latter groups as treatment failures.

Three patients ended worse than they began. One completed treatment, but was clearly worse than at the outset. This patient had major affective disorder, which continued to deteriorate, despite additional conventional treatment. Both of the other failures also had mood disorder on entry, and both dropped out of treatment after being unable to tolerate antidepressants. Three

Table 3 Individual scores (mean, 95% confidence interval)

	Before	After
Ability to work	6.31 (5.57–7.05)	2.71 (1.77–3.65)*
Home management	5.96 (5.04–6.34)	1.54 (0.78–2.17)*
Social leisure activities	5.72 (5.08–6.35)	2.08 (1.17–2.99)*
Private leisure activities	5.19 (4.52–5.86)	1.65 (0.89–2.41)*
Total functional impairment	22.61 (20.42–24.8)	7.96 (4.92–11.00)*
GHQ-12 Score	7.7 (5.7–9.04)	2.09 (0.31–3.87)†
Mental fatigue	5.82 (4.82–6.82)	1.79 (0.62–2.96)†
Physical fatigue	12.48 (11.16–13.8)	2.00 (0–4.91)†
HAD score	17.91 (14.59–21.23)	9.21 (5.73–12.69)‡
Somatic symptoms	14.33 (12.61–16.65)	8.12 (5.53–10.71)‡

* Wilcoxson matched-pairs signed ranks test: $P < 0.01$.
† Wilcoxson matched-pairs signed ranks test: $P < 0.001$.
‡ Paired t test (df = 26), $p < 0.001$.

reported no change in overall health (although all had increased their functional abilities, there had been no change in symptoms). One patient completed the entire treatment, but was unchanged both symptomatically and functionally. Finally, one dropped out because of distance, but was already improved.

The principal cause of failure is untreatable mood disorder. The average duration of symptoms in our series prior to referral was 4.8 years. In those in whom mood disorder was part of the clinical picture, there is some, albeit retrospective, evidence that this was present throughout the illness (Kruesi *et al.*, 1989; Manu *et al.*, 1989a: Taerk *et al.*, 1987), although this is disputed (Hickie *et al.*, 1990). It is not therefore surprising that many have affective disorder which proves to be treatment-resistant.

Refusal

Treatment refusal is the major obstacle we have encountered. In our own practice, admittedly a highly specialised referral centre, just under half of eligible patients refuse the offer of treatment, either immediately, or after an assessment interview. There was no doubt that most patients refused either because they thought our treatment had nothing to offer them, or requested therapies we were unable to provide (e.g. diet, antibiotics, etc.). The accuracy of the former perception is impossible to determine, but there were no clinical or symptomatic factors associated with treatment refusal—for example, the same proportion of those accepting treatment reported post-exercise myalgia. Instead, those refusing treatment were more likely to attribute all their symptoms to a purely physical problem, and less likely to accept an interaction between the physical and psychological. We believe this reflects the external social pressures that complicate so much of PVFS (David *et al.*, 1988; Wessely, in press). These will now be considered further.

Non-therapeutic factors

A further reason for either the refusal of treatment or its failure is the existence of powerful maintaining factors. ME, PVFS and related diagnoses have not been readily accepted by the medical profession, and one may accuse doctors of adding substantially to the burden of morbidity associated with PVFS. Doctors either indicate their disbelief in the reality of suffering, or, just as deleterious in the long term, react to such unhelpful views by totally denying the possibility of psychological distress. Such attitudes have led to anxiety, annoyance and ultimately a polarisation of attitudes between doctors, and also between patients and doctors. A sufferer has noted that in an effort to prove the reality of distress, and to convince the doctor to take them seriously, some patients resort to more and more extremes of behaviour (Jeffreys, 1982), which merely convinces the doctor of 'manipulation'. Finally, some develop an intense commitment to the 'cause', and inexorably find that their lives revolve more and more around the illness. This is an unforeseen, unintended, unwanted, but often insurmountable barrier to effective rehabilitation. A further barrier is that any improvement on the part of the patient that is not the result of antiviral or immune therapy may be interpreted by others (including doctors) as proof that the whole problem was psychological after all (and not ME). We note with regret that this is precisely what some of our patients have been told after the successful outcome of treatment. Patients also received conflicting advice, some of it ill-informed, from other professionals, a further obstacle to effective therapy (Salkovskis, 1989).

Factors affecting outcome

The inflexibility and polarisation of attitudes already discussed adversely influences not only acceptance of treatment, but also outcome. In our series, even of those patients who participated in treatment, those who did not feel that there was any role *at all* for psychological factors (rather than believing that psychological factors may play a role, albeit less than physical factors) tended to do worse.

Once again, clinical and symptomatic factors were not associated with outcome. Such symptoms as post-exercise myalgia, the severity of fatigue or the presence of depression or other psychiatric disorder did not affect the outcome, nor, in contrast to the anecdotal literature, did length of illness or severity of disability. The most gratifying, and dramatic, improvements occurred in five of the six patients who had previously been 'written off' as being beyond help, and confined to a bed or a wheelchair.

Relapse

Many of the current guides to the treatment of ME suggest that the course outlined above will cause relapse. However, a leading American authority on the subject has written: 'There is no evidence that forced rest or inactivity ameliorates the illness or that physical activity worsens the underlying process' (Schooley, 1988). Our results favour the American view.

It is difficult to be certain what 'relapse' means in PVFS. There are several possibilities. One is the rapid onset of symptoms that occurs when patients undertake too much too early, thus triggering muscular pain and restarting the cycle as before. Another is the known tendency of both mood and phobic disorders to relapse, perhaps triggered by infection, and thus set the entire PVFS cycle in motion again. We have also observed deterioration following discontinuation of tricyclics or when psychosocial situations change. In no case have we seen evidence of induced muscle damage. Finally, we anticipate that future research will uncover many as yet unsuspected mechanisms associated with relapse. Time alone will also tell if the programme outlined above offers prophylaxis against developing the extremes of disability that we, and others, currently encounter.

CONCLUSION

The results show that not only do many PVFS patients get better despite prolonged, severe disability, but also that such improvements occur on a programme which others have suggested would cause serious damage. Our design is inadequate to determine what exactly contributed to improvement. Although spontaneous improvement is most unlikely, given the duration of illness, we cannot rule out the nonspecific effect of either therapist time or simply taking the patient seriously. Instead, the most important finding is that something can be done for many people currently diagnosed as suffering from PVFS. Any treatment depends upon an assessment of the risk–benefit equation. We feel that cognitive behavioural therapy passes that test.

Does this cure PVFS? Probably not. Cognitive behavioural therapy as outlined above is intended to increase functional activity, and to decrease the profound restrictions imposed by the illness. In practice, as with the treatment of chronic pain, improvements in fatigue and myalgia do occur, and may be dramatic. Nevertheless, as in so much of medicine, our approach remains a rehabilitative, rather than a directly curative, one.

The programme outlined above is thus a pragmatic attempt to help patients with the clinical diagnosis of PVFS. There is little doubt that PVFS is a heterogeneous condition (Swartz, 1988), so it is to be expected that our approach will not be relevant to all. Further work will be needed to ensure that the appropriate patient receives the appropriate treatment. We are aware of the innovative work outlined in this volume implicating viral persistence in PVFS, and we do not yet know whether the programme we outline is less suitable for patients with such pathology. However, we must not forget that such work will not explain the illnesses of most of those who currently carry the diagnosis of PVFS, nor is there at present a way of clinically distinguishing the two groups. Finally, given our ignorance of how the central nervous system controls movement and mood in health, let alone disease, and our inadequate knowledge of the links between brain and immune system, it will require many years before more direct therapeutic approaches are developed.

ACKNOWLEDGEMENTS

SW is supported by the Wellcome Trust, AD by the Medical Research Council.

REFERENCES

Abramson, L., Seligman, M. and Teasdale, J. (1978) Learned helplessness in humans: critique and reformulation. *Journal of Abnormal Psychology*, **87**, 49–74.

Allan, F. (1945) The clinical management of weakness and fatigue. *Journal of the American Medical Association*, **127**, 957–960.

Alvarez, W. (1935) What is wrong with the patient who feels tired, weak and toxic? *New England Journal of Medicine*, **212**, 96–104.

Archer, M. (1987) The post-viral syndrome; a review. *Journal of the Royal College of General Practitioners*, **37**, 212–214.

Astrom, A., Friman, G. and Pilstrom, L. (1976) Effects of viral and mycoplasma infections on ultrastructure and enzyme activities in human skeletal muscle. *Acta Pathologica et Microbiologica Scandinavica (A)*, **84**, 113–122.

Bannister, B. (1988) Post-infectious disease syndrome. *Postgraduate Medical Journal*, **64**, 559–567.

Bayliss, R. (1988) Quoted in Dawson, J. (1988) Brainstorming the postviral fatigue syndrome. *British Medical Journal*, **297**, 1151–1152.

Beal, J. (1989) *Psychological Features of Patients with Post Viral Fatigue Syndrome*, Unpublished M.Sc. Thesis, University of London.

Beck, A. (1976) *Cognitive Therapy and the Emotional Disorders*. International Universities Press, New York.

Beck, A., Rush, J., Shaw, B. and Amery, Y. (1979) *Cognitive Therapy of Depression*. Guildford Press, New York.

Behan, P. and Behan, W. (1988) The postviral fatigue syndrome. *CRC Critical Reviews in Neurobiology*, **42**, 157–178.

Bennett, R. (ed.) (1986) The fibrositis/fibromyalgia syndrome; current issues and perspectives. *American Journal of Medicine*, **81**, 1–115.

Butler, S., Chalder, T., Ron, M. and Wessely, S. (1991) Cognitive behaviour therapy in the chronic fatigue syndrome. *Journal of Neurology, Neurosurgery and Psychiatry* (in press).

Carette, S., McCain, G., Bell, D. and Fam, A. (1986) Evaluation of amitriptyline in primary fibrositis: a double-blind placebo controlled study. *Arthritis and Rheumatism*, **29**, 655–659.

Clark, D., Salkovskis, P. and Chalkley, A. (1985) Respiratory control as a treatment for panic attacks. *Journal of Behavior Therapy and Experimental Psychiatry*, **16**, 23–30.

David, A., Wessely, S. and Pelosi, A. (1988) Postviral fatigue syndrome: time for a new approach. *British Medical Journal*, **296**, 696–699.

Dobkin, B. (1989) Ill, or just the Blahs? *New York Times Magazine*, 16 July, 36–37.

Editorial (1987) Aching muscles after exercise. *Lancet*, **ii**, 1123–1125.

Edwards, R. (1986) Muscle fatigue and pain. *Acta Medica Scandinavica*, Suppl. 711, 179–188.

Evans, W., Meredith, C., Cannon, J., Dinarello, C., Frontera, W., Hughes, V., Jones, B. and Knuttgen, H. (1986) Metabolic changes following eccentric exercise in trained and untrained men. *Journal of Applied*, **61**, 1864–1868.

Farmer, M., Locke, B., Moscicki, E., Dannenberg, A., Larson, D. and Radloff, L. (1988) Physical activity and depressive symptoms: the NHANES 1 Epidemiologic Follow-up Study. *American Journal of Epidemiology*, **128**, 1340–1351.

Folgering, H. and Snik, A. (1988) Hyperventilation syndrome and muscle fatigue. *Journal of Psychosomatic Research*, **32**, 165–171.

Folkman, S. (1984) Personal control and coping processes: A theoretical analysis. *Journal of Personality and Social Psychology*, **46**, 839–852.

Follick, M., Zitter, R. and Ahern, D. (1983) Failure in the operant treatment of chronic pain. In E. Foa and P. Emmelkamp (eds) *Failures in Behaviour Therapy*, pp. 311–334. John Wiley, New York.

Frank, J. (1946) Emotional reactions of American soldiers to an unfamiliar disease. *American Journal of Psychiatry*, (Vol) 102, 631–640.

Friman, G., Schiller, H. and Schwartz, M. (1977) Disturbed neuromuscular transmission in viral infections. *Scandanavian Journal of Infectious Diseases*, 9, 99–103.

Friman, G., Wright, J., Ilback, N. *et al.* (1985) Does fever or myalgia indicate reduced physical performance capacity in viral infections? *Acta Medica Scandinavica*, 217, 353–361.

Gibson, H., Carroll, N., Coakley, J. and Edwards, R. (1990) Recovery from maximal exercise in chronic fatigue states. *Abstract presented at European Society for Clinical Investigation*, Maastricht, 25th–28th April, 1990.

Gold, D., Bowden, R., Sixbey, J., Riggs, R., Katon, W., Ashley, R., Obrigewitch, R. and Corey, L. (1990) Chronic fatigue: a prospective clinical and virologic study. *Journal of the American Medical Association*, 264, 48–53.

Goldenberg, D. (1988) Fibromyalgia and other chronic fatigue syndromes: is there evidence for chronic viral disease? *Seminars in Arthritis and Rheumatism*, 18, 111–120.

Goldenberg, D., Felson, D. and Dinerman, H. (1986) Randomised, controlled trial of amitriptyline and naproxen in treatment of patients with fibrositis. *Arthritis and Rheumatism*, 29, 1371–1377.

Goldman, J. (1988) Chronic fatigue syndrome. *Annals of Internal Medicine*, 109, 166–167.

Havard, C. (1985) Lassitude. *British Medical Journal*, 290, 1161–1162.

Hawton, K., Salkovskis, P., Kirk, J. and Clark, D. (eds) (1989) *Cognitive Behaviour Therapy for Psychiatric Problems: A Practical Guide*. Oxford Medical Publications, Oxford University Press.

Helman, C. (1978) Feed a cold and starve a fever. *Culture, Medicine and Psychiatry*, 7, 107–137.

Hickie, I., Lloyd, A., Wakefield, D. and Parker, G. (1990) The psychiatric status of patients with chronic fatigue syndrome. *British Journal of Psychiatry*, 156, 534–540.

Hodgkinson, L. (1988) M.E. The mystery disease. *Woman's Journal*. November, 57–63.

Hoehn-Saric, R. and Mcleod, D. (1985) Locus of control in chronic anxiety disorders. *Acta Psychiatrica Scandinavica*, 72, 529–535.

Hough, T. (1902) Ergographic studies in muscular soreness. *American Physical Education Review*, 7, 1–17.

Hughes, J., Crow, R., Jacobs, D., Mittelmark, M. and Leon, A. (1984) Physical activity, smoking and exercise-induced fatigue. *Journal of Behavioral Medicine*, 7, 217–230.

Imboden, J. (1972) Psychosocial determinants of recovery. *Advances in Psychosomatic Medicine*, 8, 142–155.

Imboden, J., Canter, A. and Cluff, L. (1959) Brucellosis. III. Psychologic aspects of delayed convalescence. *Archives of Internal Medicine*, 103, 406–414.

Jeffreys, T. (1982) *The Mile-High Staircase*, p. 205. Hodder & Stoughton, Auckland.

Jenkins, M. (1989) Thoughts on the management of myalgic encephalomyelitis. *British Journal of Homeopathy*, 78, 6–14.

Jones, J. and Miller, B. (1987) The postviral asthenia syndrome. In E. Kurstak, Z. Lipowski and P. Morozov (eds) *Viruses, Immunity and Mental Disorder*, pp. 441–451. Plenum, London.

Jones, J., Williams, M., Schooley, R., Robinson, C. and Glaser, R. (1988) Antibodies to Epstein–Barr virus specific DNase and DNA polymerase in the chronic fatigue syndrome. *Archives of Internal Medicine*, 148, 1957–1960.

Keefe, F. and Gil, K. (1986) Behavioural concepts in the analysis of chronic pain syndromes. *Journal of Consulting and Clinical Psychology*, **54**, 776–783.

Kirmayer, L. (1988) Mind and body as metaphors: hidden values in biomedicine. In M. Lock and D. Gordon (eds) *Biomedicine Examined*, pp. 57–93. Kluver Academic Publishers, Dardrecht.

Kroenke, K., Wood, D., Mangelsdorff, D., Meier, N. and Powell, J. (1988) Chronic fatigue in primary care: prevalence, patient characteristics and outcome. *Journal of the American Medical Association*, **260**, 929–934.

Kruesi, M., Dale, J. and Straus, S. (1989) Psychiatric diagnoses in patients who have chronic fatigue syndrome. *Journal of Clinical Psychiatry*, **50**, 53–56.

Laudenslager, M. (1987) Psychosocial stress and disease. In E. Kurstak, Z. Lipowski and P. Morozov (eds) *Viruses, Immunity and Mental Health*. pp. 391–402. Plenum, London.

Lerner, A. (1988) A new continuing fatigue syndrome following mild viral illness: a proscription to exercise. *Chest*, **94**, 901–902.

Lethem, J., Slade, P., Troup, J. and Bentley, G. (1983) Outline of a fear-avoidance model of exaggerated pain perception—I. *Behaviour Research and Therapy*, **21**, 401–408.

Levi-Straus, C. (1963) *Structural Anthropology*, pp. 186–205. Basic Books, New York.

Lloyd, A., Hales, J. and Gandevia, S. (1988) Muscle strength, endurance and recovery in the post-infection fatigue syndrome. *Journal of Neurology, Neurosurgery and Psychiatry*, **51**, 1316–1322.

Manu, P., Matthews, D. and Lane, T. (1988). The mental health of patients with a chief complaint of chronic fatigue: a prospective evaluation and follow-up. *Archives of Internal Medicine*, **148**, 2213–2217.

Manu, P., Lane, T. and Matthews, D. (1989a) Prospective diagnostic evaluation of 200 patients with a chief complaint of chronic fatigue. *Clinical Research*, **37**, 820a.

Manu, P., Matthews, D., Lane, T., Tennen, H., Hesselbrock, V., Mendola, R. and Affleck, G. (1989b) Depression among patients with a chief complaint of fatigue. *Journal of Affective Disorders*, **17**, 165–172.

Matthews, D., Manu, P. and Lane, T. (1989) Diagnostic beliefs among patients with chronic fatigue. *Clinical Research*, **37**, 820A.

Mayou, R. (1981) Effectiveness of cardiac rehabilitation. *Journal of Psychosomatic Research*, **25**, 423–427.

McCain, G. (1986) Role of physical fitness training in the fibrositis/fibromyalgia syndrome. *American Journal of Medicine*, **81** [3A], 73–77.

Millon, C., Salvato, F., Blaney, N., Morgan, R., Mantero-Atienza, E., Klimas, N. and Fletcher, M. (1989) A psychological assessment of chronic fatigue syndrome/chronic Epstein Barr virus patients. *Psychology and Health*, **3**, 131–141.

Milner-Brown, H. and Miller, R. (1988) Muscle strengthening through high-resistance weight training in patients with neuromuscular disorders. *Archives of Physical Medicine and Rehabilitation*, **69**, 14–19.

Moldofsky, H. (1989) Nonrestorative sleep and symptoms after a febrile illness in patients with fibrositis and chronic fatigue syndromes. *Journal of Rheumatology*, **16**, Suppl. 19, 150–153.

Montague, T., Marrie, T., Bewick, D., Spencer, A., Kornreich, F. and Horacek, B. (1988) Cardiac effects of common viral illnesses. *Chest*, **94**, 919–925.

Montague, T., Marrie, T., Klassen, G., Bewick, D. and Horacek, M. (1989) Cardiac function at rest and with exercise in the chronic fatigue syndrome. *Chest*, **95**, 779–784.

Montgomery, G. (1983) Uncommon tiredness among college undergraduates. *Journal of Consulting and Clinical Psychology*, **51**, 517–525.

Muir, P., Nicholson, F., Tilzey, A., Signy, M., English, T. and Banatvala, J.

(1989) Chronic relapsing pericarditis and dilated cardiomyopathy: serological evidence of persistent enterovirus infection. *Lancet*, **i**, 804–807.

Nelson, E., Kirk, J., McHugo, G., Douglass, R., Ohler, J., Wasson, J. and Zubkoff, M. (1987) Chief complaint fatigue: a longitudinal study from the patient's perspective. *Family Practice Research Journal*, **6**, 175–188.

Newham, D. (1988) The consequences of eccentric contractions and their relationship to delayed onset muscle pain. *European Journal of Applied Physiology*, **57**, 353–359.

Partridge, C. and Johnson, M. (1989) Perceived control of recovery from disability: measurement and prediction. *British Journal of Clinical Psychology*, **28**, 53–59.

Peel, M. (1988) Rehabilitation in postviral syndrome. *Journal of Social and Occupational Medicine*, **38**, 44–45.

Philips, H. (1987) Avoidance behaviour and its role in sustaining chronic pain. *Behaviour Research and Therapy*, **25**, 273–279.

Philips, H. (1989) Thoughts provoked by Pain. In *Abstracts of the World Congress of Cognitive Therapy*, Oxford. June 28–July 2nd.

Pill, R. and Stott, N. (1982) Concepts of illness causation and responsibility: some preliminary data from a sample of working class mothers. *Social Science and Medicine*, **16**, 43–52.

Powell, R., Dolan, R. and Wessely, S. (1990) Attributions and self esteem in depression and the chronic fatigue syndrome. *Journal of Psychosomatic Research*, **34**, 665–673.

Ramsay, M. (1986) *Postviral Fatigue Syndrome: The Saga of Royal Free Disease*. Gower Medical, London.

Repsher, L. and Freebern, R. (1969) Effects of early and vigorous exercise on recovery from infectious hepatitis. *New England Journal of Medicine*, **281**, 1393–1396.

Riley, J., Ahern, D. and Follick, M. (1988) Chronic pain and functional impairment: assessing beliefs about their relationship. *Archives of Physical Medicine and Rehabilitation*, **69**, 579–582.

Riley, M., O'Brien, C., McCluskey, D., Bell, N. and Nicholls, D. (1990) Aerobic work capacity in patients with chronic fatigue syndrome. *British Medical Journal*, **301**, 953–956.

Robbins, J., Kirmayer, L. and Kapusta, M. (1990) Illness worry and disability in fibromyalgia. *International Journal of Psychiatry in Medicine*, **20**, 49–64.

Rosen, S., King, J., Wilkinson, J. and Nixon, P. (1990) Is chronic fatigue syndrome synonymous with effort syndrome? *Journal of the Royal Society of Medicine*, **83**, 761–764.

Salit, I. (1985) Sporadic post-infectious neuromyasthenia. *Canadian Medical Association Journal*, **133**, 659–663.

Salkovskis, P. (1988) Hyperventilation and anxiety. *Current Opinion in Psychiatry*, **1**, 72–82.

Salkovskis, P. (1989) Somatic problems. In K. Hawton, P. Salkovskis, J. Kirk and D. Clark (eds) *Cognitive Behaviour Therapy for Psychiatric Problems: A Practical Guide*, pp. 235–276. Oxford Medical Publications, Oxford University Press.

Schiller, H., Schwartz, M. and Friman, G. (1977) Disturbed neuromuscular transmission in viral infection. *New England Journal of Medicine*, **296**, 884.

Schooley, R. (1988). Chronic fatigue syndrome: a manifestation of Epstein–Barr virus infection? In J. Remington and M. Swartz (eds) *Current Clinical Topics in Infectious Diseases*, Vol. 9, pp. 126–146. McGraw-Hill, New York.

Sharpe, M. (1990) Chronic fatigue syndrome: can the psychiatrist help? In K. Hawton and P. Cowen (eds) *Difficulties and Dilemmas in the Management of the Psychiatric Patient*, pp. 231–240. Oxford University Press, Oxford.

Shepherd, C. (1987) Fatigue that's viral, not hysterical. *MIMS Magazine*, 15 October, 45–49.

Shepherd, C. (1989) *Living with ME: a Self-Help Guide*. Heinemann, London.

Smith, D. (1989) *Understanding ME*. Robinson, London.

Stephens, T. (1988) Physical activity and mental health in the United States and Canada: Evidence from four population surveys. *Preventive Medicine*, **17**, 35–47.

Stokes, M., Cooper, R. and Edwards, R. (1988) Normal strength and fatigability in patients with effort syndrome. *British Medical Journal*, **297**, 1014–1018.

Straus, S. (1988) The chronic mononucleosis syndrome. *Journal of Infectious Diseases*, **157**, 405–412.

Straus, S., Dale, J., Tobi, M., Lawley, T., Preble, O., Blaese, M., Hallahan, C. and Henle, W. (1988) Acyclovir treatment of the chronic fatigue syndrome: lack of efficacy in a placebo-controlled trial. *New England Journal of Medicine*, **319**, 1692–1698.

Swartz, M. (1988) The chronic fatigue syndrome—one entity or many? *New England Journal of Medicine*, **319**, 1726–1728.

Taerk, K., Toner, B., Salit, I., Garfinkel, P. and Ozersky, S. (1987) Depression in patients with neuromyasthenia (benign myalgic encephalomyelitis). *International Journal of Psychiatry in Medicine*, **17**, 49–56.

Taylor, J. (1907) Management of exhaustion states in men. *International Clinics*, **17**, 36–50.

Valdini, A., Steinhardt, S. and Jaffe, A. (1987) Demographic correlates of fatigue in a university family health centre. *Family Practice*, **4**, 103–107.

Valdini, A., Steinhardt, S. and Feldman, E. (1989) Usefulness of a standard battery of laboratory tests in investigating chronic fatigue in adults. *Family Practice*, **6**, 286–291.

Vollestad, N. and Sejersted, O. (1988) Biochemical correlates of fatigue: a brief review. *European Journal of Applied Physiology*, **57**, 336–347.

Wagenmakers, A., Coakley, J. and Edwards, R. (1988) Metabolic consequences of reduced habitual activities in patients with muscle pain and disease. *Ergonomics*, **31**, 1519–1527.

Waterman, G. (1909) The treatment of fatigue states. *Journal of Abnormal Psychology*, **4**, 128–139.

Watts, F. (1982) Attributional aspects of medicine. In C. Antaki and C. Brewin (eds) *Attributions and Psychological Change*, pp. 135–155. Academic Pres, London.

Weisenberg, M. (1987) Psychological intervention for the control of pain. *Behaviour Research and Therapy*, **25**, 301–312.

Wessely, S. (1990a) The natural history of chronic fatigue and myalgia syndromes. In D. Goldberg, N. Sartorius *et al.* (eds) *Psychological Disorders in General Medical Settings*, pp. 82–97. Hans Huber, Bern.

Wessely, S. (1990b) Old wine in new bottles: neurasthenia and ME. *Psychological Medicine*, **20**, 35–53.

Wessely, S. and Powell, R. (1989) Fatigue syndromes: a comparison of chronic 'postviral' fatigue with neuromuscular and affective disorders. *Journal of Neurology, Neurosurgery and Psychiatry*, **52**, 940–948.

Wessely, S. and Thomas, P. K. (1990) The chronic fatigue syndrome ('myalgic encephalomyelitis' or 'postviral fatigue'). In C. Kennard (ed.) *Recent Advances in Neurology*, Vol. 6, pp. 85–131. Churchill Livingstone, London.

Wessely, S., David, A., Butler, S. and Chalder, T. (1989) The management of the chronic 'post-viral' fatigue syndrome. *Journal of the Royal College of General Practitioners*, **39**, 26–29.

Wheeler, E., White, P., Reed, E. and Cohen, M. (1950) Neurocirculatory asthenia (anxiety neurosis, effort syndrome, neurasthenia). *Journal of the American Medical Association*, **142**, 878–889.

Yunus, M. (1988) Diagnosis, etiology and management of fibromyalgia syndrome: an update. *Comprehensive Therapy*, **14**, 8–20.

Yunus, M. (1989) Fibromyalgia syndrome: new research on an old malady. *British Medical Journal*, **298**, 474–475.

23

Chronic Fatigue States in Children

Harvey Marcovitch

Horton General Hospital, Banbury, UK

Children are not exempt from suffering a chronic fatigue syndrome (Jones *et al.*, 1985) and all paediatricians see cases sporadically (Dillon, 1978). Surprisingly, no childhood clusters have been specifically studied and reported in the literature to date, although they have certainly occurred—such as in Dalston, Cumbria in 1955 (Wallis, 1957) and in West Wales in 1986 (Lever *et al.*, 1988). An outbreak within a children's hospital affected 145 members of staff but no patients (Dillon *et al.*, 1974).

Presentation in children is little different from that in adults. Prominent symptoms include headache, back and limb pains and occasionally abdominal pain and nausea. More consistent and, so far as patients are concerned, more disabling are the extreme lethargy and fatiguability. For example, children who have hitherto been able to cycle without rest for several miles find that they are unable to pedal for more than a few hundred yards before needing a rest. Walking becomes slow and interrupted. When asked if it is pain or tiredness that limits exercise, children are often uncertain, but if pressed tend to emphasise fatigue rather than discomfort. Difficulty in concentration and lapses in short-term memory are a common experience, such that schoolwork deteriorates. Sometimes the children demonstrate a minor degree of expressive dysphasia, in which they use the wrong word and appear immediately puzzled by the error. An alteration in sleep pattern is common but maintenance of normal appetite is the rule and weight gain, sometimes excessive, common.

Most cases reported in adults comment on the existence of an apparently provocative illness with fever, sore throat and adenopathy. The acute signs and symptoms resolve, only to merge into the manifestations of post-viral

Post-viral Fatigue Syndrome. Edited by R. Jenkins and J. Mowbray
© 1991 John Wiley & Sons Ltd

fatigue syndrome (PVFS). It is always more difficult to be certain about such provocative illnesses in children, if only because they are relatively common and retrospective enquiry is very likely to provoke mention of them as precipitating events. Nonetheless, it is not uncommon in the outpatient clinic, where the child is seen several weeks after the illness has started, to receive a history of a 'glandular fever-like' illness having already been fruitlessly investigated by the general practitioner.

The plethora of symptoms is accompanied by a minimum of abnormal signs: mood is variable and can most accurately be described as 'frustrated' in many children. While a few display the apathy and immobility associated with depression, the majority are alert, can be persuaded to smile and register irritation at their disability rather than hopelessness. Signs of any precipitating respiratory infection, such as pharyngitis, tender adenopathy and fever, are not usually seen except as coincidental findings. The presence of palpable, non-tender cervical nodes or even of minimal splenomegaly are non-diagnostic since they are both common in normal children.

Unlike in adult patients, such as those described in the Royal Free epidemic (Medical Staff of the Royal Free Hospital, 1957), neurological signs are absent or inconsistent: minor asymmetries in tendon reflexes and minor deficits in co-ordination or balance are not unusual in small children and no coherent pattern of neurological abnormality has been described. Cranial nerve pulses are unusual but nystagmus is occasionally seen. Muscle tenderness is not a general feature and fatigue cannot be demonstrated by the type of manoeuvres used in the clinical diagnosis, for example, of myasthenia.

INITIAL MANAGEMENT

At the first consultation, the primary aim should be to exclude life- or health-threatening treatable conditions while reserving judgement on the eventual label to be offered. There is a sensible reason for this approach: public knowledge, or lack of it, of PVFS is such that merely mentioning it as part of a differential diagnosis is likely to be taken as a dogmatic statement. This may have a number of results: it may imprint upon the mind of the family that this is the diagnosis and such diagnostic labels tend to stick for years, possibly hindering accurate understanding and treatment of symptoms which subsequently develop. Furthermore, making a firm diagnosis at an early interview denies the clinician his or her opportunity to 'stage manage' the handling of the situation in as constructive a way as possible for the family.

A second aim should be the standard one in all paediatric consultations, of defining the eventual diagnosis not just in physical, but also in emotional, social and family terms. In doing so, the doctor will have to reach a firm or tentative conclusion as to how much emotional factors might be important in defining a patient's clinical state. The manifestations of this disease (or response to disease) are not easy to distinguish from the somatising behaviour of distressed children and this must continue to be borne in mind while working towards a diagnostic formulation. Simply accepting the patient's or parent's diagnosis without critical evaluation of its validity may cause great harm (Harris and Taitz, 1989).

INVESTIGATIONS

In dealing with the primary aim a certain number of investigations are warranted. Careful judgement is required because it is easy to adopt a policy of blindly performing a series of investigations looking for more and more unlikely possibilities. Bearing in mind the possible need to repeat tests on a number of occasions, I would strongly recommend a painless method of venepuncture using Emla* cream.

Particular diagnoses to be ruled out will depend upon the various presenting features but may include:

(a) Depression.
(b) Somatising disorder reflecting family pathology (e.g. child abuse).
(c) Substance abuse.
(d) Sleep apnoea syndrome.
(e) Chronic infection, e.g. Epstein–Barr viral disease, brucellosis, Q fever, Lyme disease, hepatitis, enteroviral and mycoplasmal infection, etc.
(f) Lymphoreticular malignancy.
(g) Myasthenia gravis.
(h) Hypothyroidism.
(i) Severe electrolyte or acid–base disturbance.
(j) Chronic renal failure.
(k) Severe anaemia.

Other conditions may sometimes have to be considered. For example, if abdominal pain and other gastrointestinal symptoms are prominent and eosinophilia present, more particularly if the family come from possibly endemic areas such as the Republic of Ireland, toxocariasis may need to be excluded (Taylor *et al.*, 1988).

The appropriate examination and investigations for this initial screen should be taken at the end of the first consultation and the family invited to return after several days when the results are to hand and can be explained.

Diagnosis of sleep apnoea syndrome is made basically by history and

---

* Lignocaine 2.5%, prylocaine 2.5% (Astra pharmaceuticals)

ENT examination which may demonstrate significant upper airway obstruction. If necessary it can be confirmed by sleep studies involving video recording and oxygen saturation monitoring (Mark and Brooks, 1984).

My own experience, and that of others, is that this diagnostic trawl, while reassuring to the doctor and of interest to parents, will rarely provide an answer. In 120 patients (including some children) investigated at Oxford during 1985–1987, a specific diagnosis was made in nine (Pasvol, personal communication). Four of these had monospot positive glandular fever, there was one diagnosis each of infection with mumps virus, parvovirus, zoster and hepatitis B, while one patient probably had a reaction to tetanus vaccine. In a US study conducted within a 'fatigue clinic', 5% of patients had organic disorder including epilepsy, asthma, and polymyalgia rheumatica (Manu *et al.*, 1988).

The problems that can arise with attempted serological diagnosis, such as with Epstein–Barr virus (EBV) are described in Chapter 3, so that the finding of apparently high titres of antibody should be discussed with a microbiologist before a firm diagnosis is offered. There is, of course, much interest in enteroviruses as a cause of PVFS but enteroviral infection in children is common and the finding of a moderately raised antibody titre to Coxsackie or echo-virus is not uncommon in childhood regardless of symptoms. Conversely, amongst 39 children with histories typical of PVFS, 22 had evidence of past or present Coxsackie infection and 17 evidence of never having encountered the organism (Wilson *et al.*, 1989).

Reported abnormal blood findings in children come from various individual case reports or very small series and too much confidence should not be invested in them. Dillon's comments (Dillon, 1978) are typical:

Two children had atypical lymphocytes in their peripheral blood and one a raised ESR. Liver function tests and serum CPK levels were normal. There were no consistent bacteriological findings. Virological investigations were non-contributory. One child had raised EB virus antibodies but of the 6 tested none had any antecomplementary activity in serum and no lymphocytes would proliferate *in vitro*. EEGs were undertaken in three, and in one the record was normal, in one compatible with [ME] and in one, slightly abnormal but not typical of [ME]. (Pampiglione *et al.*, 1978)

Electroencephalography, like serology, demonstrates some minor non-diagnostic abnormalities: in 12 children with presumed PVFS, Pampiglione and colleagues reported excess irregular intermediate slow activity, more prominent in one or another region without constant focal distribution. At times there was an excess of sharp components but no short-duration spikes or complex waveforms at any stage of the disease or after partial or complete recovery. The authors pointed out that the type and distribution of these relatively modest abnormalities were quite different from the EEG findings of acute encephalomyelitis or acute toxic disturbances such as from drugs, electrolyte imbalance, etc., which might affect the CNS.

MAKING THE DIAGNOSIS OF PVFS

At the second visit, results from the investigations will be available and most of the differential diagnostic possibilities will have been excluded. The doctor may still feel unsure as to whether he regards the presenting complaint as primarily physical or primarily psychiatric. In other words, he may find it difficult to decide whether to ascribe a primary diagnosis such as depression, malingering, family sick role pattern, etc., or whether to make a presumptive diagnosis of PVFS. In general, such compartmentalisation is likely to be unhelpful: by this time, the doctor should have collected sufficient information to be in a position to assess physical symptoms, psychological state, personality and illness behaviour. He should assess how much he thinks each of these is contributing towards the child's illness.

US investigators have attempted to refine this decision-making by providing a working case definition for chronic fatigue syndrome (Holmes *et al.*, 1988). The working group commissioned to develop a consensus included paediatricians so that its criteria are possibly appropriate to this age group. By analogy, presumably, with a diagnostic method used in rheumatic fever, the authors demand for diagnosis two compulsory major criteria and either six or more of 11 symptoms criteria and two or more of three physical criteria or alternatively at least eight of the symptom criteria.

Major criteria include the presence for at least six months of debilitating fatigue together with exclusion of a list of possible diagnoses. The minor criteria include persisting or recurring mild fever, sore throat, adenopathy, muscle weakness, myalgia, exercise fatigue, headache, arthralgia, neuropsychological complaints and sleep disturbance. The physical criteria include physician-documented fever, pharyngitis and adenitis. There is a problem with applying these criteria to children: those relating to respiratory infection are common to childhood and the remainder are all possible manifestations of psychiatric illness.

That the doctor may remain uncertain is not an uncommon issue in paediatrics, being equally true of such symptoms as recurrent abdominal pain, headache or any other variety of periodic syndrome.

AIMS OF FOLLOW-UP

Multiaxial approach

Having excluded obvious or less obvious organic disease during the initial two or three consultations, the most constructive approach is to refuse to recognise any mutual exclusivity of physical and emotional aetiologies and to deal with both possibilities while attempting to keep an open mind. My experience is that this method is most likely not to alienate parents whose resentment of psychiatric labelling may negate the doctor's best therapeutic or relationship-building endeavours (Wessely *et al.*, 1989). I try to be open with both child and parents in admitting my own uncertainties in this direction, frankly laying before them certain of the indicators of organic disease, such as the finding of abnormal enterovirus antigen in the stools of a proportion of patients (Yousef *et al.*, 1988), and at the same time pointing out that depression, anxiety and the effects of certain traumatising events in a child's life—including abuse—present with similar symptoms.

In essence, parents should be helped to understand that physical and psychological symptoms are very likely to be present together whatever the basic cause of the illness in question. It could be pointed out to them that children with a debilitating physical illness almost inevitably develop psychological symptoms and that children with primarily psychological disorders very frequently demonstrate these by exhibiting physical symptoms. This is certainly the case in PVFS, where some children become depressed, hardly surprisingly when one considers the effects of the illness. Similarly, parental reaction and the child's own response to the symptoms may well result in sick role behaviour which simply potentiates the problem.

This approach paves the way towards parents accepting consultations both of a typically 'medical' and typically 'psychiatric' nature side by side. There is a choice about how these should be organised. If the paediatrician or GP feels confident in his or her skills at eliciting emotional problems in children, then the family should be offered two separate types of consultation. Firstly, a series of interviews are carried out between child and doctor with or without participation of other members of the family, to explore whether there are emotional skeletons in the cupboard. The doctor should be honest with parents about the purpose of these consultations. It is likely that these can be terminated once the situation is clearer, and the second type of consultation will continue alone—namely a more typical outpatient-style discussion and physical examination. This should serve several purposes: the family need the time to discuss developments with the doctor and to report on therapeutic endeavours; the doctor needs to reassure himself, from time to time, that he is not missing some hitherto undiagnosed but treatable condition; problems relating to education and socialising or the lack of it have to be dealt with.

Some doctors will not feel confident in their listening or psychotherapeutic interventional skills or are not able to find the time for this process. In this case they may prefer either to hand over management to a child psychiatrist, clinical psychologist or family therapist, or embark on a joint enterprise, seeing the patient or family together or separately as seems appropriate at different times. It is sometimes a question of 'horses for courses', the personality characteristics or health beliefs of the family suiting them to a particular individual regardless of specialty.

Whatever method is followed, the aims should be to work with the family on how to keep morale high whilst the illness continues; to work with Education Authorities on how best to provide teaching for children who may be unable to attend school regularly or full-time; and to deal with enquiries about such issues as permissible exercise levels, 'alternative' or 'fringe' practitioners and questions that arise in parents, or children's, minds as a result of contact with fellow sufferers or self-help groups.

Attempts at treatment with drugs such as steroids, anti-depressants and intravenous immunoglobulin have been reported but only on an anecdotal basis. No placebo-controlled trials have been conducted. This is hardly surprising considering the difficulty of entry criteria for any such trial, though perhaps adoption of the US consensus criteria (Holmes *et al.*, 1988) may help.

Explanation

Once the doctor is as confident as he or she can be in ascribing symptoms to PVFS, they should share with the family their own understanding, including their own uncertainties about the condition. It is reasonable to offer an optimistic prognosis since the majority of children are likely to recover in 6–12 months although there are obviously exceptions to this.

Planning daily life

Advice must be offered about how much the disease should be allowed to affect the children's lifestyle. They should not be allowed to become permanent invalids from a condition which may offer reward in terms of staying at home and being cosseted. Instead a programme is devised with parents which includes the following, largely adapted from Wessely *et al.* (1989).

(a) Daily exercise to a level less than that which causes extreme fatigue.
(b) Plan specific exercise such as walking or swimming with attempts to steadily increase distances over time.
(c) Discussion about behaviour which the patient has tried to avoid in an attempt to re-introduce it gradually.
(d) Recognition that acute infections may cause exacerbation of the condition.

Education

If at all possible, children should remain at school. Where children apparently find this impossible, the doctor will have to consider school-phobia as part of the differential diagnosis. Alternative arrangements may need to be made about getting to school. For example, one of my patient's journeys involved a four-mile round-trip cycle ride as well as one and half hours on school buses. The co-operation of the school may be needed in altering the child's PE or sports programme. Sometimes it may be necessary to accept part-time attendance or, as a last resort, home tuition.

All of this needs careful co-ordination, so the doctor needs to contact the child's headteacher or tutor at the earliest opportunity, as well as involving an educational psychologist. It is better to do this by means of a case conference, hopefully with parents invited, rather than by telephone or letter. This is particularly apposite to PVFS since the teaching, psychological and administrative staff may all have personal views on the validity or otherwise of this condition. At the very least the doctor should attempt to seek a consensus view on the subject.

The problem may be most acute when children are in an examination year, say for GCSE or A-level. It is tempting to ascribe symptoms to avoidance activity for some as yet undisclosed reason. My experience with teenage sufferers of PVFS has been quite the opposite—a determination to continue despite debilitating fatigue and difficulty in concentration with consequent frustration and a risk of secondary depression. The timecourse of PVFS is such that some patients may end up largely missing an entire school year and serious discussion may be needed with the family on whether public examinations are best postponed and the year repeated.

Alternative therapies

It is a rare family that does not entertain the idea of consulting an alternative therapist or, at least, indulging in some unorthodox therapy. If the doctor has made clear in advance his contempt for these then it is unlikely that he will be told about them. The issue should be pre-empted by deliberately raising it for discussion at a consultation. Patients will be well served if the doctor protects them from harmful, expensive or useless methods while accepting their faith in those he adjudges harmless, possibly helpful and within their means. It is as well to be humble in accepting that our own methods of dealing with this disease are not exactly exemplary.

Self-help groups

Most paediatricians have ambivalent attitudes towards such groups. Some will be well known to them as constructive and sensible and they will be well used to deliberately putting patients in their way. Others may seem more dubious, particularly those associated with conditions which are both fashionable (in terms of patients actively pursuing them self-diagnostically) and hard to characterise with precision and therefore hard to treat (e.g. food allergy, PVFS). Doctors dealing with children with PVFS should make it their business to seek out literature produced by self-help groups so that they can decide whether they wish to recommend them to their patients.

Psychological management

As already stated, there is a choice as to who should be the therapist. Assessment of whether any psychiatric or emotional symptoms are secondary to viral infection or whether the latter is red herrings in a disturbed child is a continuous process. Sometimes the results are inconclusive.

Children with PVFS may become depressed, so the question of specific treatment should be considered. Most paediatricians have little experience of anxiolytics or antidepressants. They hope the same is true of GPs when dealing with children. This is one particular point when expert child psychiatric advice should be sought. Relaxation techniques may be helpful for some patients; in some hospitals, there may be a physiotherapist skilled in this area and if so her help should be sought.

Second opinion

When requested this should never be refused although the doctor should seek a veto if he does not trust the individual to whom referral is proposed. Where the doctor is unsure of his ground—particularly where he is anxious that he has diagnosed a basically untreatable condition without considering other possibilities in full—a second opinion may be good for him as well as the patient.

Prognosis

At the present time there is no published material on prognosis in children. My own experience is that patients are referred when they have already been unwell for three months or more. All but one of those I have dealt with have recovered within a further 12 months. What proportion of children will suffer prolonged invalidity is unknown although the indications are that it will be fewer than in adults. This allows paediatricians to offer an optimistic prognosis to families. Nonetheless, because of the uncertainties inherent in the diagnosis, the doctor should at all times be prepared to revise his view or reinvestigate if the situation changes. It is particularly important that he does not take a dogmatic view on the physical or psychiatric basis of this condition since dogmatism is surely unjustified in what is clearly an evolving understanding of a widespread problem.

REFERENCES

Dillon, M. J. (1978) Epidemic neuromyasthenia at the Hospital for Sick Children, Great Ormond Street, London. *Postgraduate Medical Journal*, **54**, 725–732.

Dillon, M. J., Marshall, W. C. Dudgeon, J. A. and Steigman, A. J. (1974) Epidemic neuromyasthenia: outbreak among nurses at a children's hospital. *British Medical Journal*, **1**, 301–305.

Harris, F. and Taitz, L. S. (1989) Damaging diagnosis of myalgic encephalitis in children. *British Medical Journal*, **299**, 790.

Holmes, G. P., Kaplan, J. E. Gantz, N. M. *et al.* (1988) Chronic fatigue syndrome: a working case definition. *Annals of Internal Medicine*, **108**, 387–389.

Jones, J. F., Ray, C. G., Minnich, L. L., Hicks, M. J. *et al.* (1985) Evidence for active Epstein–Barr virus infection in patients with persistent unexplained illness; elevated anti-early antigen antibodies. *Annals of Internal Medicine*, **102**, 1–7.

Lever, A. M. L., Lewis, D. M., Bannister, B. *et al.* (1988) Interferon production in post viral fatigue syndrome. *Lancet*, **ii**, 101.

Manu, P., Matthews, D. A. and Lane, T. J. (1988) The mental health of patients with a chief complaint of chronic fatigue. A prospective evaluation and follow-up. *Archives of Internal Medicine*, **148**, 2213–2217.

Mark, J. D. and Brooks, J. G. (1984) Sleep-associated airway problems in children. *Pediatric Clinics of North America*, **31** (4), 907–918.

Medical Staff of the Royal Free Hospital (1957) An outbreak of encephalomyelitis in the Royal Free Hospital group, London, in 1955. *British Medical Journal*, **2**, 895–899.

Pampiglione, G., Harris, R. and Kennedy, J. (1978) Electroencephalograph investigations in myalgic encephalomyelopathy. *Postgraduate Medical Journal*, **54**, 752–754.

Taylor, M. R. H., Keane, C. T., O'Connor, P. *et al.* (1988) The expanded spectrum of toxocarial disease. *Lancet*, **i**, 692–694.

Wallace, A.L. (1957) *An investigation into an unusual disease seen in epidemic and sporadic form in general practice in Cumberland in 1955 and subsequent years*. MD Thesis, Universityy of Edinburgh.

Wessely, S., David, A., Butler, S. *et al.* (1989) Management of chronic (postviral) fatigue syndrome. *Journal of the Royal College of General Practitioners*, **39**, 26–29.

Wilson, P. M. J., Kusumkumar, V., McCartney, R. A. and Bell, E. J. (1989) Features of Coxsackie B virus infection in children with prolonged physical and psychological morbidity. *Journal of Psychosomatic Research*, **33**, 29–36.

Yousef, G. E., Bell, E. J. Mann, G. F. *et al.* (1988) Chronic enteroviral infection in children with post viral fatigue syndrome. *Lancet*, **i**, 146–149.

24

The Post-viral Fatigue Syndrome in Athletes

R. Budgett

Northwick Park Hospital, London, UK

INTRODUCTION

Loss of form, underperformance and fatigue are frequent complaints of competitors in many sports. Newspaper sports pages carry frequent reports of underperforming and fatigued elite competitors (Brasher, 1987), often labelled as suffering from a viral illness. Unfortunately there is often little objective evidence for a viral cause of their problem, and the majority of reports are anecdotal.

There are occasional reports of epidemics of chronic fatigue in athletes (Kevles, 1988), but the majority of cases described, and all the cases I have seen, occur sporadically in athletes from different squads under different coaches using different training regimes. Their peers are generally tolerating the training load and performing well, so that there must be some unique factors which make these athletes vulnerable. There is probably a combination of intrinsic and extrinsic factors, which may include a viral infection, but will also include psychological stresses and physical stresses such as poor diet.

There are some suggestions that viral infections may predispose to fatigue; for example, four out of 12 athletes complaining of an unexplained deterioration in performance in Glasgow did have serological evidence of a recent viral infection (Epstein–Barr and Coxsackie B) which was subclinical in two of the cases. However, no cause was found in the other eight (Roberts, 1985).

The role of post-viral illness in these athletes is controversial, but there is growing acceptance that the extreme training stress suffered by elite athletes

Post-viral Fatigue Syndrome. Edited by R. Jenkins and J. Mowbray
© 1991 John Wiley & Sons Ltd

may affect immune function, leading to a susceptibility to infections (Keast, 1988). The study of chronic fatigue in athletes is bedevilled by synonyms and the terms overtraining syndrome, ME, post-viral fatigue syndrome, staleness and chronic fatigue syndrome have all been used (Eichner, 1989a; Kuipers and Keizer, 1988).

DEFINITION OF TERMS

Athlete

The term athlete will be used to include all sportsmen and sportswomen who undergo physical training.

Fatigue

Fatigue is a common symptom in all branches of medicine, and means different things to different specialists. The exercise physiologist will define fatigue as the failure to sustain the expected or required muscular force, and there are different mechanisms of fatigue depending on the duration of exercise. A sprinter will become fatigued in seconds in association with high lactic acid levels, and a marathon runner after nearly two hours when muscle glycogen stores may be depleted.

Others will use synonyms such as tiredness, lethargy and listlessness and include symptoms such as poor concentration, poor sleep, and tiredness before and poor tolerance of activity. This is essentially a subjective condition (Eichner, 1989b). Fatigue may be expected and accepted after hard exercise, and only when it becomes abnormally severe or prolonged in the eyes of the sufferer will he complain. The fatigue discussed here in athletes refers to this subjective condition associated with poor performance, and not to the short-lived normal physiological fatigue after exercise.

Overtraining

Athletes will overtrain for short periods as part of their normal training programme, hoping for an extra adaptive response and increased fitness. The term 'overtraining syndrome' is used when the athlete fails to adapt and becomes fatigued. They are described as overtrained despite there being no hard evidence that excessive training is causative, as they show signs of recovery with rest (Koutedakis et al., 1989).

PRESENTATION, INVESTIGATION, DIAGNOSIS AND EXAMINATION IN A SPORTS MEDICINE CLINIC

Presentation

False impressions

The chronically fatigued athlete sometimes bounds into the surgery looking fitter than any of the other patients, exuding an aura of false cheerfulness, and it is easy to dismiss their problems as trivial. Unlike other sufferers from chronic fatigue or ME athletes are often able to function well in their life outside sport, and so in this sense their problems are less severe. To them, however, the situation seems dire and they may feel anxious, depressed and disturbed by what is happening. This hidden agenda is easily uncovered if the competitor feels their underperformance is being treated seriously and then a full history can be taken. There are a small number of athletes who present with a more severe picture, complaining of lethargy, malaise and loss of concentration affecting their daily life. These individuals have a worse prognosis, and may be affected for over a year, but fortunately are a small minority.

Symptoms

Fatigue is part of the expected response to training, and so an athlete may accept it as normal, or his complaints may fall on unsympathetic ears, inhibiting him from communicating this sign of supposed weakness. However, both coach and athlete will sit up and take notice when performance suffers, and it is then that help is sought, with an unexplained performance slump as the main complaint. Competitors are different from other patients complaining of fatigue in that they have an objective measure of the symptom, their performance. As underperformance is so important to them and is an acceptable complaint in the eyes of their peers and coaches, other symptoms will often only become apparent on direct questioning.

Several weeks of deteriorating performance may precede total breakdown and cessation of training. These individuals can put up with almost anything except losing, and will train conscientiously through injury and illness as long as they feel positive about their future competitions, and performance does not suffer. Unfortunately the response to any setback is often to increase the volume and intensity of training in a misguided attempt to recover form.

Noakes (1986) describes a medical professor who could not understand why his legs felt so sore, he had a persistent throat infection, he was sleeping poorly, he had lost his zest for life, and his marathon was 30 minutes slower than three weeks previously despite the fact that he was training harder than ever before!

It is only when there seems to be no hope of a quick recovery that medical help is sought, by which time the athlete is in a crisis from which he or she sees no escape. These are very difficult individuals to deal with. They are aggressive, anxious, unused to being ill (as opposed to injured), and desperately want a treatable cause to be found.

Investigation and diagnosis

Hidden problems

Symptoms reported by these athletes, often only after direct questioning, include fatigue during exercise and rest, with a loss of purpose, energy and competitive drive (Costill, 1986). They tire easily, and complain of feelings of helplessness, incompetence and being trapped in a routine. Anxiety, depression, irritability, emotional lability and loss of libido have been described (Kinderman, 1986). Loss of appetite, weight loss, excess sweating and poor sleep, including difficulty getting to sleep, restlessness, vivid dreams and getting up early in the morning to pass urine, are also reported (Burke, 1981; Kuipers and Keizer, 1988). There may be increased thirst and fluid intake after exercise (Ryan, 1983), and athletes have also been noted to complain of an increased susceptibility to infections (Costill, 1986; Keast, 1988; Peters, 1983; Roberts, 1986) and injuries (Barron and Mellerowicz, 1971). Extreme muscle pain is part of an athlete's daily routine, and will not be a primary complaint; however, heavy, tired muscles which do not perform as expected will prompt immediate concern and anxiety (Noakes, 1986).

As well as asking for the symptoms listed above, a routine systematic enquiry is helpful. For instance, coughing post-exercise and at night may be a clue to the diagnosis of exercise-induced asthma, which is surprisingly common in athletes. On direct questioning 30% of the international rowing squad reported experiencing post-exercise wheeze (P. Thomas, personal communication), and this is a frequently missed cause of underperformance, tiredness and 'recurrent colds', since the symptoms are often difficult to reproduce in the surgery or laboratory (McCarthy, 1989).

Training history

The training and competition history are often helpful. Chronically fatigued athletes have often increased the intensity and volume of their training in an attempt to improve their performance. They may also admit to one or more similar episodes in the previous season, often coinciding with periods of increased training load. This load may be much less than in previous years and athletes are frustrated by their inability to reach and maintain a high level of training or competition without breaking down.

Physical stress

For example, an international 400-metre runner had a one-year history of developing a feeling of malaise, tiredness and heavy legs every time she increased her training up to a certain volume and intensity. After resting for two weeks she would start training again, but one to three months later the problem would recur and she would have to stop again. She was aware of this recurrent cycle but so determined to succeed that she would increase her training to the maximum she could manage as quickly as possible, and said she felt anxious and guilty if she did not.

Another athlete was a professional racquet sports player who suffered from symptoms of fatigue, depression, minor skin infections and poor sleep coinciding with periods of increased training and other stresses. Before presentation she had increased her training to four to five hours per day in an attempt to catch up on missed training, ignoring feelings of fatigue, and became irritable, fed up and exhausted. She felt that she 'had to try', and was worried about the imminent championships and her sponsorship contracts. The skin infections returned and her performance deteriorated.

Psychological stress

In addition to the stress of training and competition other stresses are important and should be explored (Eichner, 1989b). One of the relapses suffered by the racquets player had followed the serious injury of her sister in a car crash, and another the break-up of a long-term relationship. It seems that in some athletes the accumulation of all physical and mental stresses, coupled with a spell of perceived poor performance, exceeds their ability to cope, leading to breakdown and a state of chronic fatigue. Whatever the underlying cause, it is important to identify these sources of stress, otherwise the athlete is at high risk of breaking down again when heavy training is restarted.

The well-validated 'profile of mood states' (POMS) questionnaire, in which the athlete is asked to rate current feelings or mood against a list of 65 words (Morgan, 1980), has been used in athletic populations for many years. By completing serial questionnaires an individual or group of athletes can be objectively evaluated, and deterioration in mood state spotted before a deterioration in performance. Exercise is well known to affect mood state and is normally beneficial, increasing vigour, and decreasing tension, depression, anger and fatigue (Morgan, 1987). These factors give a characteristic 'iceberg profile' in healthy athletes when represented graphically (Morgan, 1985).

This iceberg profile may become inverted due to an increase in depression, anger and fatigue and a decrease in vigour in exhausted, overtrained athletes (Costill and Morgan, 1988). This pattern was recently confirmed in a study of underperforming fatigued athletes (Koutedakis *et al.*, 1989) with a normal 'iceberg profile' in controls which was inverted in the subjects (Figure 1).

Dietary history

It is important to enquire for a poor diet and weight loss since athletes need to consume huge quantities of calories, ideally in the form of complex carbohydrates (pasta, bread, cereals, potatoes and rice) to meet training demands (Wheeler, 1989), and many place a misguided emphasis on protein and glucose. Thus a dietary history is also helpful, with full assessment by a dietician in selected cases. Occasionally an inadequate or inappropriate diet appears to be the sole cause of chronic fatigue and underperformance, worsened by the fact that appetite falls with any accompanying depression.

Cyclists in the Tour de France need to consume up to 8000 kcal/day to replace energy expenditure, and those that fail to do this drop out (F. Brunosl, personal communication). A poor diet may lead to muscle glycogen deficiency, especially if the athlete is attempting to train hard (Costill, 1988a). This results in an inability to sprint (produce an anaerobic response), and there is rapid fatigue after the anaerobic threshold is reached. The

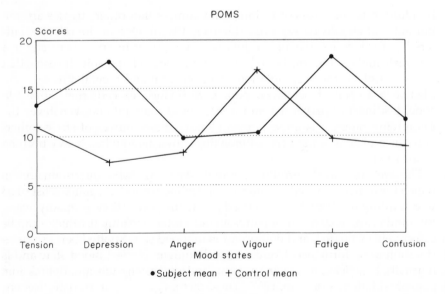

Figure 1 'Iceberg' profile

anaerobic threshold is the level of exercise at which there is significant accumulation of lactic acid because it is being produced faster than it can be metabolised, generally taken to be 4 mmol/l. Less lactate is produced because there is less glycogen, and high-intensity repetitions at or near the anaerobic threshold lead to rapid fatigue. However, long low-intensity work may be relatively well tolerated (Costill, 1988b), since this may be performed by burning fatty acids rather than glycogen.

Fluid intake should also be estimated, since dehydration is an important cause of fatigue and underperformance which may only become apparent on routine testing of urea and electrolytes. If necessary a diary of food and drink consumed can be kept, which will serve the dual purpose of alerting the investigator to any deficiencies and educating the athlete.

Dangerous symptoms

Occasionally the history points to a serious illness. One athlete felt embarrassed to admit that he was suffering from palpitations at the end of any particularly hard training session or race. He continued training, but performed poorly, being unable to push himself at the end of races, and eventually presented with unexplained underperformance and fatigue, but admitted to breathlessness and palpitations even on climbing stairs. Investigation by cardiologists showed that he had trained through a viral infection, and suffered from a Coxsackie B viral myocarditis which had damaged his myocardium, resulting in the arrhythmias. Fortunately this type of serious cause is extremely rare, and the history normally points to a picture of fatigue described as the overtraining syndrome or staleness.

Examination

There is often very little to find on physical examination, but a careful search should be made for evidence of chronic infection such as lymphadenopathy. There may be an increased postural drop in blood pressure in fatigued athletes associated with an unusually high pulse rate during exercise which returns more slowly to normal (Ryan, 1983).

Early-morning and resting pulse rates have been used for many years to monitor the effect of heavy training. A rate of around 40 beats/min is not unusual in a well-trained person, due to a combination of increased vagal tone and changes to the heart itself. Any illness or exhaustive heavy training can raise this baseline rate (Dressendorfer, 1985). If this is raised by more than 10 beats/min it is said to be significant, and can be used as a warning that training should be greatly reduced or to monitor recovery (Ryan, 1983; Czajkowski, 1982).

Muscle power

Normal muscle strength and fatiguability in patients with chronic fatigue was demonstrated by Stokes *et al.* (1988), but this has not yet been shown in athletes.

Cardiorespiratory tests

It is difficult to separate the complex psychology and physiology that make up a good performance but chronically fatigued athletes do tend to reach maximum heart rates (Koutedakis *et al.*, 1989), unlike the untrained patients who only reached 89% of their predicted heart rate in a test to exhaustion. It seems there is a difference in the response to exercise, presumably due to the physical and psychological effects of previous hard training.

Lung function tests may be appropriate before and after exercise, and a 25% drop in forced expiratory volume in one second (FEV1) and peak flow is considered diagnostic of exercise-induced asthma. An electrocardiogram (ECG) may also be appropriate to exclude serious disease such as myocarditis, but an athletes' ECG is frequently abnormal with inverted T waves, cardiomegaly and ventricular ectopics which disappear on exercise when vagal tone is reduced. This is normal in well-trained individuals, and no change has been demonstrated during periods of heavy training or underperformance (Hollman, 1980). Thus an ECG should be interpreted with caution in these patients.

Physiological testing

Exercise testing on an appropriate ergometer to measure performance (such as a treadmill or cycle ergometer), with ECG monitoring and measurement of oxygen consumption and carbon dioxide production, is a luxury available to only a few elite athletes. Such procedures enable the contribution of aerobic and anaerobic metabolism to performance, and the study of the athlete's response to exhaustive exercise, to be assessed in laboratory conditions. Ideally, results should be compared to previous tests, and recovery monitored by retesting every two months.

It is often apparent that the muscles are extracting and using oxygen inefficiently during aerobic work, and there may be rapid exhaustion within a minute of passing the anaerobic threshold, when the athlete has previously managed to continue for three to four minutes. The results form a useful quantitative confirmation of fatigue and underperformance, and enable recovery to be objectively followed.

Laboratory tests and anaemia

Routine blood tests have been used as markers to try and warn of impending collapse and follow recovery in fatigued athletes. Haemoglobin and haematocrit fall with heavy training when athletes are artificially fatigued (Rushall, 1980; Burke, 1981), but there is wide individual variation and changes are probably physiological due to increased plasma volume. There is no correlation with performance (which is an objective measure of fatigue), and some investigators have found no changes in haematocrit (Costill, 1986).

It is important to distinguish between true anaemia, which may be due to iron deficiency, particularly in female athletes (Haymes, 1986), and the reduction in haemoglobin and haematocrit due to increased plasma volume which has no effect on performance. There was a vogue in the mid-1980s for ascribing underperformance to mild anaemia due to low iron stores measured by plasma ferritin levels, but many of the cases described had levels which are now known to be normal in elite endurance athletes (Eichner, 1986). Even levels as low as 12 ng/ml are not associated with underperformance and there is no advantage in raising this with iron supplements (Newhouse *et al.*, 1989).

However, there is evidence that athletes, particularly long-distance runners and women (due to their low iron stores), are susceptible to gastrointestinal blood loss and subsequent iron deficiency anaemia (Nickerson *et al.*, 1989; Eichner, 1989), with haemoglobins below 10 g/100 ml. Thus it is probably worth checking the iron status of athletes with low haemoglobins since this is such an easily treatable cause of fatigue. However, even with adequate dietary iron they may remain iron deficient due to transferrin saturation leading to poor absorption and a slow loss as intestinal cells are shed. Transferrin saturation has been shown to be high during periods of heavy stressful training, only falling during periods of relative rest (Bannister and Hamilton, 1985). Many competitors have already treated themselves with vitamin and iron supplements, which raises the intriguing possibility that it is these iron supplements which have compromised the efforts of the immune system to eradicate infection, so leading to a chronic illness (Hershko *et al.*, 1988). The evidence is that vitamin supplements should only be given in cases of proven deficiency, and a healthy balanced diet be encouraged in all other individuals.

Liver function tests are usually within the normal range, but creatine kinase (CK) may be raised in athletes who have been training hard or are injured. There is a wide individual variation in CK (50-fold) and levels do not correlate with underperformance and fatigue (Noakes, 1987), so this muscle enzyme cannot be used to follow recovery or diagnose a fatigued state.

Virology tests

Viral titres can be helpful in diagnosing subclinical infection. The series of 12 fatigued athletes seen in Glasgow (Roberts, 1985) produced two positive monospots with atypical mononuclear cells and two with increases in Coxsackie B viral titres. However, no viral cause was found in the other eight, although four were undergoing the stress of medical examinations. In a series in London, serological tests provided a diagnosis in two out of 14 elite athletes. One had an Epstein–Barr virus infection and the other a raised Coxsackie B titre (Budgett *et al.*, 1989). The subjects for this study were selected if they were objectively shown to be underperforming for no apparent reason, and were feeling fatigued for at least two weeks. Several potential subjects were withdrawn from the study when a cause was found for their symptoms, such as dehydration, poor diet, viral myocarditis or the change in body shape of a female swimmer who had put on weight. Several had a history of prolonged or recurrent minor infections, but this was by no means a universal finding. Subsequent samples have shown a positive VP1 titre in three out of 29 subjects, two of whom suffered from prolonged fatigue, and one control (Budgett, unpublished data).

Thus viral infections, both clinical and subclinical, are probable causes of a minority of cases of prolonged fatigue in athletes. However, this cannot be assumed to be the case solely on the basis of viral titres. A general practice based study in Scotland showed a high incidence of raised Coxsackie B titres with no difference between subjects and controls (Dawson, 1987).

RESEARCH AREAS

Other tests are more esoteric, and involve many measures of immune function such as secretory IgA, natural killer (NK) cell activity, T helper/T suppressor cell ratio, and lymphocyte function, all of which may fall with exhaustive exercise (Keast, 1988; Gmunder, 1988; Burke and Tan, 1985), and similar changes have been shown with psychological stress (Baker, 1987).

The functional significance of these changes is not yet proven, and Nash (1986) actually showed that training enhanced immune function. Nevertheless, many reports have linked periods of prolonged fatigue and underperformance with an increased susceptibility to infections (Roberts, 1986; Peters, 1985). There are many factors which may affect immune function in these athletes, such as poor nutrition as discussed above, a reduced level of glutamine, or a fall in the cortisol/testosterone ratio. These variables can be measured, but are not diagnostic tests, and have not yet been shown to be objective markers of the overtraining syndrome or correlated with an increased vulnerability to infection or post-viral fatigue.

Steroids

Many studies have shown a fall in testosterone and a rise in cortisol with exhaustive exercise over several days, especially when combined with sleep and calorie deprivation (Aakvag, 1985; Opstad, 1980; Harkonnen, 1984), and this has been proposed as the underlying mechanism leading to prolonged fatigue in athletes (Adlercreutz, 1986). This would lead to an increase in catabolism and a decrease in anabolism, resulting in a failure to recover after exercise with muscle breakdown rather than growth. There is not yet good evidence for this mechanism but work underway on chronically fatigued elite competitors (Budgett *et al.*, 1989) shows lower testosterone levels and higher cortisol levels in nine subjects when compared to six controls, but these differences were not significant, and a larger study is planned.

Amino acids

Glutamine is an amino acid synthesised by and released from skeletal muscle. It is an essential fuel for all rapidly dividing cells and has been shown to provide 35% of the energy for lymphocyte metabolism (Ardawi and Newsholme, 1983). Glutamine has been shown to rise after brief or moderate exercise but fall after prolonged exhaustive exercise (Parry-Billings *et al.*, 1990) in a similar way to testosterone. It has been proposed that low levels in athletes would increase susceptibility to infection and chronic fatigue, and also provide an objective marker of the problem. A group of 13 chronically fatigued male and female athletes have been studied and compared to nine controls and the results are encouraging. Plasma glutamine levels were significantly lower in the underperforming fatigued subjects when compared to the controls matched for sport, ability and training (Budgett *et al.*, 1989). However, it is difficult to be sure of the role of glutamine in the fatigue of these athletes, and studies of immunological function are planned to see if there is a correlation.

PREVENTION AND MANAGEMENT

The underlying cause and pathophysiology of chronic fatigue in athletes is not known and so there is no specific or curative treatment available. The criteria for diagnosis vary in different studies, and there is as yet no diagnostic test. Thus prevention and management are difficult and controversial.

Prevention

Prevention strategies are hampered by the lack of known precipitating factors and causes, but there is some evidence that careful monitoring of physical and mental health can provide an early warning of prolonged underperformance (Ryan, 1983).

Early detection

If it is accepted that increased psychological and physical stress from hard training and competition may play a part in increasing an athlete's susceptibility to prolonged fatigue then an immediate reduction of these stresses may help prevent a more prolonged syndrome developing.

Pulse rate. The early-morning resting pulse rate is used by many athletes and is simple and cheap. A rise of more than 10 beats per minute is considered significant and requires an immediate cut in the training load and investigation for any underlying infection or illness.

Psychological mood state. Morgan (1987) followed 200 swimmers for 10 years using the POMS questionnaire and claimed that 5–10% became chronically fatigued and depressed each year with reduced performance and an inability to train at customary levels, which he called staleness. The questionnaire was useful in warning of impending fatigue and then following recovery.

Laboratory tests. Biochemical markers of imminent staleness, such as haematocrit, urea, creatine kinase, cortisol and sex hormones, are unreliable and tend to correlate with training intensity rather than the response of individuals to the training. Thus athletes at present can only measure their resting pulse and keep a close eye on their general health and how they feel after exercise, taking notice and reacting to any changes from their norm.

Prevention strategies

Training regimes. Apart from early detection there are other preventative strategies which may help. Training schedules should be well balanced and increase only gradually in a wave-like way, with alternate days of intensive and endurance work. An increasing proportion of coaches and commentators feel that athletes are better off under- than overtraining (Ryan, 1983), but the need to reach ever higher peaks of achievement encourages competitors and coaches to push harder if improvement slows. It is sensible to take account of extra stresses outside sport, and reduce the training load at times of exams and other obvious crises.

It is also advisable to have at least a one month break from hard training each year, to allow full recovery. This may be particularly important in women, who have highly saturated transferrin and are unable to absorb adequate iron, since it is only during periods of reduced training stress that the saturation will fall (Bannister and Hamilton, 1985). Interestingly, those women who are most stressed by training often become oligo- or amenorrhoeic (Sanborn and Wagner, 1986), so being partially protected from iron deficiency.

Diet and weight loss. An adequate diet is also important, and expert help may be needed if a competitor is trying to lose weight in order to make a weight category while training hard. Some individuals have unrealistic expectations of their ability to lose weight and have to be told that this is dangerous for their health. A simple objective way of assessing the feasibility of a proposed weight loss is to measure percentage body fat by skin-fold thicknesses. The weight reduction requires partial starvation, and should be carried out during a period of light training when no competitions are planned. Unfortunately, all too often weight reduction is sudden and rushed as a championship approaches, with resultant fatigue due to the inadequate replacement of glycogen stores.

The message that complex carbohydrates and not snack bars are the ideal fuel for training needs to be constantly reinforced (Wheeler, 1989). Athletes may not find time to eat these types of foods, which are less convenient, but must make the attempt or else they run the risk of becoming fatigued and unable to tolerate their training due to glycogen depletion (Costill, 1988c).

Dehydration may also cause fatigue during exercise in warm weather. Studies have shown a 2% slowing of running pace for each percentage point of weight loss due to dehydration (Costill, 1988a). Thirst is a poor indicator of the extent of dehydration because the drive in man is weak compared to animals, so athletes must be encouraged to drink more than they think they need. If there is any evidence of dehydration, athletes can supplement laboratory measurements with their own monitoring of the colour of their urine.

Viral illness. A proportion of cases will be due to viral infection and so it seems sensible to take precautions to avoid transmission of infection. This is often difficult in a sports situation, and since it seems that the individual's response is the most important factor in the development of post-viral fatigue, a vigorous campaign to sterilise the club changing room is unlikely to have much impact on chronic fatigue. However, it is likely to prevent much acute infection, and reduce morbidity from the common minor illnesses that athletes suffer from.

Management

Problems

The treatment of chronic fatigue in athletes, whether from a post-viral cause or the so-called overtraining syndrome, is even more difficult than in non-athletes. These individuals do not want to rest, and as soon as they feel partially recovered will attempt to restart training. They also feel guilty about missing training and may try to make up the deficit by training even harder in their convalescence. The underlying pathophysiology is unknown in most cases and so treatment is empirical rather than scientific.

Complete or relative rest?

Cases need to be assessed on severity and duration. In general, the longer the history of fatigue before training was stopped, the longer recovery takes. In the absence of a cure, rest is the basis of treatment (Koutedakis *et al.*, 1989), and can be combined with a reduction in all stresses and a positive 'regeneration' programme. The prognosis is likely to be worse in those with severe symptoms and positive viral titres including Coxsackie and a positive VP1, and these athletes need to be persuaded to rest completely from training and competition.

There are those who, being less severely affected, are impossible to stop, and it is sometimes possible to compromise in these cases. The athlete can be advised to exercise gently and non-competitively at a different sport with no measures of performance available. This has the advantage of maintaining some degree of cardiovascular fitness, while reducing the stress of exercise to a minimum and providing a break from the grind of training. Often these low levels of exercise are easily tolerated, and the psychological and physical benefits help speed recovery (Szabadi, 1988) while the athlete feels more in control of his progress.

Regeneration

Regeneration strategies are much talked about in coaching magazines, but unfortunately have not been convincingly shown to prevent staleness or speed recovery from chronic fatigue (Crampton, 1987). Sufficient rest, sleep, relaxation and nutrition are central to this strategy (Kinderman, 1986), which has been widely used in the Soviet Union and eastern Europe to try and speed the recovery of underperforming competitors.

Massage, sauna, spa/hydrotherapy, physiotherapy, relaxation tanks and counselling have all been used and were reported to speed recovery in one study from the Soviet Union (Paikov, 1985). There is certainly good evidence of a positive psychological effect (Fox, 1986), with increased calmness, well-being and promotion of sleep. An important benefit is likely to be that the athlete feels that positive action is being taken to speed recovery.

Rehabilitation

Resumption of training should be slow and careful. Each athlete will recover at a different rate and so each week should be taken as a small step. If there is a recurrence of fatigue the training must be cut and started again at a much lower level with a slow build-up again. Other stresses are important and should be reduced as far as is possible even if a regeneration programme is not available.

There seems to be a vulnerable stage at three months when an athlete increases his training and is in danger of relapse. In the majority of athletes there is full recovery by four months, but this does not guarantee freedom from a recurrence. Thus care must be advised in all future training and competition. The use of the term 'overtraining syndrome' implies causation which is unproven, but is a useful label for the athlete since it implies that rest is the cure for their underperformance, and not increased training as they might otherwise assume.

CONCLUSION

It seems likely that most of these athletes are different from patients generally diagnosed as suffering from myalgic encephalomyelitis and so the results of investigations and subsequent diagnosis will also be different. Whether or not the stress of hard training plays a role is not yet proven, but athletes do seem more vulnerable to fatigue, and will notice levels of incapacity which sedentary patients might shrug off without inconvenience. Inevitably, selection criteria will be different when individuals in hard training are studied, and in general their prognosis will be better because they were not so badly affected in the first place. However, there are a small minority who fit into the picture of severe post-viral fatigue and these may have a positive VP1 titre.

SUMMARY

Chronic fatigue is a common problem seen in a sports medicine clinic, but the presenting complaint is often underperformance. Investigations should aim to identify treatable or serious disease, and it is important to assess the whole individual without artificially separating the mind and body in order to identify avoidable stresses. In many athletes no firm diagnosis can be made, and they are labelled as suffering from the overtraining syndrome, staleness, the chronic fatigue syndrome, ME, or the post-viral fatigue syndrome. If no treatable cause is found, treatment is empirical and does not depend on the label given to the fatigued athlete. Only a small percentage will be truly post-viral, and management depends on the severity, duration and response to relative or absolute rest.

REFERENCES

Aakvag, A. (1985) Hormonal response to prolonged physical strain, effect of calorie deficiency and sleep deprivation. In Fotherby and Pal (eds) *Exericise Endocrinology*, pp. 25–64. de Gruyter, Berlin.

Adlercreutz, H. (1986) Effect of training on plasma anabolic and catabolic steroid hormones and their response during physical exercise. *International Journal of Sports Medicine*, **7**, 27–28.

Ardawi, S. and Newsholme, E. A. (1983) Glutamine metabolism in lymphocytes of the rat. *Biochemical Journal*, **212**, 835–842.

Baker, G. H. (1987) Psychological factors and immunity. *Journal of Psychosomatic Research*, **31**, 1–10.

Bannister, E. W. and Hamilton, C. L. (1985) Variations in iron status with fatigue modelled from training in female distance runners. *European Journal of Applied Physiology*, **54**, 16–23.

Barron, D. K. and Mellerowicz, H. (1971) Overtraining. In Larson and Leonard (eds) *Encyclopedia of Sports Sciences and Medicine*, pp. 1310–1312. Macmillan, New York.

Budgett, R. *et al.* (1989) The overtraining syndrome/staleness. In *Proceedings of the First International Olympic Committee World Congress on Sports Sciences*, Colorado Springs, USA, pp. 118–119. US Olympic Committee, Colorado Springs.

Burke, E. (1981) Blood testing to determine overtraining in swimmers. *Swimming Technique*, 18 November, 29–33.

Burke, L. S. and Tan, S. A. (1985) The suppressive effect of stress from acute exhaustive exercise on T lymphocyte helper/suppressor cell ratio in athletes and non-athletes. *Medicine and Science in Sports and Exercise*, **17**, 706.

Brasher, C. (1988) The under-achievers who overtrain. *Observer*, 17th January, 1988.

Costill, D. L. (1986) *Inside Running*, pp. 123–132. Benchmark Press Inc., Indianapolis.

Costill, D. L. (1988a) Nutrition and dietetics. In A. Dirix, H. Knuttgen and K. Tittel (eds) *Olympic Book of Sports Medicine*, pp. 603–634. Blackwell Scientific Publications, Oxford.

Costill, D. L. (1988b) Physiological response to successive days of intense training in competitive swimmers. *Medicine and Science in Sports and Exercise*, **20** (3), 255–259.

Costill, D. L. (1988c) Effects of repeated days of intensified training on muscle glycogen and swimming performance. *Medicine and Science in Sports and Exercise*, **20** (3), 249–254.

Costill, D. L. and Morgan, W. P. (1988) Mood disturbance following increased training in swimmers. *Medicine and Science in Sports and Exercise*, **20** (4), 408–414.

Crampton, J. (1987) Regeneration vs burnout: prevention is better than cure! *Sports Coach*, April/June, 7–11.

Czajkowski, W. (1982) A simple method to control fatigue in endurance training. In P. V. Komi (ed.) *Exercise and Sport Biology*, International Series on Sport Sciences, vol. 10, pp. 207–212. Human Kinetic Publishers, Champaign, Illinois.

Dawson, J. (1987) Royal Free disease: perplexity continues. *British Medical Journal*, **294**, 327–328.

Dressendorfer, R. H. (1985) Increased morning heart rate in runners: a valid sign of overtraining? *Physician and Sports Medicine*, **13** (8), 77–86.

Eichner, E. (1986) The anaemias of athletes. *Physician and Sports Medicine*, **14** (9), 122–130.

Eichner, E. (1989a) Chronic fatigue syndrome: how vulnerable are athletes? *Physician and Sports Medicine*, **17** (6), 157–160.

Eichner, E. (1989b) Chronic fatigue syndrome: searching for the cause and treatment. *Physician and Sports Medicine*, **17** (6), 142–152.

Eichner, E. (1989c) Gastrointestinal bleeding in athletes. *Physician and Sports Medicine*, **17** (5), 128–140.

Fox, J. (1986) The effect of the intentional usage of various forms of regenerative procedures on mood state in Australian athletes. Unpublished graduation paper, Footscray Institute of Technology.

Gmunder, F. K. (1988) Effect of long term physical exercise on lymphocyte reactivity: similarity to spaceflight reactions. *Aviation Space and Environmental Medicine*, **59**, 146–151.

Harkonnen, M. (1984) Biochemical indicators in diagnosis of overstrain condition in athletes. *Sp Med and Ex. Sci.* Proceedings of the Olympic Scientific Congress, Eugene, Oregon, USA.

Haymes, E. M. (1986) Nutrition for the female distance runner. In B. L. Drinkwater (ed.) *Female Endurance Athletes*. Human Kinetics Publishers, Champaign.

Hershko, C., Peto, T. and Weatherall, D. (1988) Iron and infection. *British Medical Journal*, **296**, 660–664.

Hollmann, W. (1980) Sportsmedizin, Arbeits und Trainingsgrundlagen. F. K. Schattauer Verlag, Stuttgart.

Keast, D. (1988) Exercise and the immune response. *Sports Medicine*, **5**, 248–267.

Kevles, B. (1988) Flat tired out. How EBV, the mysterious chronic fatigue syndrome, has brought a group of women cyclists to a grinding halt. *City Sports Magazine*, **14**(9), 17–22.

Kinderman, W. (1986) Das Ubertraining-Ausdruck einer vegitativen Fehlsteuerung. *Deutsche Zeitschrift fur Sportmedizin*, **H8**, 138–145.

Koutedakis, Y., Budgett, R. and Faulmann, L. (1989) The role of physical rest for underperforming elite competitors. *Proceedings of the First International Olympic Committee World Congress on Sports Sciences*, pp. 140–141. Colorado Springs, USA. US Olympic Committee, Colorado Springs.

Kuipers, H. and Keizer, H. A. (1988) Overtraining in elite athletes. *Sports Medicine*, **6**, 79–92.

McCarthy, P. (1989) Wheezing or breezing through exercise-induced asthma *Physician and Sports Medicine*, **17** (7), 125–130.

Morgan, W. P. (1980) Test of champions: the iceberg profile. *Psychology Today*, July, 92–108.

Morgan, W. P. (1985) Affective beneficence of vigorous physical activity. *Medicine and Science in Sports and Exercise*, **17**, 94–100.

Morgan, W. P. (1987) Psychological monitoring of overtraining and staleness. *British Journal of Sports Medicine*, **21**, 107–114.

Nash, H. L. (1986) Can exercise make us immune to disease? *Physician and Sports*, **14**, 250–253.

Newhouse, I. Clement, D., Taunton, J. and McKenzie, D. (1989) The effects of prelatent/latent iron deficiency on physical work capacity. *Medicine and Science in Sports and Exercise*, **21** (3), 263–268.

Nickerson, H. *et al.* (1989) Causes of iron deficiency in adolescent athletes. *Journal of Paediatrics*, **114** (4), 657–663.

Noakes, T. (1986) *Lore of Running*. Oxford University Press, Cape Town.

Noakes, T. (1987) Effect of exercise on serum enzyme activities in humans. *Sports Medicine*, **41**, 245–267.

Opstad, P. K. (1980) Altered physical response to short-term bicycle exercise in young men after prolonged physical strain, calorific deficiency, and sleep deprivation. *European Journal of Applied Physiology*, **45**, 51–62.

Paikov, V. B. (1985) Means of restoration in the training of speed skaters. *Soviet Sports Review*, **20** (1), 9–12. (Translated from *Konkobezhniv Sport*, 1982, **1**, 39–43.)

Parry-Billings, M. *et al.* (1990) A communication link between skeletal muscle, brain and cells of the immune system. *International Journal of Sports Medicine*, **11** (Suppl. 2), S122–128.

Peters, E. M. (1983) Ultramarathon running and upper respiratory tract infections: an epidemiological survey. *South African Medical Journal*, **64**, 582–584.

Roberts, J. A. (1985) Loss of form in young athletes due to viral infection. *British Medical Journal*, **290**, 357–358.

Roberts, J. A. (1986) Virus illness and sports performance. *Sports Medicine*, **31**, 298–303.

Rushall, B. S. (1980) Haematological responses to training elite swimmers. *Canadian Journal of Applied Sports Sciences*, **5**, 164.

Ryan, A. (1983) Overtraining in athletes: a round table. *Physician and Sports Medicine*, **11**, 93–110.

Sanborn, C. F. and Wagner, W. W. (1986) Athletic amenorrhea. In B. L. Drinkwater (ed.) *Female Endurance Athletes*. Human Kinetics Publishers, Champaign.

Stokes, M., Cooper, R. and Edwards, R. (1988) Normal muscle strength and fatigability in patients with effort syndromes. *British Medical Journal*, **297**, 1014–1017.

Szabadi, E. (1988) Physical exercise and mental health. *British Medical Journal*, **296**, 259–260.

Wheeler, K. (1989) Sports nutrition for the primary care physician: the importance of carbohydrate. *Physician and Sports Medicine*, **17** (5), 106–117.

Part IV

A Multiaxial Approach to Immunity

25

Psychological Factors that May Lower Immunity

Jeremy Chase

Watford General Hospital, Watford, UK

INTRODUCTION

Affects and passions of the mynde annoye the body and shorten the life.

(Sir Thomas Elyott, 1539)

It is comments such as this that bear witness to the long-held belief that emotional life determines what happens to our bodies. Shakespeare has romanticised the image of a broken heart and drawn attention to the need to express emotion. In Macbeth he writes, 'Give sorrow words: the grief that does not speak, Whispers the o'er fraught heart and bids it break.' In the nineteenth century consumptives were romanticised, often being seen as victims of their own passions, longings and depression. The discovery of the tuberculis bacillus cut through such thinking, though the physically mal-nourished, who are unable to mount a satisfactory immune response, re-main vulnerable to the secondary phase of this illness. This chapter seeks to assess the underlying validity of these romantic ideas in the light of the current available data on stress and immunity, and to provide an explana-tion for observations such as the following. The Greek physician Galen observed some 2000 years ago that depressed women were more likely than others to develop cancer. It remains a puzzle why bereaved spouses have a higher mortality than the general population (Jacobs and Ostfeld, 1977; Jones *et al.*, 1984), and why life events are associated with the recurrence of breast tumours (Ramirez *et al.*, 1989).

The description of psychological mechanisms that shape the onset and development of illness has been a focus of psychosomatic medicine for

Post-viral Fatigue Syndrome. Edited by R. Jenkins and J. Mowbray

© 1991 John Wiley & Sons Ltd

much of this century. Three major themes in psychosomatic medicine have contributed to and strengthened these popular beliefs. With the highly influential writings of Selye (1936), scientific respectability was given to the idea that stress and disease were intimately related. Adrenocortical hypertrophy was the explanation given for the general adaptation syndrome, and a variety of quite different stress events were given equivalent aetiological importance. Though the nonspecificity of the body's response has subsequently been found to be quite unsubstantiated, the idea has remained, guiding contemporary researchers to follow similarly deterministic arguments, but looking for other neuroendocrine pathways.

Secondly, Alexander's theories of organ specificity (Alexander, 1950) linked certain psychological profiles with particular diseases. Subsequent reviews have cast much doubt on the strength of this model in predicting illness (Grinker, 1969; Lipowski, 1984), but its impact has produced interesting research into psychological profiles and recurrence of tumours (Greer, 1979; Pettingale et al., 1981; Funch and Marshall, 1983).

Lastly, during the 1970s, advances in neuroendocrinology and immunology have pointed towards the biological connections between these systems, and these have again generated much speculation about the role of emotional states and physical disorders. The field of psychoneuroimmunology has largely been established through studying subjects during physical or emotional stress, and measuring some component of their immune system and mental state. The extent to which this has been documented will be reviewed in this chapter, which may leave the reader with many unanswered questions about the clinical relevance of such changes in the immune system.

Psychosomatic medicine has helped in the understanding of the multifactorial aetiology of many diseases, such as asthma, heart disease and infections, e.g. appendicitis. This book is largely about an illness, ME, which is characterised by excessive muscle and mental fatiguability, which recent research evidence is linking to the persistence of active viral infection. However, ME is also associated with a relatively high incidence of psychological symptoms, as are many severe disabling illnesses. This chapter does not seek to disentangle the precise aetiology of ME, and the relative contributions of physical and psychological causes of this syndrome. It does set out to draw attention to the effects of stress on the immune system, which in turn could predispose to a wide variety of illnesses.

IMMUNITY AND ILLNESS

The normal defences against infections fall into two main categories. Nonspecific mechanisms, sometimes called 'innate' immunity, operate without the need for previous contact with the infectious agent. Specific mechanisms are initiated by the recognition of a specific infectious agent by the immune system, and it is these that will be given attention. The principal defence mechanisms are listed in Table 1.

True immune deficiency diseases are uncommon and classified as either primary or secondary. The latter are those not arising congenitally or resulting from intrinsic abnormalities in development of T or B cells. Such acquired states arise from malnutrition, cytotoxic drugs, X-rays or, less commonly, protein-losing enteropathy, and intestinal lymphangiectasia. Whether physical or psychological stress has a clinically significant effect on the immune system is not clear, and some eminent physicians would argue that the evidence is thin (Denman, 1986). The bulk of research to date has concentrated on a comparatively few functional tests, notably T lymphocyte responses to mitogen *in vitro*, natural killer (NK) cell activity and helper suppressor cell ratios.

Infections, particularly in adults, are still poorly understood in relation to minor changes in these functional assays, and their aetiological importance is therefore not discussed in this chapter.

NEUROENDOCRINOLOGY AND THE IMMUNE SYSTEM

Whilst neuroendocrinology has long been a focus for biologically minded psychiatrists, the relationship between brain function and the immune system has only emerged in the last decade, and remains largely unexplored. However, there is good reason to study these systems together.

Table 1 Principal nonspecific and specific host defence mechanisms. (From Irving *et al.*, 1985. Reproduced by permission of Current Medical Literature)

Nonspecific	Specific

Prevention of entry
  Intact integument
  Secretions
  Ciliary movement
  Commensal flora
	Cytotoxic mechanisms
	  T lymphocytes
	  K cells

Humoral mechanisms
  Acute phase response
  Complement system
  Interferon
	Immunoglobulin production
	  B lymphocytes

Cellular mechanisms
  Neutrophils
  Mononuclear phagocytes
  Natural killer cells	

Anatomically the brain stem nuclei are connected to the thymus gland by direct preganglionic nerve pathways (Bulloch and Moore, 1981). Lymph nodes and the spleen are innervated through the autonomic nervous system and lesioning of limbic cortex and anterior hypothalamus has major effects on the immune system. Neuropeptides released into the circulation, and binding to specific receptors, influence the function of lymphocytes (Blalock et al., 1985).

Psychic and autonomic arousal releases a wide variety of hormones, including adrenal corticosteroids, which are controlled by levels of pituitary ACTH. This hormone, like β-endorphin and β-lipotrophin, is derived from the same precursor pro-opiomelanocortin (POMC), and together these have come to be regarded as stress hormones. The general effect of hypercortisolism on the immune system is suppression, resulting in lymphopenia (Claman, 1972; Dougherty et al., 1964), decreased cytotoxic function and lymphokine production. The effect of opioids on immune function is less well understood. Opiate receptors have been found on normal human T lymphocytes (Wybran et al., 1979), and this was confirmed, describing their specificity (Hazum et al., 1979). Similar receptors have been found on leukocytes (Mehrishi and Mills, 1983). The effect of opioids, in vitro, on functional studies of T cell proliferation followed, and there have been conflicting results. In vitro addition of β-endorphin suppresses T cell blastogenesis (McCain et al., 1982; Berk et al., 1983), but the response is donor-dependent (Heijnen, 1987). The effect on NK cell activity of B-endorphin is stimulatory (Mathews et al., 1982; Kay and Morely, 1983), although low doses may have the reverse effect (Williamson et al., 1987). Opiate dependence suppresses in vitro mitogen-stimulated blastogenesis (Law et al., 1978; Ho and Leung, 1979). The existence of ACTH receptors on lymphocytes (Bost et al., 1987) has led to similar investigations indicating that ACTH had a variable effect depending on both donor and concentration (Heijnen, 1987). Catecholamines mediate lymphocyte function through both χ- and β-receptors (Hadden et al., 1970), and a wide range of neurotransmitters and hormones, e.g. growth hormone, histamine, parathyroid hormone and prostaglandins (Coffey and Hadden, 1985), inhibit differentiation of mature lymphocytes.

Until comparatively recently the influence of brain function on the immune system was thought to be unidirectional. There are several important pieces of evidence that challenge this assumption, and suggest that peripheral immune activity signals hypothalamic nuclei. Lymphocytes produce soluble proteins, or lymphokines, e.g. interferons and interleukin-2, which stimulate growth in certain T lymphocytes and mononuclear phagocytes, but also demonstrate properties of some hormones. There is strong antigenic relatedness between interferon, ACTH and endorphins (Blalock and Smith, 1980). Moreover, lymphocytes produce corticotropin

(Smith and Blalock, 1981), which is identical to the pituitary hormone. In addition to the pro-opiomelanocortin-derived hormones, lymphocytes also produce immunoreactive thyrotropin (TSH) (Smith *et al.*, 1983), vasoactive intestinal polypeptide (VIP) (Giachetti *et al.*, 1978) and somatostatin (Lygren *et al.*, 1985). These findings strongly suggest the presence of a lymphoid adrenal axis (Blalock and Smith, 1985). In animal studies an afferent pathway from peripheral immune responses to the central nervous system is suggested by the work of Besedofsky *et al.* (1977), who demonstrated increased hypothalamic firing rates in rats following intraperitoneal immunisation. Later work, again in rats, demonstrated decreased noradrenergic turnover in the hypothalamus at the peak of the immune response to red sheep blood cells or lympholines (Besedofsky *et al.*, 1983).

STRESS AND IMMUNE CHANGES

The aim of this section is to review the evidence that a wide range of stressful events have an effect on immune function. Attention will be given to studies that report changes in lymphocyte numbers, *in vitro* T lymphocyte responses (or transformation) to plant mitogens, helper suppressor cell ratios, interferon levels and viral antibody titres. Brief reference will first be made to the behaviourally conditioned immune response in animals, as these observations were important in generating questions about the links between stress, behaviour and immune function.

Behavioural conditioning in animals

Behavioural conditioning of the immune response in animals began in France in the 1920s, with the presentation of various antigens, e.g. tapioca and staphylococcal filtrates, and measurement of leukocyte counts of exudate at the site of injection (Metal'nikov and Chorine, 1926). The results disappeared into obscurity and through serendipity were reproduced in America (Ader and Cohen, 1975). Mice began to die after experiments that attempted to develop taste aversion (conditioned response) after exposure to saccharin (conditioned stimulus) paired with cyclophosphamide injections (unconditioned stimulus). They found that repeated exposure to the saccharin alone was depressing the immune system after exposure to pathogens. Subsequent exposure of animals to antigens revealed antibody titres to be lowest in the conditioned animals. In these experiments adrenocorticosteroids did not appear to play a major role in the immunosuppression of humoral immunity (Ader *et al.*, 1979). However, corticosteroids can be conditioned and might prove immunosuppressive.

The clinical implications of these findings have been mooted. It may be possible to reduce drug dosage if conditioned stimuli are paired with drug presentation (Bovbjerg *et al.*, 1982). Direct conditioned enhancement of host resistance is demonstrated in animals, whose NK cell activity increases when exposed to camphor, previously paired with an immunostimulating drug (Ghanta *et al.*, 1985).

The influence of stress on human immune function

Methodology in this field varies considerably. Studies of stress and immunity performed in the early 1970s focused on extraordinary circumstances, e.g. space flight, 72 hours of sleep deprivation and marathon running, but no measures of emotional state were recorded. The next broad category includes the study of essentially middle-class American students at times of examinations. Associated psychological and behavioural changes, the ingestion of drugs, particularly alcohol, and eating and sleep patterns were, to varying degrees, controlled for. Early studies of bereaved people faced the criticism that affective changes were assumed but not measured. However, those studies did arouse interest in the relationship between depression and immunity. These studies are quite different. Though few of them describe preceding standardised life events, they do have the advantage of one clear independent variable, the mental and biological state recorded over time. For these reasons studies of depression and immunity will be dealt with separately from studies of stress and immunity.

Space flight

Concern about the health of astronauts led NASA to include immune parameters in the medical evaluation of space flight, and this resulted in some of the earliest reports of immune changes during the most stressful periods of the missions. Fischer *et al.* (1972) reported lymphocytosis in the immediate post-recovery phase of flight, but no change in lymphocyte transformation. Later reports suggested that transformation was diminished during the immediate recovery phase (Kimsey, 1975), judged to be the most stressful time as shown by neuroendrocrine changes (Leach and Rambaut, 1974).

Sleep

Observations of healthy subjects enduring extremes of sleep deprivation (44–72 hours) suggested that phagocytosis was reduced during this time (Palmblad *et al.*, 1976), and lymphocyte transformation (as measured by a reduction in the counts of radioactive thymidine per minute) diminished by 15% (Palmblad *et al.*, 1979). Regrettably, mental states were not evaluated, as they may have acted as an intermediate variable and differentiated subjects' reactions. More recently, reduced NK cytotoxicity has been related to the degree of sleep disturbance in a cohort of severely depressed inpatients (Irwin *et al.*, 1989). These findings should not be surprising as there is a circadian rhythmn in lymphoyte transformation, with an enhancement in the early hours of the morning, a sharp increase in interleukin-1 (Il-1) activity near midnight and a similar decline in NK cell activity between 1 a.m. and 3 a.m. (Moldofsky *et al.*, 1986). These changes are related to the onset of slow-wave sleep, which is disrupted during periods of emotional turmoil and depression. Whether sleep deprivation, as found in affective disorder, is deleterious remains an open question. Jabaay's study (Jabaay *et al.*, 1989) of immune function and varied lifestyles, which included duration of sleep, did not indicate that sleep alone was correlated with any of a range of immune variables.

Exercise

Prolonged exercise results in a leukocytosis which reverts to normal within 48 hours (Dickson *et al.*, 1982). Marathon running reduces lymphocyte transformation (counts are reduced to half their value), but recovery occurs within 24 hours (Eskola *et al.*, 1978). No such changes were found in runners of comparable fitness who only exercised moderately for 30 minutes. Though this is barely analogous to the state found in agitated depression, certain levels of exercise play a role in modifying body defences, which begs questions about motor activity during anxiety and depressive states. These changes may be clinically relevant, as, amongst marathon runners, infections are reported to be more common after racing (Peters and Bateman, 1983).

Bereavement

The increase in mortality among bereaved spouses has been observed for two centuries, and this attributable risk may be as high as 50% (Jacobs and Ostfeld, 1977). In Britain, 2% of men and 8% of women between 45 and 59 are widowed. These figures rise to 30% of the men and 60% of women over the age of 75 (McAvoy, 1986). This at-risk population was thought to be four million in 1968 *Office of Population Censuses and Surveys*, 1986) and a proportion of them die from infectious diseases and cancer. It was therefore of considerable interest that Bartrop *et al.* (1977) observed decreased lymphoblast transformation in 33 pairs of bereaved spouses when compaired with controls at eight weeks, despite normal levels of thyroxine, prolactin, growth hormone and cortisol. These findings were confirmed by Schleifer *et al.* (1983), who prospectively studied male spouses of women dying of breast cancer, and found suppression of lymphocyte transformation as early as four weeks post-bereavement, but normal T and B cell numbers. In both these studies mood was not measured, but clinical depression in the second month post-bereavement might be expected in the majority of cases. Sleep disturbance would very probably be present in these circumstances, but the authors claim that they did not observe such changes, though no measurements were undertaken. A study following a similar design found that amongst 34 women experiencing differing levels of social adjustment after a range of life events, moderate levels of depression (Hamilton Rating Scale for Depression between 12 and 14) and high social readjustment scores were associated with lower NK cell activity (Irwin *et al.*, 1987b). The intensity of depressive symptoms and insomnia were related to reduced NK cell activity and an absolute loss of T suppressor cells.

Unemployment

Unemployment has wide social and psychological consequences, and some studies report an increase in morbidity and mortality (Brenner, 1979). A Swedish study measured lymphocyte transformation and helper and suppressor T cells and B cells in a small group ($n = 17$) of unemployed women over a 14-month period (Arnetz *et al.*, 1987). Subject selection was not described and they did not report changes in affective state, but they reported that there was no difference in scores on the GHQ (General Health Questionnaire) when compared with their healthy, fully employed, age- and sex-matched controls. Despite a comparable psychological profile, lymphocyte transformation declined significantly in the experimental group, in response to both phytohaemagglutinin and purified protein derivative of tuberculin.

Marital disruption

There is much evidence to suggest that during separation partners experience substantial emotional turmoil, and as such are disproportionately represented in psychiatric inpatient and outpatient populations. Feelings of anger and depression are frequently reported, and the incidence of clinical depression is higher than in controls (Blumenthal, 1967). When recently separated and divorced women were compared with healthy married women, poorer responses on two qualitative measures of immune function were found (Kiecolt-Glaser *et al.*, 1987). In subjects they found raised antibody titres to Epstein–Barr virus (EBV), and diminished percentages of NK cells. The same group found comparable results in a cohort of recently divorced men (Kiecolt-Glaser *et al.*, 1988), in whom the less distressed men performed best on functional immune assays.

Examination stress

Sitting and studying for examinations is anxiety-provoking and results in altered patterns of sleep, eating and drug ingestion. Investigators have frequently chosen college students as subjects, who over the course of a year have been studied before and after their examinations. A wide range of immune variables have been measured, and the studies will be reviewed in relation to the immune variable measured. Dorian *et al.* (1982) in Canada demonstrated alterations in lymphocyte responses to mitogen stimulation, and impaired antibody formation in residents prior to their examinations. This study has been repeated with greater degrees of sophistication by workers at Ohio State University on four occasions. These studies (see below) have all used healthy medical students, who were investigated psychologically and immunologically, at times of high and low stress. A similar design was used by a British group (Baker *et al.*, 1985), comparing anxiety levels and immune states in medical students who were either in their first or second year. Dental students (Jemmott *et al.*, 1983) have also been studied at times of examinations, with subjects defined as high or low motivation as judged by the degree of inhibited power.

Immunoglobulins. In the study of Jemmott *et al.*(1983) salivary IgA was measured, as it constitutes part of the first-line defence against upper respiratory tract infections. Subjective ratings confirmed that the low- and high-stress times were experienced as being different, and salivary IgA was significantly lower on all three occasions of high stress. Measurement at the end of the vacation after the examinations revealed the group characterised by inhibited power motivation to have low IgA levels. They inferred that this group, akin to type A personalities, did not relax in the vacations, and no recovery in immune state was observed. A further study reported total plasma IgA, IgM and IgG and salivary IgA in 44 medical students one month before, and on the day of, their examinations (Kiecolt-Glaser *et al.*, 1984). All three plasma isotypes had increased on the day of the examination, although significance was only achieved for plasma IgA. However, no change was found in salivary IgA levels, throwing doubt on Jemmott's earlier findings.

These results may have little clinical relevance, but it is interesting to note that children taught deep relaxation, during which they are requested to elevate their immunity, show appreciable increases (mean of 8.2 mg to a mean of 12.6 mg per decilietr) in their salivary IgA levels, as compared with controls (Olness *et al.*, 1989).

Lymphocyte transformation. Psychiatric residents studied a fortnight before and after their major qualifying examinations had diminished lymphocyte transformation in the pre-examination period, as compared with healthy controls (Dorian et al., 1982). Two weeks after the stressor, transformation was higher in the experimental group. A similar decline in transformation has been reported in students at the time of their examinations (Glaser et al., 1985).

T cell subsets. Subpopulations of T cells help regulate the immune response (Guillemin et al., 1985), though it is not yet clear to what extent the phenotypic characteristics of lymphocytes, e.g. OKT4 and OKT8, correlate with their function, e.g. helper or suppressor activity. In some syndromes numbers of T helper cells predict the emergence of illness, e.g. acquired immunodeficiency syndrome (Creemers et al., 1985), and may be associated with infectious disease (Blumberg and Schooley, 1985).

As part of a study to demonstrate the effect of relaxation on the psychological and immune states of medical student volunteers, Kiecolt-Glaser et al. (1986) found low levels of helper cells (OKT4) in the month before their examinations, when compared with healthy laboratory staff. On the day of their examination there was a significant decline in percentage of helper cells, and in the helper/suppressor cell ratio. Change in the percentage of suppressor cells was not significant. Those randomly assigned to relaxation training between the two sampling times showed lower anxiety on the day of their examinations, and the frequency of practice was a significant predictor of the subset ratio. A particular strength of this study was careful control of drug and alcohol intake, sleep and eating patterns. Three biochemical nutritional assays (albumin, transferrin and total iron-binding protein) were within normal limits on both samples. These results are, however, not consistent with the findings of an English study (Baker et al., 1985), that demonstrated an increase in helper cells and decrease in suppressor cells at times of high anxiety in medical students.

NK cell cytotoxicity. In three separate studies, reduced NK cell lysis has been observed at the time of examinations. The first study, containing 75 first-year medical students (Kiecolt-Glaser et al., 1984), demonstrated decreased lysis on the day of examinations compared with the preceding month. Target cells used in the assay were K-562 cells, a myeloid cell line. These results were then replicated in a second study (Kiecolt-Glaser et al., 1986), using the same cell line but at three different concentrations. The final study (Glaser et al., 1986) produced similar results using a different cell line as target cell.

The capacity of T lymphocytes to recognise virus antigen on the surface of B cells, and then lyse these cells, is a more specific antiviral test. Attempts have been made to monitor T-cell-mediated immunity to EBV-transformed autologous B lymphocytes in students during examinations (Glaser et al., 1987). A decline in T cell killing by memory T lymphocytes was found during the examination period. As expected, T cells of the EBV seronegative students showed no cell-killing activity, confirming the hypothesis that it was particularly the memory function that was impaired during examination stress.

Viral antibody titres. The relationship between stress and the recurrence of latent virus, e.g. herpes simplex, EBV and cytomegalovirus, has attracted considerable public attention. Anecdotal evidence suggests that recurrence of herpes infection occurs at times of stress. Researchers have reported that altered psychological states, as measured by the GHQ, at the time of first presentation, predicts the time of recurrence (Goldmeier *et al.*, 1986) and recurrence rates (Goldmeier and Johnson, 1982; Kemeny *et al.*, 1989).

Not only may state changes be important in determining the clinical course of viral infection, but personality traits may also affect the duration of the common cold. Experimentally induced rhinovirus infection is worse in introverts and in those who have experienced life events that substantially affected their activity levels (Totman *et al.*, 1980; Broadbent *et al.*, 1984).

It is possible that these clinical observations may be explained, in part, by changes in certain hormones. Stress-related hormones, nor adrenaline and adrenaline, commonly raised with anxiety, block the capacity of gamma-interferon to activate murine macrophages to kill herpes simplex virus-2 (HSV-2)-infected cells *in vitro* (Koff and Dunegan, 1986), and the cellular immune response is thought to be an important factor in controlling the expression of latent infection (Klein *et al.*, 1981; Rickinson *et al.*, 1981). Reactivation of infection, for whatever reason, would be reflected in raised titres. It is therefore of interest that the viral capsid antigen (VCA) and early antigen (EA) to EBV were raised at times of examination stress (Glaser *et al.*, 1985), as were antibodies to HSV-1 and cytomegalovirus (CMV). What is also interesting about this study is the fairly small change in anxiety symptoms across the sampling points one month pre-examination and on the day of examination (e.g. a mean of 56 and 67 on the Brief Symptom Inventory anxiety scale). In their later study (Glaser *et al.*, 1987), which repeated the measurements at three high and three low stress points, EBV VCA titres were again higher at the time of examination. These results were highly significant ($F < 0.0001$) with increases in titres of between two- and four-fold.

Interferon assays. Interferons are part of a large family of regulatory proteins, whose functions have recently been reviewed (Balkwill, 1989). Whilst there are three main types, the two most widely studied are alpha- and gamma-interferon. The former has the widest clinical use in treating viral infection, and in specific tumours. They have a limited role in altering the course of an already established acute viral illness, but short-term prophylaxis in family contacts of an infected individual reduced the risk of rhinovirus colds by

78% (Gordon-Douglas, 1986). Gamma-interferon is produced by T cells _in vitro_ when stimulated by plant mitogens, and the production is readily measurable. At the time of their examinations, gamma-interferon levels are diminished in otherwise healthy students (Glaser _et al._, 1986). In a subsequent study, Glaser _et al._ (1987) demonstrated that the virus cytopathic effect of interferon dropped sharply during examinations.

A major criticism of the stress paradigm arises from the observation that identical life events may evoke quite different responses in different subjects. The measurement of the response to events has been absent from much of the earlier 'stress immunity' literature, which may have produced false negatives by aggregating the immunological data from subjects with variable stress responses. Subsequent studies attempted to standardise life events using the Holmes–Rahe scale of social adjustment (Holmes and Rahe, 1967), which is a self-report scale, and rated symptoms on, for example, the Brief Symptom Inventory (BSI). There are as yet few British studies in this field, but it is likely that they would use the much respected objectively measured life event ratings (Brown _et al._, 1973). If we are to answer the question 'Do emotional factors play a role in determining immunity?', then it is important that future research continues to measure the emotional state independently of the events that may have preceded that state, and correlate these measures with immune variables.

DEPRESSION AND IMMUNITY

Anxiety states usually emerge in the face of threatening circumstances, such as have been described in the section on stress. Depression is a state of mind, frequently accompanied by physical symptoms that may result from psychological trauma, frequently loss, or be associated with physical illness. Anxiety and agitation are frequently associated with depression, but the presence of these symptoms with depression varies enormously. The characteristics of the depressive state are important as it may not be the depth of mood disturbance but rather the accompanying symptoms, e.g. sleep pattern, motor activity or vegetative signs, that determine the immune change. Independently, these can all influence immune state, and they will therefore be given special attention in the following pages.

Depression frequently follows viral infections, and efforts have been made to link the prevalence of severe depression with viruses known to have an affinity with the central nervous system. Serological observations of viral antibody titres in psychotic depressed patients demonstrated higher titres and incidence of HSV antibodies than in healthy controls (Cappel _et al._, 1978; Rimon and Halonen, 1969; Lycke _et al._, 1974; Rimon _et al._, 1971). These findings were probably state markers, as subsequent observations of patients with psychotic depression on relapse and in remission (Cappel *et al.*, 1978) demonstrated high HSV titres during the depression, which subsequently fell to the level of controls once the depression resolved. Measels, CMV and rubella antibodies were largely stable across the sampling times, and did not differ from controls. This, they inferred, was due to reactivation of infection, with consequences for monoamine metabolism and thus the emergence of depression. A subsequent study of large groups of psychiatric patients (King *et al.*, 1985) has not confirmed high HSV titres.

Following the observation that bereaved spouses had diminished lymphocyte transformation (Bartrop *et al.*, 1977), cellular responses in depression became a focus in the early 1980s. Initial studies suggested that depressed males, mean age 54, when compared with less depressed groups who had also experienced a bereavement, had lower lymphocyte responses (Linn *et al.*, 1982). This study lacked a control group, and psychological scores were not given. Sengar *et al.* (1982) reported normal lymphocyte transformation in a group of manic depressives, studied during remission. This emphasised that cellular immune changes are probably state and not trait markers. The first study of patients with major depressive disorder, whose subjects had a mean age of 41 and a Hamilton Rating Scale for Depression (HRSD) of 16.2, demonstrated a marked decrease in lymphocyte transformation to three different mitogens (Kronfol *et al.*, 1983). In an older and more depressed sample of patients (mean age 52 and mean HRSD of 28), a similar decrease in three different mitogen-driven transformations was found (Schleifer *et al.*, 1984). When the same group repeated their study looking at younger outpatients with less severe depression (mean age 43 and HRSD of 19), they were unable to reproduce their earlier positive findings (Schleifer *et al.*, 1985). They concluded that the severity of depression was accounting for the changes, but they had not controlled for sleep disturbance or other vegetative signs, included in the HRSD. In another group of inpatients with major depression, of similar age (mean age 35) and severity (HRSD of 20), no difference was found in lymphocyte transformation, as compared with controls (Albrecht *et al.*, 1985). Once again, the vegetative signs had not been described.

By this time searches for possible modulators of immune changes were being undertaken. Kronfol and colleague's second study (Kronfol *et al.*, 1986), though it again demonstrated impaired lymphocyte function in a group of marginally more depressed and older patients (mean age of 46), found no association between urinary free cortisol excretion over 48 hours and immune changes. Calabrese *et al.* (1986) demonstrated diminished lymphocyte transformation in a sample of severely depressed and older patients (mean age of 55 and HRSD of 26), and reported that prostaglandin E2 (PGE2) was significantly elevated. PGE2 levels showed an inverse

correlation with mitogen responses, but helper and suppressor T cell percentages did not differ from that of controls.

The association between depression and immune changes has thus been
demonstrated in five of the seven major studies. However, age and severity
seemed to be important variables, and most studies did not include more
than 30 patients. It was therefore of great interest that Schleifer et al. (1989)
repeated their earlier work on a large sample of 91 subjects of widely differing age and severity of symptoms. Unlike in the earlier studies, age- and sex-
matched controls were paired from the outset and blood was obtained from
each pair on the same day. Immune measures included mitogen responses,
T cell subsets and NK cell activity. Ages ranged from 18 to 76, with a mean
of 41.2 (SD 14.9), and HRSD ranged from 14 to 40, with a mean of 25.9 (SD
6.5). Two-thirds were outpatients. No differences were found between
patients and controls in the means of any of the immune measures. There
were, however, significant age- and severity-related differences between
patients and controls in mitogen responses and T4 lymphocytes. Unlike
those of controls, patients' T4 lymphocytes and mitogen responses decreased with age, a finding which several but not all studies have demonstrated in healthy controls (Foad et al., 1974; Weksler and Hutteroth, 1974;
Portaro et al., 1978). Supporting the findings of their previous study, they
found severity of symptoms to be associated with mitogen responses, and
that morning plasma cortisol levels, though elevated, did not predict a
change in any immune variable. They concluded that depression as a state is
not the determining variable but rather that older patients with more severe
depression have appreciably altered mitogen responses.

CONCLUSION

In this chapter there is much to suggest that immune changes do occur
during times of adversity, depression and extremes of behaviour. In general,
studies demonstrate diminished immunity, with the most consistent finding
being reductions in lymphocyte transformation, NK cell activity and reactivation of latent viral infection. Further work may shed light on more
specific changes in lymphokine production during transformation, and
should continue to measure multiple immune variables, particularly as we
remain uncertain about the clinical value of individual measures. More attention should be given to the biological concomitants of emotional disorders, as simple factors like disturbed sleep and levels of agitation may
account for much of the variance.

In two decades substantial advances have been made in understanding
the complexity of the immune system which have emphasised its close
biological connections with neuroendocrine function. Whilst this is of great

academic interest, observers of human behaviour, psychologists and psychiatrists have been quick to adopt this new knowledge to draw attention to its explanatory potential. In doing so major assumptions may be made about the clinical relevance of minor immune changes, a subject in which we are barely advancing. That people may be driven into decline by adversity is a widespread belief, and the search for evidence to support this has encouraged researchers into the field of psychoneuroimmunology. Close liaison with multidisciplinary teams, greater experimental control, and prospective designs in high-risk groups, will advance our knowledge in this interesting field.

REFERENCES

Ader, R. and Cohen, N. (1975) Behaviourally conditioned immunosuppression. *Psychosomatic Medicine*, **37**, 333–340.

Ader, R., Cohen, N. and Grota, L. J. (1979) Adrenal involvement in conditioned immunosuppression. *International Journal of Immunopharmacology*, **1**, 141–145.

Albrecht, J., Hilderman, J. H., Schlesser, M. A,. and Rush, A. J. (1985) A controlled study of cellular immune function in affective disorders before and during somatic treatment. *Psychiatry Research*, **15**, 185–193.

Alexander, F. (1950) *Psychosomatic Medicine*, Norton, New York.

Arnetz, B. B., Wasserman, J., Petrini, B., Brenner, S. O., Levi, L., Eneroth, P., Salovaara, H., Hjelm, R., Salovaara, L., Theoerell, T. and Petterson, I. L. (1987) Immune function in unemployed women. *Psychosomatic Medicine*, **49** (1), 3–12.

Baker, G. A., Sautalo, R. and Blumenstein, J. (1977) Effect of psychotropic drugs upon the blastogenic response of human T-lymphocytes. *Biological Psychiatry*, **12**, 159.

Baker, G. H. B., Irani, M. S., Byrom, N. A., Nagvekar, N. M., Wood, R. J., Hobbs, J. R. and Brewerton, D. A. (1985) Stress, cortisol concentrations, and lymphocyte subpopulations. *British Medical Journal*, **290**, 1393–1394.

Balkwill, F. R. (1989) Interferons. *Lancet*, **i**, 1060–1063.

Bartrop, R. W., Luckhurst, E., Lazarus, L., Kiloh, L. G. and Penny, R. (1977) Depressed lymphocyte function after bereavement. *Lancet*, **i**, 834–836.

Berk, L. S., Tan, S. A., Carmona, M. and Eby, W. C. (1983) Beta-endorphin suppresses pokeweed induced blastogenesis of human lymphocytes. *Clinical Research*, **31**, 23A.

Besedovsky, H. O., Sorkin, E., Felix, D. and Haas, H. (1977) Hypothalamic changes during the immune response. *European Journal of Immunology*, **7** (5), 325–328.

Besedovsky, H. O., del Ray, A., Sorkin, E., DaPrada, M., Burri, M. and Honneger, C. (1983) The immune response evokes changes in brain noradrenergic neurones. *Science*, **221**, 564–566.

Besedovsky, H. O., Adriana, E. R. and Sorkin, E. (1985) Immune–neuroendocrine interactions. *Journal of Immunology*, **135**, 750–754.

Blalock, J. E. and Smith, E. M. (1980) Human leukocyte interferon: structural and biological relatedness to adrenocorticotropic hormone and endorphins. *Proceedings of the National Academy of Sciences of the USA*, **78**, 7530.

Blalock, J. E., Harbour-McMenamin, D. and Smith, E. M. (1985) Peptide hormones shared by the neuroendocrine and immunologic systems. *Journal of Immunology*, **135**, 858–861.

Blumberg, R. S. and Schooley, R. T. (1985) Lymphocyte markers and infectious diseases. *Seminars in Hematology*, **22**, 31–114.

Blumenthal, M. D. (1967) Mental health among the divorced: A field study of divorced and never divorced persons. *Archives of General Psychiatry*, **16**, 603–608.

Bost, K. L., Smith, E. M., Wear, L. B. and Blalock, J. E. (1987) Presence of ACTH and its receptors on a B lymphocytic cell line: A possible autocrine function of a neuroendocrine hormone. *Journal of Biological Regulation and Homeostasis Agents*, **1**, 23.

Bovbjerg, D., Cohen, H. and Ader, R. (1982) The central nervous system and learning: a strategy for immune regulation. *Immunology Today*, **3** (11), 287–291.

Brenner, M. H. (1979) Mortality and the national economy. *Lancet*, **ii**, 568–573.

Broadbent, D. E., Broadbent, M. H. P., Phillpotts, R. J. and Wallace, J. (1984) Some further studies on the prediction of experimental colds in volunteers by psychological factors. *Journal of Psychosomatic Research*, **28** (6), 511–523.

Brown, G. W., Sklair, F., Harris, T. O. and Birley, J. L. T. (1973) Life events and psychiatric disorders. Part 1: Some methodological issues. *Psychological Medicine*, **3**, 74.

Bulloch, K. and Moore, R. Y. (1981) Innervation of the thymus gland by brain stem and spinal cord in mouse and rat. *American Journal of Anatomy*, **162** (2), 157–166.

Calabrese, J. R., Skwerer, R. G., Barna, B., Gulledge, A. D., Valenzuela, R., Butkus, A., Subichin, S. and Krupp, N. E. (1986) Depression, immunocompetence, and prostaglandins of the E series. *Psychiatry Research*, **17**, 41–47.

Cappell, R., Gregoire, F., Thiry, L. and Sprecher, S. (1978) Antibody and cell mediated immunity to herpes simplex virus in psychotic depression. *Journal of Clinical Psychiatry*, **39**, 266–268.

Claman, H. (1972) Corticosteroids and lymphoid cells. *New England Journal of Medicine*, **287**, 388–397.

Coffey, R. G. and Hadden, J. W. (1985) Neurotransmitters, hormones, and cyclic nucleotides in lymphocyte regulation. *Federation Proceedings*, **44**, 112–117.

Creemers, P. C., Stark, D. F. and Boyko, W. Y. (1985) Evaluation of natural killer cell activity in patients with persistent generalised lymphadenopathy and acquired immunodeficiency syndrome. *Clinical Immunology and Immunopathology*, **36**, 141–150.

Denman, A. M. (1986) Immunity and depression. *British Medical Journal*, **293**, 464–465.

Dickson, D. N., Wilkinson, R. L. and Noakes, T. D. (1982) Effects of ultra-marathon training and racing on haematological parameters and serum ferritin levels in well trained athletes. *International Journal of Sports Medicine*, **2**, 111–117.

Dorian, B., Garfinkel, P., Brown, C., Shore, A., Gladman, D. and Keystone, E. (1982) Aberration in lymphocyte subpopulations and function during psychological stress. *Clinical Experimental Immunology*, **50**, 132–138.

Dorian, B. J., Garfinkel, P. E., Keystone, E. C., Brown, G., Shore, A. and Gladman, D. (1986) Stress, immunity and illness. *Psychosomatic Medicine*, **48**, 304.

Dougherty, T., Berliner, M. and Schneebeli, G. (1964) Hormonal control of lymphatic structure and function. *Annals of the New York Academy of Science*, **113**, 825–843.

Eskola, J., Ruuskanen, O., Soppi, E., Viljanen, J., Jarvinen, M. and Toivonem, H. (1978) Effects of sports stress on lymphocyte transformation and antibody formation. *Clinical and Experimental Immunology*, **32**, 339–345.

Fischer, C. L., Daniels, J. C. and Levin, W. C. (1972) Effects of the space flight environment on man's immune system: lymphocyte counts and reactivity. *Aerospace Medicine*, **43**, 1122–1125.

Foad, B. S. I., Adams, L. E., Yamauchi, Y. and Litwin, A. (1974) Phytomitogen responses of peripheral blood lymphocytes in young and older subjects. *Clinical and Experimental Immunology*, **17**, 657–664.

Funch, D. P. and Marshall, J. (1983) The role of stress, social support and age in survival from breast cancer. *Journal of Psychosomatic Research*, **27**, 77–83.

Ghanta, V. K., Hiramoto, R. N., Solvason, H. B. and Spector, N. H. (1985) Neural and environmental influences on neoplasia and NK activity. *Journal of Immunology*, **135** (Supplement 2), 848s–852s.

Giachetti, A., Goth, A. and Said, S. I. (1978) Vasoactive intestinal polypeptide (VIP) in rabbit platelets and rat mast cells. *Federation Proceedings*, **37**, 657.

Glaser, R., Kiecolt-Glaser, J. K., Stout, J. C., Tarr, K. L., Speicher, C. E. and Holliday, J. E. (1985) Stress related impairments in cellular immunity. *Psychiatric Research*, **16**, 233–239.

Glaser, R., Rice, R., Speicher, C. E., Stout, J. C. and Keicolt-Glaser, J. C. (1986) Stress depresses interferon production by leukocytes concomitant with a decrease in natural killer cell activity. *Behavioural Sciences*, **100**, 675–678.

Glaser, R., Rice, J., Sheridan, J., Fertel, R., Stout, J., Speicher, C., Pinsky, D., Kotur, M., Post, A., Beck, M. and Kiecolt-Glaser, J. (1987) Stress-related immune suppression: health implications. *Brain, Behaviour, and Immunity*, **1**, 7–20.

Goldmeier, D. and Johnson, A. (1982) Does psychiatric illness affect the rate of genital herpes? *British Journal of Venereal Diseases*, **58**, 40–43.

Goldmeier, D., Johnson, A., Jeffries, D., Walker, G. D., Underhill, G., Robinson, G. and Ribbans, H. (1986) Psychological aspects of recurrence of genital herpes. *Journal of Psychosomatic Medicine*, **30** (5), 601–608.

Gordon-Douglas, R. (1986) The common cold—relief at last? *New England Journal of Medicine*, **314**, 114–115.

Greer, S. (1979) Psychological enquiry: a contribution to cancer research. *Psychological Medicine*, **9**, 81–89.

Grinker, R. R. (1969) An editor's farewell. *Archives of General Psychiatry*, **21**, 641–646.

Guillemin, R., Cohn, M. and Melnechuk, T. (eds) (1985) *Immunity*. Raven Press, New York.

Hadden, J. W., Hadden, E. M. and Middleton, E. (1970) Lymphocyte blast transformation. I. Demonstration of adrenergic receptors on human peripheral lymphocytes. *Cellular Immunology*, **1**, 583–595.

Hazum, E., Chang, K. J. and Cuatrecasas, P. (1979) Specific non-opiate receptors for beta-endorphin. *Science*, **205**, 1033–1035.

Heijnen, C. J. (1987) Modulation of the immune response by POMC-derived peptides. *Brain, Behaviour and Immunity*, **1**, 284–291.

Ho, W. K. K. and Leung, A. (1979) Effect of morphine addiction on con-A mediated blastogenesis. *Pharmacology Research Communications*, **11**, 413–419.

Holmes, T. H. and Rahe, R. H. (1967) The social readjustment rating scale. *Journal of Psychosomatic Research*, **11**, 213.

Irving, W., Donnely, P. and Starke, I. (1985) Normal defences against infection. In A. Geddes (ed.) *Infection and the Immunocompromised Patient*, p. 3. Current Medical Literature Ltd.

Irwin, M., Daniels, M., Bloom, E. T., Smith, T. L. and Weiner, H. (1987a) Life events, depressive symptoms and immune function. *American Journal of Psychiatry*, **144** (4), 437–441.

Irwin, M., Smith, T. L. and Gillin, J. C. (1987b) Low natural killer cell cytotoxity in major depression. *Life Sciences*, **41**, 2127–2133.

Irwin, M., Gillin, C., Caldwell, C. and Smith, T. L. (1989) Electroencephalographic sleep measures and immune function in depression. *Psychosomatic Medicine*, **51**, 245.

Jabaay, L., Vingerhoets, A., Menges, L., Ballieux, R. and van Houte, A. J. (1989) Life style and immunologic parameters. *Psychosomatic Medicine*, **51**, 257.

Jacobs, S. and Ostfeld, A. (1977) An epidemiological review of the mortality of bereavement. *Psychosomatic Medicine*, **39** (5), 344–357.

Jemmott, J. B., Borysenko, J. Z., Borysenko, M., McCelland, D. C., Chapman, R., Meyer, D. and Benson, H. (1983) Academic stress, power motivation, and decrease in secretory rate of salivary immunoglobulin A. *Lancet*, **i**, 1400–1402.

Jones, D. R., Goldblatt, P. O. and Leon, D. A. (1984) Bereavement and cancer: some data on death of spouses from the longitudinal study of Office of Population Censuses and Surveys. *British Medical Journal*, **289**, 461–464.

Kay, N. E. and Morley, J. E. (1983) B endorphin enhances human natural killer (NK) cell activity. *Clinical Research*, **31**, 346A.

Kemeny, M. E., Cohen, F., Zegans, L. S. and Conant, M. A. (1989) Psychological and immunological predictors of genital herpes recurrence. *Psychosomatic Medicine*, **51**, 195–208.

Kiecolt-Glaser, J. K., Garner, W., Speicher, C., Penn, G.M., Holliday, J. and Glaser, J. (1984) Psychosocial modifiers of immunocompetence in medical students. *Psychosomatic Medicine*, **46**, 7–14.

Kiecolt-Glaser, J. K., Glaser, R., Strain, E. C., Stout, J. C., Tarr, K. L., Holliday, J. E. and Speicher, C. E. (1986) Modulation of cellular immunity in medical students. *Journal of Behavioural Medicine*, **9**, 5–21.

Kiecolt-Glaser, J. K., Fischer, L. D., Ogrocki, P., Stout, J. C., Speicher, C. E. and Glaser, R. (1987) Marital quality, marital disruption, and immune function. *Psychosomatic Medicine*, **49** (1), 13–34.

Kiecolt-Glaser, J. K., Kennedy, S., Malkoff, S., Fischer, L., Speicher, C. E. and Glaser, R. (1988) Marital discord and immunity in males. *Psychosomatic Medicine*, **50**, 213–229.

Kimsey, S. L. (1975) The effects of extended space flight on haematological and immune systems. *Journal of the American Medical Women's Association*, **30**, 218–232.

King, D. J., Cooper, S. J., Earle, J. A. P., Martin, S. J., McFerran, N. V., Rima, B. K. and Wisdom, G. B. (1985) A survey of serum antibodies to eight common viruses in psychiatric patients. *British Journal of Psychiatry*, **147**, 137–144.

Klein, E., Ernberg, I., Masuuci, M. G., Szigeti, R., Wu, Y. T., Mascutti, G. and Svedmeyr, E. (1981) T-cell response to B-cells and Epstein Barr virus antigens in infectious mononucleosis. *Cancer Research*, **41**, 4210–4215.

Koff, W. C. and Dunegan, M. A. (1986) Neuroendocrine hormones suppress macrophage-mediated lysis of herpes simplex virus-infected cells. *Journal of Immunology*, **136**, 705–709.

Kronfol, Z., Silva, J., Greden, J., Dembinski, S., Gardner, R. and Carroll, B. (1983) Impaired lymphocyte function in depressive illness. *Life Sciences*, **33**, 241–247.

Kronfol, Z., House, J. D., Silva, J., Greden, J. and Carroll, B. J. (1986) Depression, urinary free cortisol excretion and lymphocyte function. *British Journal of Psychiatry*, **148**, 70–73.

Law, J. S., Watanabe, K. and West, W. L. (1978) Morphine effects on the responsiveness of lymphocyte to Con-A. *Pharmacologist*, **20**, 231.

Leach, C. S. and Rambaut, P. C. (1974) Biochemical responses of the Skylab crewman. *Proceedings of the Skylab Life Sciences Symposium*, **2**, 425–454.

Linn, B. S., Linn, M. W. and Jensen, J. (1982) Degree of depression and immune responsiveness. *Psychosomatic Medicine*, **44** (1), 128–129.

Lipowski, Z. (1984) What does the word psychosomatic really mean? A historical and semantic enquiry. *Psychosomatic Medicine*, **46**, 153–171.

Lycke, E., Norrby, R. and Roos, B. E. (1974) A serological study of mentally ill patients. *British Journal of Psychiatry*, **124**, 273–279.

Lygren, I., Revhaug, A., Burhol, P. G., Giercksky, K. E. and Jennsen, T. G. (1985) Vasoactive intestinal polypeptide and somatostatin in leukocytes. *Scandinavian Journal of Clinical and Laboratory Investigations*, **44**, 347.

Mathews, P. M., Sibbitt, W. L. and Bankhurst, A. D. (1982) The modulation of natural killer cells by endorphins. *Clinical Research*, **30**, 54A.

McAvoy, B. R. (1986) Death after bereavement. *British Medical Journal*, **293**, 835–836.

McCain, H. W., Lamster, I. B., Bozzone, J. M. and Grbic, J. T. (1982) B-endorphin modulates human immune activity via non-opiate receptor mechanisms. *Life Sciences*, **31**, 1619–1624.

Mehrishi, J. N. and Mills, I. H. (1983) Opiate receptors on lymphocytes and platelets in man. *Clinical Immunology and Immunopathology*, **27**, 240–279.

Metal'nikov, S. and Chorine, V. (1926) Roles de reflexes conditionnels dans l'immunite. *Annals de L'Institut Pasteur (Paris)*, **40** (11), 893–900.

Moldofsky, H., Lue, F. A., Eisen, J., Keystone, E. and Gorczinski, R. M. (1986) The relationship between interleukin-1 and immune functions to sleep in humans. *Psychosomatic Medicine*, **48**, 309–318.

Murphy, D., Gardner, R., Greden, J. F. and Carroll, B. J. (1987) Lymphocyte numbers in endogenous depression. *Psychological Medicine*, **17**, 381–385.

Office of Population Censuses and Surveys (1968) *Social Trends*, **16**, HMSO, London.

Olness, K., Culbert, T. and Uden, D. (1989) Self-regulation of salivary immunoglobulin A by children. *Paediatrics*, **83** (1), 66–71.

Palmblad, J., Cantell, K., Strander, H., Froberg, J., Karlson, C. G., Levi, L., Grangstrom, M. and Under, P. (1976) Stressor exposure and immunological response in man: interferon producing capacity and phagocytosis. *Psychosomatic Research*, **20**, 193–199.

Palmblad, J., Petrini, B., Wasserman, J. and Akerstedt, T. (1979) Lymphocyte and granulocyte reactions during sleep deprivation. *Psychosomatic Medicine*, **41** (4), 273–278.

Peters, E. and Bateman, E. (1983) Ultra-marathon running and upper respiratory tract infection. An epidemiological survey. *South African Medical Journal*, **65**, 582–584.

Pettingale, K. W., Philalithis, A., Tee, D. E. H. and Greer, H. S. (1981) The biological correlates of psychological responses to breast cancer. *Journal of Psychosomatic Research*, **25** (5), 453–458.

Portaro, J. K., Glick, G. I. and Zighelboim, J. (1978) Population immunology: Age and immune cell parameters. *Clinical Immunology and Immunopathology*, **11**, 339–345.

Ramirez, A. J., Craig, T. K. J., Watson, J. P., Fentiman, I. S. and Noerth, W. R. S. (1989) Stress and relapse from breast cancer. *British Medical Journal*, **298**, 291–293.

Rickinson, A. B., Moss, D. J., Wallace, I. F., Rowe, M., Misko, I. S., Epstein, M. A. and Pope, J. H. (1981) Long-term T-cell mediated immunity in Epstein Barr virus. *Cancer Research*, **41**, 4216–4221.

Rimon, R. and Halonen, P. (1969) Herpes simplex virus infection and depressive illness. *Diseases of the Nervous System*, **30**, 338–340.

Rimon, R., Halonen, P., Anttinen, E. and Evola, E. (1971) Complement fixing antibody to herpes simplex virus in patients with psychotic depression. *Diseases of the Nervous System*, **32**, 822–824.

Schleifer, S. J., Keller, S. E., Camerino, M., Thornton, J. C. and Stein, M. (1983) Suppression of lymphocyte stimulation following bereavement. *Journal of the American Medical Association*, **250** (3), 374–377.

Schleifer, S. J., Keller, S. E., Myersen, A. T., Raskin, M. J., Davis, K. L. and Stein, M. (1984) Lymphocyte function in major depressive disorder. *Archives of General Psychiatry*, **41**, 484–486.

Schleifer, S. J., Keller, S. E., Siris, S. G., Davis, K. L. and Stein, M. (1985) Depression and immunity. *Archives of General Psychiatry*, **42**, 129–133.

Schleifer, S. J., Keller, S. E., Bond, R. N., Cohen, J. and Stein, M. (1989) Major depressive disorder and immunity. *Archives of General Psychiatry*, **46**, 81–87.

Selye, H. (1936) The general adaptation syndrome and the diseases of adaptation. *Journal of Clinical Endocrinology*, **6** (2), 117–230.

Sengar, D. P. S., Waters, B. G. H., Dunne, J. V. and Bouer, I. M. (1982) Lymphocyte subpopulations and mitogenic responses of lymphocytes in manic-depressive disorders. *Biological Psychiatry*, **17** (9), 1017–1021.

Shekelle, R. B., Raynor, W. J. and Ostfeld, A. M. (1981) Psychological depression and 17-year risk of death from cancer. *Psychosomatic Medicine*, **43** (2), 117–125.

Smith, E. M. and Blalock, J. E. (1981) Human leukocyte production of ACTH and endorphin like substances: association with leukocyte interferon. *Proceedings of the National Academy of Sciences of the USA*, **78**, 7530.

Smith, E. M., Phan, M., Coppenhaver, D., Kruger, T. E. and Blalock, J. E. (1983) Human leukocyte production of immunoreactive thyrotropin. *Proceedings of the National Academy of Sciences of the USA*, **80**, 6010.

Totman, R., Kiff, J., Reed, S. E. and Craig, J. W. (1980) Predicting experimental colds in volunteers from different measures of recent life stress. *Journal of Psychosomatic Research*, **24**, 155–163.

Weksler, M. E. and Hutteroth, T. H. (1974) Impaired lymphocyte function in aged humans. *Journal of Clinical Investigations*, **53**, 99–104.

Williamson, S. A., Knight, R. A., Lightman, S. L. and Hobbs, J. R. (1987) Differential effects of B endorphin fragments on human natural killing. *Brain, Behaviour and Immunity*, **1**, 329–335.

Wybran, J., Appleboom, T., Famey, J. P. and Govaerts, A. (1979) Suggestive evidence for receptors for morphine and methionine-encephalin on normal human blood T lymphocytes. *Journal of Immunology*, **123** (3), 1068–1070.

26

Nutrition and the Post-viral Fatigue Syndrome

Alan Stewart

Biolab Medical Unit, London, UK

INTRODUCTION

Over the past 30 years, there has been increasing interest in the post-viral fatigue syndrome (PVFS) or myalgic encephalomyelitis (ME), as it is also known.

Over this same period, there has also been a substantial growth of interest, by both the medical and scientific communities, as well as the general public, in the role that nutritional factors may play in mortality and morbidity of many common diseases. The majority of this interest has centred upon diseases such as coronary artery disease and cancer, but attention has also turned to less serious, and less immediate, disorders that particularly affect the quality of life, rather than its duration.

Nutrition has been a popular subject, at least with the general public. Many popular texts have hailed the use of both diet and nutritional supplements as the answer to many of our ills. To the PVFS sufferer it has at least offered a non-toxic method of self-help. To the psychologically dependent, hypochondriacal 'sufferer', it may provide an intellectual refuge.

But what is the evidence that nutritional factors might be important in PVFS?

This brief chapter will look at the relationship between nutrition and immune function and how this might be of value in PVFS. The author's experience in a small number of patients will also be presented.

Post-viral Fatigue Syndrome. Edited by R. Jenkins and J. Mowbray
© 1991 John Wiley & Sons Ltd

POST-VIRAL FATIGUE SYNDROME: SYMPTOMS AND PATHOLOGY

A variety of descriptions of post-viral fatigue syndrome (PVFS) have been made over the years (Ramsay, 1986). The characteristic symptom is fatigue, which is frequently made worse by exercise or effort. The fatigue classically occurs following on from an acute infection, or perhaps a series of infections, and may be accompanied by a whole host of physical and mental symptoms. These may include muscular aches and pains, muscular weakness, headaches, malaise, depression, anxiety, etc.

Whilst there have been numerous reports of both sporadic and epidemic cases, it is only in recent years that pathological characteristics in sufferers with PVFS have been described.

Nuclear magnetic resonance has been used (Arnold *et al.*, 1984) to show a disturbance in muscle metabolism, with the production of excessive intracellular acidosis on exercise, in one subject with PVFS. Furthermore, electromyographic disturbance has been shown in a high percentage of PVFS patients (Jamal and Hansen, 1985).

Persistent Epstein–Barr infection has also been demonstrated in some patients with PVFS (Jones *et al.*, 1985).

More recently, there has been evidence of continuing enteroviral infection in many PVFS patients, though it is also present in a small number of healthy controls (Yousef *et al.*, 1988).

Persistent immune abnormalities have also been described in patients with PVFS. Such changes include reduction in the suppressor/cytotoxic T lymphocyte ratio in patients in the acute phase of PVFS (Behan *et al.*, 1985), and higher levels of interferon when compared with controls (Ho-Yen *et al.*, 1988). Such changes in pathology could be due to nutritional factors.

POST-VIRAL FATIGUE SYNDROME AND NUTRITION

Unfortunately there have not been any systematic studies looking at the nutritional status of patients with PVFS. Features that would suggest a substantial compromise of nutritional status, such as major changes in appetite and dietary intake, weight loss or diarrhoea due to malabsorption, are not common features of PVFS.

There is, however, some similarity between nutritional deficiency states and the symptoms of PVFS, as well as some of the pathological changes. How common subclinical or clinical deficiencies are in the general population is also not entirely clear, though they would be expected to occur infrequently in those who eat a well-balanced diet, and are usually free of illness.

Classically, certain nutrient deficiency states produce a symptom picture that includes fatigue. This includes deficiencies of vitamins C (ascorbic acid)

B_1 (thiamine), B_3 (niacin), B_6 (pyridoxine), B_5 (pantothenic acid, biotin), B_{12} (folate), iron, magnesium, potassium and sodium. Usually a single nutrient deficiency would have to be severe to produce significant fatigue (Passmore and Eastwood, 1986; Goodhart and Shils, 1980).

Furthermore, many nutrients affect both humoral and cell-mediated immunity, including vitamins A, D and E, most of the B group, C, iron, zinc, copper, magnesium, selenium and possibly some other trace elements, and essential fatty acids (Beisel *et al.*, 1981; Gershwin *et al.*, 1985).

The possibility exists, also, that some nutrients, when given in doses either above the recommended daily allowance (RDA), or to individuals who are not actually deficient, may serve to reduce the rate of infection, or stimulate immune function.

Thus, subclinical or clinical nutritional deficiencies could contribute to either the symptomatology or pathology of PVFS.

ASSESSMENT OF NUTRITIONAL STATE IN SUBJECTS WITH PVFS

Subjects

During the two years 1988 and 1989, a number of patients with fatigue attended a holistic medical practice for assessment and treatment of their symptoms. From more than 50 patients with fatigue, 16 were identified as likely to be suffering from post-viral fatigue. This diagnosis was made if fatigue, often with other symptoms, followed on from a clearly defined single episode of infection or a series of infections. If other identifiable causes for fatigue could be determined or there was no clear association with infection, then they were excluded. During this time period, five subjects presented with fatigue which they or their referring general practitioner had diagnosed as post-viral fatigue, who were excluded because a different serious illness was diagnosed. They included one case each of carcinoma of the colon and anaemia (haemoglobin 6.9 g/dl), Addison's disease, dystrophia myotonica, pyrexia of unknown origin (PUO), and psychogenic diabetes insipidus with hyponatraemia—which had followed an infective episode. In all but the patient with Addison's disease, the diagnosis was made following examination and investigation by the author.

Investigations, results and outcome

After a standard history and examination, blood was taken by venepuncture, without or with minimal use of a tourniquet; the patients had not eaten for at least four hours previously.

The following laboratory assessments were made, though not all were

Table 1 Nutritional status and

No.	Name	Age (years)	Sex	Duration of symptoms (months)	Serum vitamin A (20–55 mg/dl)	Vitamins (enzyme activation < 15% = normal 15–25% = borderline > 25% = deficient)			Serum vitamin C (0.4–2.0 mg/dl)
						B_1	B_2	B_3	
1	CA	27	F	4	—	—	—	—	—
2	RB	41	M	8	37	15	—	20	—
3	SD	18	M	1	19	—	26	21	—
4	KE	12	F	4	29	—	—	7	—
5	AH	35	F	12	20	—	—	—	—
6	LH	14	F	11	20	9	—	11	—
7	PH	41	M	12	—	26	—	34	—
8	NP	80	F	28	—	25	—	40	0.4
9	MR	45	M	42	29	—	—	—	—
10	GS	24	F	6	82	19	—	30	—
11	WS	51	M	6	—	22	—	12	—
12	SS	41	F	6	—	—	—	—	—
13	MT	19	M	38	40	—	—	14	0.3
14	CV	15	M	18	—	—	—	—	—
15	SW	21	M	3	19	—	—	31	—
16	SW	39	F	1	—	13	—	22	—
Mean		32.7		12.5	32.8	18.4		22.0	
± SD		± 17.2		± 12.3	± 18.9	± 5.9		± 10.1	

performed in each patient—serum vitamins A (retinol) and C by colorimetric methods, vitamins B_1, B_2 and B_6 by erythrocyte enzyme activation (red cell transketolase, glutathione reductase and glutamic-oxalacetic transaminase activities respectively), and serum zinc, copper and erythrocyte magnesium by use of an atomic absorption spectrophotometer (Pye-Unicam 9000).

Other tests that were sometimes performed included immunoglobulins G, A and M, and VP1 antigen (Yousef *et al.*, 1988).

Subject details, results of investigations and outcome are given in Table 1.

Of the 16 subjects, eight were female and eight male. The average age was 32.7 ± 17.2 years, with a mean duration of symptoms of 12.5 ± 12.3 months.

Nine subjects had an assessment of serum vitamin A, and four of them had values at, or just below, the lower limits of normal.

Vitamin B_1 and B_6 states were borderline or deficient in over half of the subjects in whom these were measured.

Serum vitamin C was below, or at the lower end of, normal in the two subjects in whom the estimation was made.

Serum zinc and copper were measured in all 16 subjects. Serum zinc outcome of patients with PVFS

Serum zinc (11.5–20 μmol/l)	Serum copper (12.5 μmol/l)	RBC magnesium (1.7–2.6 mmol/l)	VP1 antigen status	Comments	Outcome
12.0	14.4	—	Negative	Mildly elevated LFTs*	No improvement
12.3	13.0	1.87	—	IgA deficient	Good improvement
9.1	15.9	1.54	—	—	Good improvement
11.4	12.5	1.56	—	—	Slight improvement
11.1	16.2	1.63	—	—	No improvement
11.3	15.1	1.72	—	IgA deficient	No improvement
16.0	16.0	1.99	Positive	—	Full improvement
7.9	15.2	1.6	Positive	—	Good improvement
12.0	12.0	1.52	Negative	—	Slight improvement
18.5	12.5	1.61	Negative	—	Good improvement
10.2	12.5	1.6	—	—	Slight improvement
11.0	14.8	2.0	Negative	Vaginal thrush and gluten intolerant	Good improvement
12.3	11.9	1.89	Negative	—	Slight improvement
13.7	14.6	2.0	—	Gluten and yeast intolerant	Good improvement
14.0	13.3	1.65	—	—	Good improvement
11.6	14.8	1.56	—	—	No improvement
12.15 ±2.45	14.0 ±1.45	1.72 ±0.17			8/16 Good/full improvement

* Liver function tests.

values were below the normal range in eight subjects and serum copper values were low in two subjects.

Erythrocyte magnesium values were assessed in 15 of the subjects, and were subnormal in nine of them.

A dietary history was taken from all subjects and none were thought to be eating a diet substantially deprived of macro-or micronutrients. Though some had noted a loss of appetite, weight loss or diarrhoea were not features in any of the subjects.

All subjects were asked to improve their diets, in particular to reduce their consumption of sucrose, foods high in refined carbohydrates, tea, coffee and alcohol, and increase consumption of high-protein foods, fresh vegetables and fresh fruit. Two subjects (12 and 14) who had a history of allergies were advised to exclude a variety of foods from their diet and, as a consequence, appeared to be intolerant of gluten-rich cereals and gluten and yeast, respectively. Both noted an improvement in the level of fatigue on restructuring their diets in this fashion in the long term.

All subjects were given a variety of vitamin and mineral preparations providing all those nutrients that had been found to be lacking from laboratory tests. The daily dosage of most vitamins was between five and 20 times the RDA, and that for minerals was between one and two times the RDA. Comprehensive multivitamin, multimineral supplements were often used, in addition.

Of the 16 subjects presented, eight had either full or good improvement as defined by complete or substantial clearance of fatigue and other symptoms to a point that allowed them to return to premorbid levels of work and social activity.

The remaining eight subjects had either no or slight improvement. The duration of follow-up was between six months and two years. The degree of improvement did not relate to either duration of symptoms or percentage of abnormal nutritional results.

Discussion

From these 16 subjects there is laboratory evidence of sporadic mild to moderate nutritional deficiencies in PVFS patients.

The reasons for these subclinical deficiencies are unclear. There are no details of the subjects' premorbid nutritional state, so such deficiencies could have existed prior to the onset of the illness. Subclinical deficiency, for example of vitamin B_6, is known to occur in the general healthy population (Ritchie and Singkamani, 1986). Intakes of some nutrients, especially zinc, may at times only just reach RDA values (Spring *et al.*, 1979). However, in general widespread deficiency is unlikely in the healthy, well-fed UK population.

Possibly the original viral illness had induced a change in appetite and nutrient intake, or caused a reduction in the absorption of nutrients from the gastrointestinal tract. Alternatively, a continuing immune response to an infective agent could have increased the demand for certain nutrients.

As functional tests of immune function were not performed it is not known whether these mild to moderate deficiencies actually affected immune function or not.

As 14 of the 16 subjects had at least one abnormal result, albeit often slight, there is the therapeutic possibility of using some nutritional supplements to improve immune function and/or symptomatology.

Other researchers (Bondestam *et al.*, 1985) have shown a reduction in serum zinc in children with recurrent infections. Zinc deficiency can affect both humoral and cell-mediated immunity (Beisel *et al.*, 1981) and zinc supplements have been shown to improve immune function in the elderly (Duchateau *et al.*, 1981) and reduce the duration of the common cold (Eby *et al.*, 1984).

Vitamin B_6 supplementation in the elderly at the level of 50 mg/day, some

25 times the RDA, has been shown to improve parameters of immune function (Talbott *et al.*, 1987).

Whilst vitamin A deficiency is rare in Western communities, supplementation at RDA levels of retinol to a group of Australian children of pre-school age, who had normal serum vitamin A levels, resulted in 19% fewer episodes suggestive of respiratory infection, when compared with those receiving placebo (Pinnock *et al.*, 1986). Vitamin A deficiency has been shown to increase bacterial binding to respiratory epithelial cells (Chandra, 1988) as well as influencing many other immune mechanisms (Beisel *et al.*, 1981).

It does seem that mild subclinical deficiencies may exist in certain populations, which in turn could influence immune function and predispose to repeated infections, and/or the development of PVFS.

Further studies are necessary to determine whether deficiencies of nutrients are more common in PVFS sufferers, compared with healthy controls, to what degree such deficiencies might contribute to the impairment of immune function, and whether supplementation, together with an improved diet, is of more benefit than placebo.

Such an approach at least offers a physiological basis for furthering our understanding of PVFS and improving its management.

REFERENCES

Arnold, D. I., Bore, P. J., Radda, G. K., Styles, P. and Taylor, D. J. (1984) Excessive intracellular acidosis of skeletal muscle on exercise in a patient with a postviral fatigue syndrome. *Lancet*, **1**, 1367–1369.

Behan, P. O., Behan, W. M. H. and Bell, E. J. (1985) The postviral fatigue syndrome: analysis of the findings in 50 cases. *Journal of Infection*, **10**, 211–222.

Beisel, W. R., Edelman, R., Nauss, K. and Suskind, R. M. (1981) Single-nutrient effects on immunologic functions. *Journal of the American Medical Association*, **245**, 53–58.

Bondestam, M., Foucard, T. and Gebre-Medhin, M. (1985) Subclinical trace element deficiency in children with undue susceptibility of infections. *Acta Paediatrica Scandinavica*, **74**, 515–520.

Chandra, R. K. (1988) Increased bacterial binding to respiratory epithelial cells in Vitamin A deficiency. *British Medical Journal*, **297**, 834.

Duchateau, J., Delepesse, G., Vrijens, R. and Collet, H. (1981) Beneficial effects of oral zinc supplementation on the immune response of old people. *American Journal of Medicine*, **70**, 1001–1004.

Eby, G. A., Davis, D. R. and Halcomb, W. W. (1984) Reduction in duration of common colds by zinc gluconate lozenges in a double-blind study. *Antimicrobial Agents and Chemotherapy*, **25**, 20–24.

Gershwin, M. E., Beach, R. S. and Hurley, L. S. (1985) *Nutrition and Immunity*. Academic Press, London.

Goodhart, R. S. and Shils, M. E. (1980) *Modern Nutrition in Health and Disease*, 6th edn, pp. 142–408. Lea and Febiger, Philadelphia.

Ho-Yen, D. O., Carrington, D. and Armstrong, A. (1988) Myalgic encephalomyelitis and alpha-interferon. *Lancet*, **1**, 125.

Jamal, G. A. and Hansen, S. (1985) Electrophysiological studies in the postviral fatigue syndrome. *Journal of Neurology, Neurosurgery and Psychiatry*, **48**, 691–694.

Jones, J. P., Ray, G., Minnich, L. L., Hocks, M. J., Kiblet, R. and Incas, D. O. (1985) Evidence for active Epstein–Barr virus infection in patients with persistent unexplained illnesses: elevated early antigen antibodies. *Annals of Internal Medicine*, **201**, 1–7.

Passmore, R. and Eastwood, M. A. (1986) *Human Nutrition and Dietetics*, 8th edn, pp. 115–167. Churchill Livingstone, Edinburgh.

Pinnock, C. B., Douglas, R. M. and Badcock, N. R. (1986) Vitamin A status in children who are prone to respiratory tract infections. *Australian Paediatric Journal*, **22**, 95–99.

Ramsay, A. E. (1986) *Postviral Fatigue Syndrome*. Gower Medical Publishing, London.

Ritchie, C. D. and Singkamani, R. (1986) Plasma pyridoxal-5-phosphate in women with the premenstrual syndrome. *Human Nutrition. Clinical Nutrition*, **40C**, 75–81.

Spring, J. A., Robertson, J. and Buss, D. H. (1979) Trace nutrients—3. Magnesium, copper, zinc, vitamin B6, vitamin B12 and folic acid in the British household food supply. *British Journal of Nutrition*, **41**, 487–493.

Talbott, M. C., Miller, L. T. and Kerkeliet, N. I. (1987) Pyridoxine supplementation: effect on lymphocyte responses in elderly persons. *American Journal of Clinical Nutrition*, **46**, 659–664.

Yousef, G. E., Mann, G. F., Smith, B. G., Bell, E. J., Murugesan, V., McCartney, R. A. and Mowbray, J. F. (1988) Chronic enterovirus infection in patients with postviral fatigue syndrome. *Lancet*, **1**, 146–150.

27

Essential Fatty Acids and the Post-viral Fatigue Syndrome

David F. Horrobin

Efamol Research Institute, Kentville, Nova Scotia, Canada

INTRODUCTION

The idea that essential fatty acids (EFAs) might be involved in post-viral fatigue syndrome (PVFS) is likely, at least initially, to seem improbable to most people. However, there is a substantial body of experimental and clinical evidence relating viral infections to abnormalities of EFA metabolism. This is now supported by a placebo-controlled trial which has demonstrated that modulation of EFA intake can produce a highly significant improvement in PVFS.

In order to understand the possible mechanisms involved, it is important to have some knowledge of EFA biochemistry. The EFAs are essential nutrients which, like vitamins, must be consumed in the diet because they cannot be made *de novo* within the body. There are two types of EFA (Figure 1), the n-6 series whose dietary parent is linoleic acid (LA), and the n-3 series whose dietary parent is alpha-linolenic acid (ALA). The two major dietary EFAs have only limited biological actions of their own. Most of their effects require onward conversion to a series of metabolites. They are converted, as shown in Figure 1, by a series of alternating desaturation (which add one double bond) and elongation (which add two carbon atoms) reactions. The first step in this process, 6-desaturation, is critical because it is slow and rate-limiting. If 6-desaturation is inadequate, there may be EFA-related abnormalities even in the presence of a normal diet as a result of deficits of the metabolites. If dietary EFAs are to be fully utilized by the body, 6-desaturation and onward metabolism of LA and ALA *must* occur.

The EFAs have two major functions in the body. First, they are required for the normal structures of all membranes, upon which they confer

Post-viral Fatigue Syndrome. Edited by R. Jenkins and J. Mowbray

properties of fluidity and flexibility. Their presence in the membrane modulates the behaviour of membrane-bound proteins, including receptors, enzymes and ion channels. Changes in the membrane composition as a result of defective EFA metabolism may therefore lead to important abnormalities in all tissues.

The second major function is that some of the EFAs, notably dihomogammalinolenic acid (DGLA) and arachidonic acid (AA), and to a lesser extent eicosapentaenoic acid (EPA) and adrenic acid, can be converted to short-acting messengers known as eicosanoids. There are many eicosanoids, but the most important are the prostaglandins (PGs) formed via the cyclooxygenase enzyme systems, and the leukotrienes (LTs) formed via the lipoxygenase systems. The eicosanoids are short-lived molecules produced in each tissue as required and then almost immediately destroyed. They regulate such factors as the levels of cyclic nucleotides and calcium within cells and are involved in the second-by-second control of cell function.

These two core actions of the EFAs mean that they exert important influences on the operations of every tissue in the body.

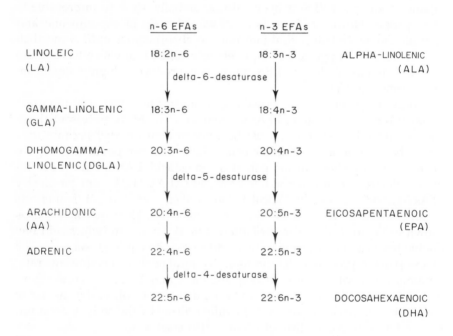

Figure 1   Outline of the metabilism of n-6 and n-3 essential fatty acids. In order to be fully utilized by the body, linoleic and alpha-linolenic acids must be 6-desaturated and further metabolized

EFFECTS OF EFAs ON VIRAL INFECTIONS

Several pieces of evidence from both clinical and laboratory medicine suggest that EFAs are important in enabling the body to resist viral infections.

Atopic eczema

People with atopic eczema are highly susceptible to viral infections (Strannegard *et al.*, 1985; Hanifin and Lobitz, 1977). Smallpox vaccination in such individuals, instead of causing a strictly localized lesion, could lead to widespread vaccinia: atopic eczema was a valid reason for not having a smallpox vaccination certificate in the days when they were required for international travel. Severe herpes simplex, warts, and molluscum contagiosum, all diseases caused by cutaneous viruses, occur more frequently and with greater severity in those with atopic eczema (Strannegard *et al.*, 1985; Hanifin and Lobitz, 1977; Currie *et al.*, 1971; Solomon and Telner, 1966).

The skin in atopic eczema is fragile and easily breaks down. It therefore used to be thought that the increased risk of viral infection was related to ease of viral penetration and was confined to cutaneous infections. However, this is not so. Systemic viral infections are also significantly commoner and/or more severe in patients with atopic eczema (Strannegard and Strannegard, 1981; Rystedt *et al.*, 1984, 1986). Atopic patients are more likely to have respiratory tract infections, more likely to have Epstein–Barr virus (EBV) infections, and more likely to have high antibody titres to EBV.

The relevance of this is that patients with atopic eczema appear to have a mild inherited abnormality of EFA metabolism. They seem unable to 6-desaturate the dietary EFAs as effectively as normal. As a result, levels of LA and ALA are normal or slightly elevated in blood, whereas concentrations of their metabolites are substantially reduced (Manku *et al.*, 1984; Strannegard *et al.*, 1987; Wright and Bolton, 1990) (Figure 2). That this is not a secondary consequence of the skin inflammation is shown by the fact that the abnormality can be detected even in umbilical cord blood of infants at risk of atopic eczema, prior to the clinical emergence of the dermatological condition (Strannegard *et al.*, 1987). It is possible, as will be elaborated below, that the EFA abnormalities are responsible for the increased risk of viral infections.

Interferon and EFAs

Interferon is one of the most important endogenous antiviral agents. Administration of interferon is associated with febrile side effects. These have been found to be due to an ability of interferon to stimulate the conversion of EFAs to PGs via the cyclo-oxygenase system (Karmazyn *et al.*, 1977). That this is not just a side effect, but is central to the mechanism of interferon action, has been shown by a number of experiments (Pottathil *et al.*, 1980; Chandrabose *et al.*, 1981). Interferon fails to exert its antiviral effects if the cyclo-oxygenase is inhibited by drugs. Particularly striking is the fact that a cell line with a genetic absence of the cyclo-oxygenase did not demonstrate any antiviral actions of interferon: a closely related cell line but with active cyclo-oxygenase responded normally to interferon (Pottathil *et al.*, 1980; Chandrabose *et al.*, 1981). Thus interferon is antiviral in conditions in which it can stimulate the conversion of EFAs to PGs, but not in situations when that conversion cannot take place normally. Interferon will therefore require normal intracellular levels of EFAs in order to function effectively. It is therefore not implausible to suggest that in atopic eczema the susceptibility to viral infections could relate to a lack of adequate concentrations of EFA precursors. This is shown in Figure 3.

Direct antiviral actions of EFAs

EFAs have direct antiviral actions, particularly against those many viruses which have a lipid envelop. At surprisingly low concentrations the viruses can disrupt this envelope and destroy the virus (Sands *et al.*, 1979; Horowitz *et al.*, 1988). It has long been known that human milk can be lethal to viruses: it now appears that this is mainly attributable to the high EFA content of

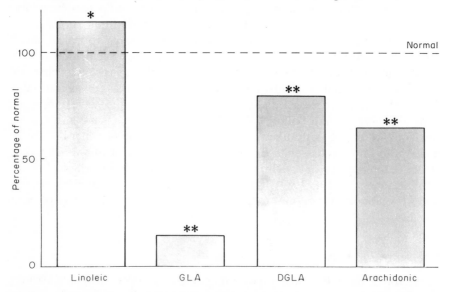

Figure 2   Comparison of the main n-6 EFAs in plasma phospholipids from patients with atopic eczema (bars) with the levels in normal individuals indicated by the dotted line. Data from Manku *et al.* (1984)

human milk (Isaacs *et al.*, 1986). Thus in the presence of inadequate EFA levels this defence against viruses would also be ineffective.

EFFECTS OF VIRAL INFECTIONS ON EFAs

Just as EFAs may modify responses to viral infections, so may viral infections change EFA levels. This was first shown by Stoesser in 1935 when, using primitive methodology, he found that the total EFA content of blood fell sharply during acute viral infections (Stoesser, 1935). Forty years later it was found that *in vitro* viral infections of cells could reduce or abolish the ability of those cells to 6-desaturate EFAs (Dunbar and Bayley, 1975; Bayley, 1977). Virally infected cells could not convert LA and ALA to their metabolites normally. Stoesser's findings were confirmed using modern methodology in 1988 (Williams *et al.*, 1988). Students with EBV infections were followed for 12 months after infection. During the first six months there was consistent lowering of the levels of both linoleic acid and its metabolites. Detailed examination of the EFA patterns indicated apparent inhibition of the desaturation but not of the elongation steps of EFA metabolism, a finding consistent with the *in vitro* work. In the second six months, many of the patients became clinically normal but in others the symptoms of illness persisted. In those who recovered, blood EFA levels returned to normal,

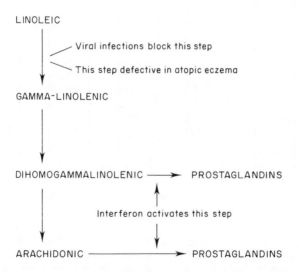

Figure 3 Outline of the interactions between viral infections, interferon effects, atopic eczema and essential fatty acids

while in those who remained ill the abnormality in EFAs persisted (Figure 4). Thus there is an association between persisting clinical disease and abnormal EFA levels. This association cannot, of course, reveal whether the clinical illness causes the abnormal EFA picture, or whether the abnormal EFAs cause the clinical illness, or whether both are due to a persisting viral infection.

In patients with AIDS there are similar reductions in EFA levels in blood but these are much more severe (Begin *et al.*, 1988). The levels of the major EFAs in this group of patients are in general only 50–70% of normal, representing a state of severe deficiency.

Just as atopic eczema is known to predispose to viral infections, so viral infections have frequently been reported to precipitate an atopic disorder (Bahna *et al.*, 1979; Frick *et al.*, 1979; Nordbring *et al.*, 1972; Parkin *et al.*, 1987; Ziegler *et al.*, 1985; Barnetson, 1981). This is particularly the case with EB and AIDS virus infections but can occur with any systemic viral illness. In most cases the atopic eczema or other atopic disorder, such as asthma or allergic rhinitis, represents a recrudescence of a past atopic state which had become dormant. However, sometimes a viral infection can lead to the development of a full-blown atopic syndrome even in an adult with no personal or family history or atopy.

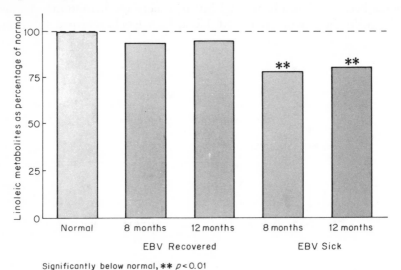

Significantly below normal, ** $p < 0.01$

Figure 4 Levels of the 6-desaturated metabolites of n-6 EFAs in the plasma lipids eight months and 12 months after EBV infection, as compared to the levels in normal individuals shown by the dotted line. In patients who recovered clinically, EFA levels were not significantly different from normal. In those who remained clinically ill after eight and 12 months, the plasma EFA levels remained significantly low. Data from Williams *et al.* (1988)

INTERACTIONS BETWEEN VIRUSES, EFAs AND ATOPY

If atopic eczema is associated with a minor defect in 6-desaturation of EFAs, and if viral infections can inhibit EFA metabolism, especially at the desaturation points, then the observed interactions between atopy and viruses can be readily explained (Figure 3). Atopic disorders will lead to susceptibility to viral infections because the flow of EFAs from dietary LA to the PG precursors, DGLA and AA, is reduced. This will mean a reduced overall capacity for PG synthesis. As a result, the rate of PG formation in response to any given level of interferon will be below normal and the antiviral potency of that level of interferon will be less than expected. Because of this reduced activity of interferon, defences against viral infections will be restricted. The reduced direct antiviral actions of the EFAs will also play a role, particularly with enveloped viruses.

On the other hand, the ability of viruses to interfere with EFA metabolism, especially at the 6-desaturation level, is likely to induce an EFA pattern which in part is characteristic of atopy. Individuals who already have an atopic tendency will be most susceptible to this effect, leading to clinical exacerbation in those who already have an atopic history. In some individuals who have no atopic history, the induced biochemical abnormality may lead to the emergence of an atopic syndrome.

Of particular interest is the possibility that these interactions make evolutionary sense from the viral point of view. If interferon actions on DGLA and arachidonic acid metabolism are important in eliminating viral infections, then it is in the interest of the virus to restrict the ability of the infected cell to make DGLA and AA. Thus any mutant which by chance had such activity would be likely to be successful and therefore conserved. This would explain why an ability to inhibit 6-desaturation may be widely distributed among viruses.

EFAs AND POST-VIRAL FATIGUE SYNDROME

The aetiology of PVFS is at present unknown but is discussed extensively elsewhere in this volume. There is almost always a history of viral infection and there may be evidence of ongoing infections with many different viruses. No specific virus has been implicated and evidence of continuing infection is not present in all patients. It is therefore not clear whether the symptoms are related to an ongoing infection or to some permanent metabolic change induced by an infection which has been resolved. The syndrome is characterized by a range of symptoms of which exhaustion, weakness, aches and pains, inability to concentrate, depression, memory loss, dizziness, vertigo and palpitations are perhaps the commonest. In almost all patients the syndrome is made worse by any form of stress.

If the syndrome is caused by an ongoing viral infection, it should be resolved by specific antiviral therapy. Unfortunately such therapies are available for few viruses and the only placebo-controlled trial, using acyclovir, failed (Straus *et al.*, 1988).

Alternatively the syndrome might be caused by an ongoing metabolic abnormality precipitated by the infection, or the clinical symptoms might be related both to an ongoing viral infection and to a metabolic abnormality.

As a hypothesis I propose that PVFS is triggered by the effects of a viral infection on EFA metabolism. This effect would lead to general reduction of EFA levels and in particular to inhibition of 6-desaturation with a reduced flow of metabolites from dietary LA and ALA. Such a change in EFA metabolism would have profound effects in itself because of the importance of EFAs and their derivatives in all tissues. Interestingly, there are a number of similarities between PVFS and carnitine deficiency: carnitine is required for the transport of EFAs intracellularly. Such a change in EFA metabolism would make it difficult for the host to eliminate viruses, leading to an increased risk of ongoing infection and persistence of the syndrome.

The effect of stress can readily be explained by this hypothesis. Both cortisol and catecholamines which are released during stress are potent inhibitors of 6-desaturation (Brenner, 1982). It has already been shown that stress-induced hypertension can be prevented by bypassing 6-desaturation by providing gammalinolenic acid (GLA, Figure 1) directly (Mills and Ward, 1986). Stress, especially if it occurs in those whose 6-desaturation is already partially impaired, is likely to have a profound effect on EFA metabolism.

The hypothesis can be tested by measuring EFA levels in patients with PVFS and by providing 6-desaturated n-6 and n-3 EFAs directly. This treatment is directed at restoring EFA levels and at eliminating those problems caused by abnormal EFA metabolism. In particular such treatment may enhance the ability of the individual to deal with viral infections by restoring a normal response to interferon.

A CLINICAL TRIAL OF EFAs IN PVFS

The trial was conducted in Glasgow by P. O. and W. M. H. Behan. Our laboratory was responsible for measuring the fatty acid levels. Sixty-three patients with well-defined PVFS entered the study. The original plan was to have three groups, double placebo, EFAs plus placebo, and EFAs plus carnitine. Unfortunately the carnitine failed to arrive in time and so the trial continued with 39 patients being assigned to receive EFAs and 24 to receive placebo. The EFA preparation was Efamol Marine, containing 80% evening primrose oil and 20% concentrated fish oil. The dose was 8×500 mg capsules providing approximately 2250 mg of LA, 280 mg of GLA, 140 mg of EPA and 90 mg of docosahexaenoic acid (DHA) per day. The trial was double blind and parallel and continued for three months with patients being evaluated at baseline and one and three months. Two methods of evaluation were used: at one and three months the patients were asked to state whether they were better, worse or unchanged as compared to the start of the trial; also, at each assessment point, they were required to note on a 0–3 scale the severity of exhaustion, muscle weakness, aches and pains, concentration problems, dizziness, vertigo, depression and memory failure. 0 meant the symptom was absent, 1 mild, 2 moderate and 3 severe (Behan and Behan, 1990; Behan *et al.*, 1990).

The results of the fatty acid analyses are summarized in Figure 5, where they are compared with the values found in normal individuals. At baseline, the levels of total n-6 EFAs, total n-3 EFAs and the major individual EFAs were all below normal while in compensation the concentrations of saturated fatty acids and of oleic acid were above normal. In those patients who received Efamol Marine, by the end of three months the values had returned close to normal for most parameters, except for the n-3 EFAS which had overshot so that they were above normal. This indicates that people with PVFS have abnormal red blood cell EFA levels which can be normalized by appropriate treatment.

With regard to clinical outcome, after three months 85% of the patients on Efamol Marine rated themselves as better than at the start, whereas only 17% of those on placebo said they were better ($2p < 0.0001$). Without exception, all the individual symptoms improved highly significantly more on Efamol Marine than on placebo. The changes in severity of some of these symptoms are shown in Figure 6. Thus there can be no doubt that the normalization of the membrane fatty acid picture was associated with a substantial clinical improvement. Much more work is required to demonstrate the mechanism of the effect.

CONCLUSIONS

Essential fatty acids are required to enable the body to resist viral infections. They have direct antiviral actions and are also needed to allow expression of the antiviral effects of interferon. People with abnormal essential fatty acid metabolism, such as those with atopic eczema, are highly susceptible to viral infections. Conversely, viral infections interfere with essential fatty acid metabolism, so reducing the body's ability to defend itself against viruses. Plasma essential fatty acid levels are abnormal in patients with post-viral fatigue syndrome. Treatment directed at normalizing the plasma fatty acid levels is also associated with a highly significant clinical improvement. It is therefore possible that EFA abnormalities could contribute to the post-viral fatigue syndrome. Since a first placebo-controlled trial aimed at testing this hypothesis has been successful, further trials are now urgently required.

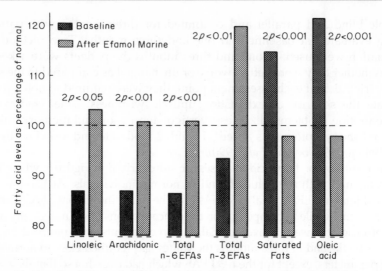

Figure 5 Levels of the main EFAs in red cell membrane phospholipids in patients with post-viral fatigue syndrome before (dark bars) and after (light bars) treatment with n-6 and n-3 6-desaturated EFAs in the form of Efamol Marine. Prior to treatment levels of both n-6 and n-3 EFAs were below normal, whereas levels of saturated fatty acids and of the mono-unsaturated oleic acid were well above normal. Treatment effectively normalized the fatty acid levels, except for those of the n-3 EFAs wich overshot to above normal. Data from Behan *et al.* (1990)

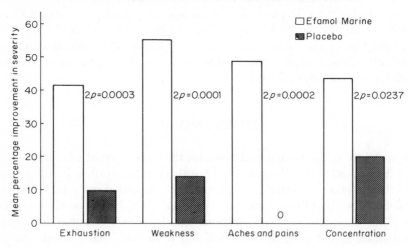

Figure 6 Changes in the main symptoms of post-viral fatigue syndrome during three months of treatment with Efamol Marine or placebo. For each symptom in each patient the change in score was expressed as a percentage of the score on starting the trial. Data from Behan *et al.* (1990)

REFERENCES

Bahna, S. L., Horowitz, C. A., Fiala, M. and Heiner, D. C. (1979) IgE response in heterophil-positive infectious mononucleosis. *Journal of Allergy and Clinical Immunology*, **63**, 228–241.

Barnetson, R. S., Hardie, R. A. and Merrett, T. G. (1981) Late onset atopic eczema and multiple food allergies after infectious mononucleosis. *British Medical Journal*, **283**, 1086.

Bayley, J. M. (1977) Lipid metabolism in cultured cells. In F. Snyder (ed.) *Metabolism in Mammals*, Vol II, pp. 352–364. Plenum Press, New York.

Begin, M. E., Ells, G., Manku, M. S. and Horrobin, D. F. (1988) Fatty acid composition of plasma from AIDS patients and normal individuals. *Archives of AIDS Research*, **33**, 159–166.

Behan, P. O. and Behan, W. M. H. (1990) Essential fatty acids in the treatment of post-viral fatigue syndrome. In D. F. Horrobin (ed.) *Omega-6 Essential Fatty Acids: Pathophysiology and Roles in Clinical Medicine*. Alan R Liss, New York.

Behan, P. O., Behan, W. M. H. and Horrobin, D. F. (1990) A placebo-controlled trial of n-3 and n-6 essential fatty acids in the treatment of post-viral fatigue syndrome. *Acta Neurologica Scandinavica*, **82**, 209–216.

Brenner, R. R. (1982) Nutritional and hormonal factors influencing desaturation of essential fatty acids. *Progress in Lipid Research*, **20**, 41–48.

Chandrabose, K. A., Cuatrecasas, P., Pottathil, R. and Lang, D. J. (1981) Interferon-resistant cell line lacks cyclo-oxygenase activity. *Science*, **212**, 329–331.

Currie, J. M., Wright, R. C. and Miller, O. G. (1971) The frequency of warts in atopic patients. *Cutis*, **8**, 243–244.

Dunbar, I. M. and Bayley, J. M. (1975) Enzyme deletions and essential fatty acid metabolism in cultured cells. *Journal of Biological Chemistry*, **250**, 1152–1154.

Frick, O. L., German, D. F. and Mills, J. (1979) Development of allergy in children. I. Association with virus infections. *Journal of Allergy and Clinical Immunology*, **63**, 228–241.

Hanifin, J. and Lobitz, W. C. (1977) Newer concepts of atopic dermatitis. *Archives of Dermatology*, **113**, 663–670.

Horowitz, B., Piet, M. P. J., Prince, A. M., Edwards, C. A., Lippin, A. and Walakovits, L. A. (1988) Inactivation of lipid-enveloped viruses in labile blood derivatives by unsaturated fatty acids. *Vox Sanguinis*, **54**, 14–20.

Isaacs, C. E., Thormar, H. and Pessolano, T. (1986) Membrane disruptive effect of human milk: inactivation of enveloped viruses. *Journal of Infectious Diseases*, **154**, 966–971.

Karmazyn, M., Horrobin, D. F., Manku, M.S. and Ally, A. I. (1977) Interferon fever. *Lancet*, **11**, 307.

Manku, M. S., Horrobin, D. F., Morse, N. L., Wright, S. and Burton, J. L. (1984) Essential fatty acids in the plasma phospholipids of patients with atopic eczema. *British Journal of Dermatology*, **110**, 643–648.

Mills, D. E. and Ward, R. P. (1986) Effects of essential fatty acid metabolism on cardiovascular responses to stress in the rat. *Lipids*, **21**, 139–142.

Nordbring, F., Johansson, S. G. O. and Espmark, A. (1972) Raised serum levels of IgE in infectious mononucleosis. *Scandinavian Journal of Infectious Diseases*, **4**, 119–124.

Parkin, J. M., Eales, L.-J., Galazka, A. R. and Pinching, A. J. (1987) Atopic manifestations in the acquired immune deficiency syndrome response to recombinant interferon gamma. *British Medical Journal*, **294**, 1185–1186.

Pottathil, R., Chandrabose, K. A., Cuatrecasas, P. and Lang, D. J. (1980) Establishment of the interferon-mediated antiviral state: role of fatty acid cyclo-oxygenase. *Proceedings of the National Academy of Sciences of the USA*, **77**, 5437–5440.

Rystedt, I., Strannegard, I.–L. and Strannegard, O. (1984) Increased serum levels of anti-bodies to Epstein–Barr virus in adults with a history of atopic dermatitis. *International Archives of Allergy and Applied Immunology*, **75**, 179–183.

Rystedt, I., Strannegard, I.–L. and Strannegard, O. (1986) Recurrent viral infections in patients with past or present atopic dermatitis. *British Journal of Dermatology*, **114**, 575–582.

Sands, J., Auperin, D. and Snipes, W. (1979) Extreme sensitivity of enveloped viruses, including herpes simplex, to long chain unsaturated monoglycerides and alcohols. *Antimicrobial Agents and Chemotherapy*, **15**, 67–73.

Solomon, L. M. and Telner, P. (1966) Eruptive molluscum contagiosum in atopic dermatitis. *Canadian Medical Association Journal*, **95**, 978–979.

Stoesser, A. V. (1935) Effect of acute infection on iodine number of serum fatty acids. *Proceedings of the Society for Experimental Biology and Medicine*, **32**, 1326–1327.

Strannegard, I.–L. and Strannegard, O. (1981) Epstein–Barr virus antibodies in children with atopic disease. *International Archives of Allergy and Applied Immunology*, **64**, 314–319.

Strannegard, O., Strannegard, I.–L. and Rystedt, I. (1985) Viral infections in atopic dermatitis. *Acta Dermato-Venereologica (Stockholm)*, Suppl. 114, 121–124.

Strannegard, I.–L., Svennerholm, L. and Strannegard, O. (1987) Essential fatty acids in serum lecithin of children with atopic dermatitis and in umbilical cord serum of infants with high or low IgE levels. *International Archives of Allergy and Applied Immunology*, **82**, 422–423.

Straus, S. E., Dale, J. K., Tobi, M. *et al.* (1988) Acyclovir treatment of the chronic fatigue syndrome. Lack of efficacy in a placebo-controlled trial. *New England and Journal of Medicine*, **319**, 1692–1698.

Williams, L. L., Doody, D. M. and Horrocks, I. A. (1988) Serum fatty acid proportions are altered during the year following acute Epstein-Barr virus infection. *Lipids*, **23**, 981–988.

Wright, S. and Bolton, C. (1989) Breast milk fatty acids in children with atopic eczema. *British Journal of Nutrition*, **62**, 693–697.

Ziegler, J. B., Cooper, D. A., Johnson, R. O. and Gold, J. (1985) Postnatal transmission of AIDS-associated retrovirus from mother to infant. *Lancet*, **i**, 896–898.

28

The Effect of Intestinal Microbes on Systemic Immunity

Leo Galland

Great Smokies Diagnostic Laboratory, Asheville, North Carolina, USA

In keeping with its immense surface area and intense exposure to foreign antigens, the intestinal tract is the largest organ of immune surveillance and response in the human body (Targan *et al.*, 1987). It should not be surprising that events occurring in its lumen or on the mucosal surface have systemic effects on immune function and disease resistance. This chapter examines the contribution made by luminal organisms commonly encountered in humans: bacteria, protozoa and yeasts. Particular attention will be given to data concerning a role for *Giardia lamblia* infestation and *Candida albicans* colonization in the pathogenesis of chronic fatigue and immune dysfunction.

BACTERIAL MICROFLORA

Over 500 species of bacteria live in the healthy human alimentary canal; in the average adult they weigh about one kilogram. The normal colonic microflora ferment soluble fibre to yield short-chain fatty acids which supply 5–10% of human energy requirements (McNeil, 1984). Endogenous flora synthesize at least seven essential nutrients, supplementing dietary intake: folic acid, biotin, pantothenic acid, riboflavin, pyridoxine, cobalamin and vitamin K (Mackowiak, 1982). They participate in the metabolism of drugs, hormones and carcinogens, including digoxin (Lindenbaum *et al.*, 1981), sulphasalazine, and estrogens (Gorbach, 1982). By demethylating methylmercury, gut flora protect mice from mercury toxicity (Rowland *et al.*, 1984). They prevent potential pathogens from establishing infection by numerous mechanisms, which include: production of short-chain fatty acids and bacteriocin, induction of a low oxidation–reduction potential,

Post-viral Fatigue Syndrome. Edited by R. Jenkins and J. Mowbray
© 1991 John Wiley & Sons Ltd

competition for nutrients, deconjugation of the bile acids (which renders them bacteriostatic), blockade of adherence receptors and degradation of bacterial toxins (Savage, 1980).

Germ-free animals have mild to moderate defects in immune function when compared to control animals. These include lower levels of natural antibodies, hyporesponsive macrophages and neutrophiles, defective production of colony-stimulating factors, leukopenia, lymphoid hypoplasia, subnormal interferon levels and weak delayed hypersensitivity (DHS) responses. They are more susceptible to infection with intracellular parasites such as *Listeria, Mycobacterium* and *Nocardia*, but are not more susceptible to viral infection (Mackowiak, 1982). Adverse effects of endogenous bacteria have also been described, indicating the complexity of the host–saprophyte relationship. In diseases where host immune response is the primary cause of pathology, such as lymphocytic choriomeningitis, germ-free animals fare better than control animals (Mackowiak, 1982).

The immunologic effects of normal gut flora are in part due to antigenic stimulation and in part to the bacterial origin of specific immune activators, such as endotoxin lipopolysaccharide (LPS) and muramyl dipeptides (Morrison and Ryan, 1979; Mackowiak, 1982; Stokes, 1984). An important role for these substances in normal immune regulation has not been established, however (Mayrhofer, 1984).

The gut flora of healthy individuals is very stable (Sears *et al.*, 1950, 1956); this stability may in part be due to interbacterial inhibition (Sprunt and Redman, 1968). Alteration in the level of normal flora by antibiotics has long been known to allow secondary infection by pathogenic bacteria and yeasts (Keefer, 1951; Seelig, 1966).

Occasional publications describe abnormal fecal flora in patients with atopic eczema. Kuvaeva *et al.* (1984) studied 60 infants in Moscow with IgE-mediated food allergy and eczema. They reported a decrease in anaerobic bacteria and lactic acid-producing aerobes and an increase of Enterobacteriaceae. Severity of eczema was directly proportional to severity of dysbiosis. No control data are given. Ionescu *et al.* (1986) studied fecal flora in children and adults with atopic eczema. Compared with healthy controls, there was a marked reduction in *Lactobacillus, Bifidobacterium* and *Enteroccoccus* species in the great majority of cases. This was associated with increased concentrations of *Candida* species, *Proteus, Klebsiella*, and *Staphylococcus aureus*, and appearance of atypical coliforms and *Clostridium innocuum*. The high frequency of hypoalbumenemia, indicanuria and steatorrhea in the eczema group suggested small bowel bacterial overgrowth with secondary malabsorption. In neither of these studies is it possible to determine whether abnormal bowel flora caused allergy or whether food-allergic disease destabilized gut flora.

Immunologic reactions to normal or abnormal components of the bacterial gut flora are implicated in the etiology of some inflammatory disorders. Reactive arthritis may occur after intestinal infection with *Salmonella typhimurium*, *Yersinia enterocolitica* serotype 3, *Shigella flexneri*, *Campylobacter jejuni* and *Clostridium difficile* (Inman, 1988). Because arthritogenic potential is strain-specific and because 60–80% of patients with reactive arthritis carry the HLA-B27 gene, it is likely that genetically determined antigenic cross-reactivity plays a role (Yu *et al.*, 1989).

Ankylosing spondylitis (AS) occurs almost exclusively in HLA-B27-positive individuals. An increased rate of intestinal colonization with *Klebsiella pneumoniae* has been described in this condition, according to some but not all studies (Kinsella, 1988). Immunologic cross-reactivity has been shown for HLA-B27 antigen expressed on the host cell membrane and antigens present in *K. pneumoniae*, *S. flexneri* and *Y. enterocolitica*, suggesting molecular mimicry in the pathogenesis of this disease (Yu, 1988). Workers in Australia have demonstrated bacteria with cross-reactive antigenic determinants in bowel flora of B27-positive AS patients; these bacteria are almost never found in B27-positive controls without AS (McGuignan *et al.*, 1986).

Endotoxemia has been described in patients with psoriasis (Rosenberg and Belew, 1982a) and cystic acne (Juhlin and Michaelson, 1984). Activation of the alternative complement pathway (APC) by gut-derived endotoxin may play a role in the pathogenesis of these disorders. Exposure of macrophages to endotoxin causes release of cytokines, such as interleukin-1 (Il-1) and tumor necrosis factor (TNF). These peptides have powerful effects on the immunologic and metabolic response to infection. Whether gut-derived endotoxins influence cytokine production *in vivo* is unknown.

GIARDIA LAMBLIA

Although it was first described by van Leuwenhoek in 1681, it is only in the past 25 years that *G. lamblia* has been acknowledged as an important pathogen (Gillon, 1984). Giardiasis is the commonest cause of parasitic disease in the United States (Myer and Jarroll, 1980) with an overall prevalence estimated at 7.4%, which is about the same as its average worldwide prevalence (Mahmoud and Warren, 1975). Prevalence in Great Britain varies from 2% to 10% (Felman and Nikitas, 1985). At least 27% of *Giardia* infections identified at the University of Edinburgh Medical School had been acquired within the UK, and a diagnosis of giardiasis had not been suspected in two-thirds of cases (Gibb, 1989).

Reports based on stool screening may underestimate the prevalence of giardiasis. Comparison of stool examination with duodenal aspiration has consistently shown that stool examination fails to identify infected patients even at the height of acute infection. Single stool specimens have a sensitivity of zero (Rosenthal and Liebman, 1980) to 50% (Kamath and Murugasu, 1974). Collecting multiple specimens over several days increases the sensitivity to 85–90% (Gillon, 1984).

To overcome the limitations of stool analysis we developed a diagnostic technique by which rectal mucus obtained at anoscopy is stained with a monoclonal antibody to *Giardia* cysts and examined by epifluorescence microscopy (Galland and Bueno, 1989). We recently conducted a two-year retrospective study of 218 patients who presented to our medical clinic with a chief complaint of chronic fatigue (Galland *et al.*, 1990). *G. lamblia* infection was identified by rectal swab in 61 patients. The symptoms of patients with and without giardiasis are shown in Table 1.

All patients with giardiasis and 86% of patients without giardiasis complained of digestive symptoms, but these were generally mild. The most interesting difference between the two groups lies in the positive association between giardiasis and symptoms such as myalgia, muscle weakness, flu-like feelings, sweats and adenopathy. In fact, 61% of fatigued patients with giardiasis had been diagnosed elsewhere as suffering from chronic fatigue syndrome (CFS) or ME, compared to only 19% of fatigued patients without giardiasis. Cure of giardiasis resulted in clearing of fatigue and related 'viral' symptoms (myalgia, sweats, flu-like feelings) in 70% of cases, some palliation of fatigue in 18%, and was of no benefit in 12%. This study shows that giardiasis can present with fatigue as the major manifestation, accompanied by minor gastrointestinal complaints and sometimes by myalgia and other symptoms suggestive of ME. It indicates that *G. lamblia* infection may be a common cause of CFS, at least in the United States. It is noteworthy that tricyclic antidepressants, a standard treatment for CFS, suppress the growth of *Giardia in vitro* (Weinbach *et al.*, 1985).

The mechanism by which *G. lamblia* causes disease is not known. Experiments with human volunteers demonstrate that the ability of *Giardia* to produce infection and to cause diarrhea depends upon the strain of

Table 1   Systemic symptoms of CFS patients

	With giardiasis (%) (N = 63)	Without giardiasis (%) (N = 157)
Depression	61	41
Muscle weakness	46	19
Headache	41	36
Sore throat	41	11
Lymphadenopathy	36	8
Arthralgia	36	27
Myalgia	34	18
Flu-like feelings	34	6
Poor exercise tolerance	30	10

G. lamblia used (Nash *et al.*, 1987), the inoculum dose (Rentdorff, 1954; Rentdorff and Holt, 1954), and previous exposure to the organism (Nash *et al.*, 1987). Heterogeneity of *Giardia* isolates from humans in the same city occurs and has been proposed as one mechanism for variability of clinical response to infection (Korman *et al.*, 1986).

The ease with which *G. muris* infections are established in mice varies with the genetic background of the host (Belosevic *et al.*, 1984). Acute murine giardiasis suppresses the response of splenic and mesenteric lymphocytes to sheep erythrocytes; susceptible mice express a greater degree of immunosuppression than do resistant mice (Belosevic *et al.*, 1985a). Acute giardiasis in rodents is associated with increased intestinal production of prostaglandins E and F (Ganguly *et al.*, 1984b) and cyclic AMP (Ganguly *et al.*, 1984a), probably a result of macrophage activation (Kanwar *et al.*, 1987). Just as production of PGE by host macrophages may contribute to diarrhea, activation of a population of suppressor macrophages in mesenteric lymph nodes contributes to immunosuppression in acute giardiasis (Belosevic *et al.*, 1985b). Disaccharidase deficiency, a frequent complication of giardiasis, may also be immunologically mediated. Sensitized gerbils develop a depression of disaccharidase activity when exposed to *Giardia* antigens; live organisms are not required (denHollander *et al.*, 1988).

In chronic infection, the immune response to the host also appears to be a critical determinant of outcome (denHollander *et al.*, 1988). Chronic giardiasis in humans has been associated with deficiency of secretary IgA (Vinayak *et al.*, 1987) and with impaired macrophage cytotoxicity (Smith *et al.*, 1982). In animals infected with *G. muris*, both T helper/inducer lymphocytes and mast cells are critical for clearance of the parasite (Heyworth *et al.*, 1987; denHollander *et al.*, 1988), whereas cytotoxic T cells and natural killer cells are not (Heyworth *et al.*, 1986). It is noteworthy that athymic mice with chronic giardiasis do not develop mucosal damage (Roberts-Thompson and Mitchell, 1978). Gillon *et al.* (1982) have proposed that the release of enteropathic lymphokines by intraepithelial T cells is the cause of the intestinal injury in chronic giardiasis. In humans, the severity of malabsorption observed with chronic giardiasis is more closely related to the presence of intraepithelial lymphocytes and the antibody titer to *Giardia* cyst antigen than to the estimated parasite burden (Solomons, 1982).

In rodents and humans, therefore, acute *Giardia* infection elicits a protective response from mast cells and T helper lymphocytes (responsible for stimulating sIGA secretion) which is essential for clearance of parasites. A macrophage response occurs as well; this is both protective (Smith *et al.*, 1982) and immunosuppressive (Belosevic *et al.*, 1985b), depending perhaps on the activity of different macrophage populations. Chronic giardiasis is a disease of immune dysregulation in which effector lymphocytes mediate tissue damage. Defective control of macrophage–lymphocyte communication in *Giardia* infection is likely, and appears to be genetically determined. Defective macrophage–lymphocyte communication is also a feature of human atopic disease (Galland, 1986) and the relationship between human giardiasis and allergy is therefore of interest.

Immunologic hypersensitivity to *G. lamblia* has been reported; the result may be asthma (Fossati, 1971; Lopez-Brea *et al.*, 1979), urticaria (Harris and Mitchell, 1949; Wilhelm, 1958; Webster, 1958; Dellamonica *et al.*, 1976; Weisman, 1979; Kennou, 1980; Farthing *et al.*, 1983), arthritis (Goobar, 1977; Farthing *et al.*, 1983; Woo and Panayi, 1984; Shaw and Stevens, 1987; Galland, 1989) and uveitis (Carroll *et al.*, 1961). Hypersensitivity reactions may occur in the absence of digestive complaints (Wilhelm, 1957; Kennou, 1980; Galland, 1989). In none of these cases was the mechanism of hypersensitivity known; eosinophilia was a feature in only two cases (Kennou, 1980; Farthing *et al.*, 1983). A high frequency of pre-existing atopic disease occurs in patients with chronic giardiasis (Chester *et al.*, 1985; Galland *et al.*, 1990) and may be a factor in susceptibility to infection. We have observed that when several members of a family are infected with *Giardia*, symptoms tend to be more prominent among those with allergy. We suspect that the immune dysregulation which underlies atopy allows the immunologic response to *Giardia* infection to favor chronic disease.

Two other features of chronic giardiasis are relevant to an understanding of CFS: the effect of *G. lamblia* infection on nutritional status and its interaction with other organisms, specifically viruses, bacteria and fungi.

G. lamblia can cause intestinal protein loss without producing diarrhea (Sherman and Lieberman, 1980). Specific micronutrient deficiencies have also been described in chronic giardiasis. Low levels of carotene and folate (Brasitus, 1983) and abnormal vitamin A and folic acid absorption curves (Solomons, 1982) occur in a large minority of patients with chronic symptoms. Serum vitamin B_{12} may be low (Cowan and Campbell, 1973), and abnormal Schilling tests occur in a substantial number of patients (Solomons, 1982). Direct competition between parasite and host for vitamin B_{12}, as suggested by Cowan and Campbell (1973), seems unlikely, as *Giardia* selectively damages the duodenum and upper jejunum, and cobalamin is absorbed in the distal ileum. Bacterial overgrowth of the small bowel has been described in giardiasis (Yardley *et al.*, 1965; Tandon *et al.*, 1977; Tompkins *et al.*, 1978; Rogers, 1979) and is associated with severity of malabsorption (Tompkins *et al.*, 1978; Tandon *et al.*, 1977). Solomons (1982) has proposed bacterial overgrowth as a possible cause of abnormal Schilling tests in giardiasis. *Bacteroides fragilis* produces a substance which binds the B_{12}-intrinsic factor complex (Mackowiak, 1982) and may cause malabsorption.

Colonization of the jejunum with *Candida albicans* was reported in 30% of patients with giardiasis and was absent in controls (Naik *et al.*, 1978). The implications of intestinal candidiasis for CFS are described later in this chapter. Some strains of *G. lamblia* contain double-stranded RNA viruses (denHollander *et al.*, 1988). The role of *Giardia* as a vector for viral infection requires further study.

AMOEBAE

Entamoeba histolytica infects 10% of the world's population (Walsh, 1986a,b). Cysts can be found in stool samples of 2% to over 40% of individuals, depending on the area and level of hygiene and sanitation (Guerrant, 1986). Amoebic antibodies, indicative of past or present invasive infection, were found in 1% of general hospital patients, 2% of random serum specimens, and 4% of healthy military recruits in the United States (Walsh, 1986b). Amoebic infection is found in about one-third of homosexual men attending clinics for sexually transmitted diseases in the United States (Petri and Ravdin, 1986). Over 90% of individuals infected with *Entamoeba histolytica* are asymptomatic.

The clinical response to amoebic infection is better understood than the clinical response to *Giardia* infection. Pathogenic strains of *Entamoeba histolytica* are able to evade lysis by both classical and alternative pathways of complement (Reed *et al.*, 1986). Intestinal bacteria, *E. coli* in particular, are necessary for this complement resistance and for amoebic virulence (Wittner and Rosenbaum, 1970). It is suggested that ingested bacteria lower the redox potential and allow the amoebae to escape destruction by oxidative enzymes (Gitler and Mirelman, 1986). Whereas amoebae of low virulence are killed by granulocytes, highly virulent amoebae resist phagocytosis and instead kill the attacking leukocytes (Guerrant *et al.*, 1981; Chadee *et al.*, 1985). Mirelman (Mirelman, 1987; Mirelman *et al.*, 1986) has reported that one can reversibly change the zymodeme patterns of *Entamoeba histolytica* isolates from non-pathogenic to invasive by culturing amoebae with the gut flora of patients who have either invasive disease or no symptoms. His work, which is controversial, suggests that pathogenicity may actually be determined by the bacterial milieu.

The immunologic effects of amoebic infection have been the focus of a recent trans-Atlantic controversy. Workers in London observed that *Entamoeba histolytica* infestation of HIV-infected homosexual men involved only non-pathogenic amoebic zymodemes; amoebic antibodies were absent and there was no association with diarrhea or increased morbidity (Allason-Jones *et al.*, 1986). Several North American groups, on the other hand, have found that AIDS patients with diarrhea are often infected with 'non-pathogenic' amoebae. Treatment with metronidazole or paromomycin produces relief of diarrhea in parallel with the disappearance of these amoebae from feces (Rolsten *et al.*, 1986; Sullam *et al.*, 1986; Pearce and Abrams, 1987).

Several researchers in the United States have advanced the notion that infection with E. *histolytica* and other parasites may promote the development of AIDS in HIV-infected individuals (Pearce, 1983; Pearce and Abrams, 1984, 1986; Archer and Glinsman, 1985; Krogstad, 1986; Petri and Ravdin, 1986; Croxson *et al.*, 1988). *Entamoeba histolytica* contains a soluble lectin which is mitogenic for T lymphocytes (Chen *et al.*, 1985; Petri and Ravdin, 1986). T helper cell activation by this lectin may induce HIV replication *in vivo*. A soluble *Entamoeba histolytica* protein, although not mitogenic itself, induced HIV replication in tissue culture of lymphocytes obtained from three out of seven men with chronic HIV infection (Croxson *et al.*, 1988).

Synergism between intestinal parasites and lymphotrophic retroviruses has also been advanced as an explanation for the pathogenesis of Burkitt's lymphoma (Burkitt, 1983) and adult T cell leukemia/lymphoma (Tajima *et al.*, 1981). It seems likely that the clinical importance of amoebic infection is related as much to the characteristics of the host as of the parasite.

Chronic *Entamoeba histolytica* infection of humans has been associated with autoimmune phenomena, including the appearance of antibodies to colonic epithelial cells (Salem *et al.*, 1973) and development of symmetrical polyarthritis very similar to rheumatoid arthritis (RA) (Zinneman, 1950; Rappaport *et al.*, 1951; Kasliwal, 1970). Singh *et al.* (1985) measured amoebic antibody levels in 41 Indian patients with a primary diagnosis of RA, 35 age- and sex-matched healthy volunteers, 162 hospital inpatients and 26 patients with other arthritides. Amoebic antibodies were elevated in 39% of RA patients and 0–11% of the various control groups. Only two patients with RA had experienced recent diarrheal disease. These authors suggest that an excessive and prolonged antibody response to *Entamoeba histolytica* or other enteric organisms may contribute to joint inflammation in RA.

Galland (1989) described a patient with rheumatoid-like arthritis and antinuclear antibodies whose arthritis went into rapid and complete remission upon treatment of *G. lamblia* infection with metronidazole. Relapse occurred when the patient acquired *Entamoeba histolytica* during a trip to Egypt; remission occurred slowly following treatment of amoebiasis. Diarrhea, polyarthritis and circulating antinuclear antibodies developed in a United States serviceman heavily infested with *Endolimax nana*, allegedly a non-pathogen (Burnstein and Liakos, 1983). Metronidazole rapidly reversed all abnormalities. The reported cases of amoebic arthritis may represent a variant of parasitic rheumatism, an inflammatory polyarthropathy produced by circulating antigen–antibody complexes (Bocanegra, 1988). The presence of autoantibodies, however, is not characteristic of parasitic rheumatism, and suggests other mechanisms of immune dysfunction: either a pre-existing disease is exacerbated by intercurrent amoebic infection or amoebic infection itself provokes autoimmunity, perhaps mediated by the action of immune response genes (Singh *et al.*, 1985).

CANDIDA ALBICANS

Candida species are part of the normal flora of the lower intestinal tract of adult humans, being cultured from stool and rectal mucus of 23.2–82.4% of healthy subjects (Odds, 1988). Serious infection with *Candida albicans* has increased dramatically over the past 40 years; this increase is largely iatrogenic and may be attributed to widespread use of antibiotics and immunosuppressive drugs (Seelig, 1966; Kirkpatrick, 1984). *Candida albicans* is an opportunist *par excellence* and its ability to exploit pre-existing immune deficiency in a host animal is well known, although the precise mechanisms involved in the switch from commensalism to parasitism remain uncertain (Odds, 1988). In contrast, little scientific attention has been focused on the *effect* of *Candida* infection or colonization on immune responses of the host.

That *C. albicans* is a potential allergen has been known for years. Over 90% of a healthy adult population has delayed skin test hypersensitivity (type IV) to antigenic extracts of *C. albicans* (Dwyer, 1984). There are numerous reports of atopic diseases, primarily asthma and allergic rhinitis, associated with type I *Candida* hypersensitivity. Positive immediate hypersensitivity reactions to intradermal or prick tests with *C. albicans* antigen are more prevalent among asthmatics than among non-atopics (Itkin and Dennis, 1966; Pepys *et al.*, 1968; Kurimoto, 1975; Kabe *et al.*, 1971). One study found no difference (Gordon and Klaustermeyer, 1986) but observed that 'strong skin test reactivity' to *Candida* was associated with atopy. El-Hefny (1968a) found *Candida* reactivity to vary directly with severity of asthma. When challenged with inhaled *Candida* antigen, asthmatics with immediate skin test hypersensitivity develop acute bronchoconstriction (Itkin and Dennis, 1966; Pepys *et al.*, 1968; Kabe *et al.*, 1971; Kurimoto, 1975; Edy and Pepys, 1980; Akiyama *et al.*, 1981). Pretreatment with inhaled cromolyn sodium prevents experimental bronchoconstriction under these conditions (Gordon and Klaustermeyer, 1986). Kurimoto (1975) concluded that type I hypersensitivity is involved in both the early and late phase responses to *Candida* antigen but that late bronchial responses may also involve type III hypersensitivity, as a transient drop in C3 and C4 levels occurred.

Candida infections can induce an Arthus reaction in guinea pigs (Kabe *et al.* 1971); Arthus-type reactivity to *C. albicans* was demonstrated in 26% of asthmatics, being positively associated with severity and duration of asthma (El-Hefny, 1968b). Kurimoto (1975) frequently provoked systemic reactions when administering *Candida* antigen by inhalation to his *Candida*-allergic subjects and attributed this to type III allergy. There are few published reports on the value of hyposensitization with *Candida* extract in asthma treatment. El-Hefny (1968a,b), who used an antigen she prepared herself, demonstrated in a controlled study that *Candida*-sensitive asthmatics undergoing hyposensitization with multiple antigens had a significantly better outcome if *C. albicans* extract was included in the antigen mixture. Other reports of improvement in asthma with *Candida* hyposensitization are uncontrolled or anecdotal (Sclafer, 1957; Charpin, 1958; Kabe *et al.*, 1971; Gumowski *et al.*, 1987).

Eczema and urticaria are also mentioned in the literature on *Candida* allergy and are also reported to respond to immunotherapy (Sclafer, 1957; Charpin, 1958; Holti, 1966; Planes *et al.*, 1972). James and Warin (1971) found positive prick tests to *C. albicans* in 36 of 100 consecutive patients with chronic urticaria; they induced hives by blind oral challenge with *Candida* extract in 25 of 33 patients. *Candida* allergy was associated with immediate skin test reactivity to inhalant molds and with positive responses to blind oral challenge with *Saccharomyces cerevisiae*. Oral antifungal therapy with nystatin tablets and amphotericin troches was combined with a yeast-free diet in treatment of all *Candida*-allergic patients and 18 patients with negative *Candida* prick tests. Clearing of urticaria occurred for 81% of *Candida* prick-test-reactive patients and 39% of prick-test-negative patients ($P < 0.01$).

Gastrointestinal manifestations of *Candida* allergy have been reported by Sclafer (1951), Liebeskind (1962), Holti (1966) and Alexander (1975). Holti studied 65 patients with irritable bowel syndrome and symptoms of explosive diarrhea and colicky abdominal pain; they had been sick for an average of five years. All 56 patients with positive skin wheals to *C. albicans* also had positive stool cultures for yeasts. *C. albicans* was isolated from none of the nine patients with a negative skin test to *C. albicans* and from 24% of a healthy control group. Sixty-one per cent of *Candida*-allergic patients also reacted to *Saccharomyces cerevisiae*. Treatment with oral nystatin was associated with permanent disappearance of symptoms in 17 of 57 patients. Thirty-two additional patients were placed on yeast-free diets and, within three days, nine were totally symptom-free and 14 were much improved. A double-blind controlled study of the effects of administering *C. albicans* extract by mouth was conducted using five patients with mucous colitis who had been free of symptoms for at least four weeks. *C. albicans* extract, but not placebo, produced diarrhea and borborygmi within 20 minutes in all five. In five control subjects with positive *Candida* skin tests but no digestive complaints, oral *Candida* extract produced no symptoms.

These studies are described in some detail because they indicate that *Candida* allergy is not a rare disease with limited symptoms, as maintained by some authorities (American Medical Association Council on Scientific Affairs, 1987), but a relatively common disorder with protean manifestations.

A relationship between *Candida* allergy and *Candida* infection is suggested by clinical research in vaginitis. *Candida* allergy has been well described in patients with chronic vaginitis (Tomsikova *et al.*, 1980). Mathur *et al.* (1977) found that total IgE was elevated in sera and cervicovaginal secretions of women with recurrent *Candida* vaginitis and that most of this IgE reacted with

Candida antigens. Witkin *et al.* (1988, 1989) found anti-*Candida* IgE in vaginal secretions of 18.8% and 27.8% of women with chronic vaginitis. Vaginal specimens with IgE antibodies also contained detectable levels of prostaglandin E2 (PGE2), an important mediator of inflammation. Witkin *et al.* (1986, 1988) suggest that production of PGE2, stimulated by vaginal allergy to *Candida* and other substances, inhibits lymphocyte responses to *Candida* in the vagina, permitting *Candida* infection to flourish. They found that macrophages of women with recurrent vaginal candidiasis inhibit response of control lymphocytes to *Candida* antigen: this inhibition is reversed by PG-synthesis inhibitors and by exogenous Il-2. This group has recently shown (Witkin *et al.*, 1989) that cervical infection with human papilloma virus (HPV) is strongly correlated with the presence of anti-*Candida* IgE; 47.4% of 19 women with HPV and only 5.9% of 17 women without HPV were positive for anti-*Candida* IgE ($p < 0.025$). Conversely, nine out of 10 women with anti-*Candida* IgE compared to 10 out of 26 women without anti-*Candida* IgE harbored HPV. They speculate that the immunosuppressive effects of *Candida* allergy permit chronic viral infection of the uterine cervix. In small, uncontrolled studies Palacios (1976) and Rosedale and Browne (1979) had demonstrated reduction in episodes of vaginal thrush by hyposensitizing injections of *C. albicans* extract, suggesting clinical utility for Witkin's findings.

There are several clinical case reports of immunosuppression occurring *in vivo* as an apparent side effect of *Candida* infection (Cuff *et al.*, 1986). Paterson *et al.* (1971) described a 20-year-old female patient with a 15-year history of chronic mucocutaneous candidiasis (CMC) who was anergic and whose plasma contained a factor capable of extinguishing the blastogenic response of normal lymphocytes to *Candida* and mumps. Treatment with intravenous amphotericin B cleared the *Candida* infection and simultaneously eliminated the circulating plasma inhibitor, slowly restoring normal cell-mediated immunity (CMI). The patient remained free of yeast infection and immunologically normal for at least seven months after discontinuation of amphotericin B. The authors speculated that the circulating inhibitor was yeast-derived.

Circulating immunosuppressive factors have been described in other cases of CMC (Valdimarsson *et al.*, 1973). The immunosuppressive factors are thought to be soluble polysaccharides, such as mannan, contained in the yeast membrane and released into the circulation (Fischer *et al.*, 1978). Mannan at high dose inhibits mitogen- and antigen-stimulated proliferation of human lymphocytes *in vitro*. Lower concentrations specifically inhibit the lymphocyte blastogenic response to *C. albicans*, probably by competing for polysaccharide–antigen binding sites (Nelson *et al.*, 1984). In that macrophages normally remove mannan from the circulation, the immunosuppressive effects of mannan *in vivo* probably depend upon defective macrophage function, which may be a factor in some cases of CMC (Fischer *et al.*, 1982).

A *Candida albicans* cell wall glycoprotein rich in mannan causes histamine release from rat mast cells *in vitro* (Nosal *et al.*, 1974; Svec, 1974). An experiment in mice suggested that some immunosuppressive effects of the glycoprotein reside in the protein moiety and are mannan-independent (Carrow and Domer, 1985). There is a case reported of refractory esophagitis caused by *C. tropicalis* in a 28-year-old nurse that was associated with cutaneous anergy and a circulating inhibitor that was not mannan but a low-molecular-weight protein derived from the yeast itself (Lee *et al.*, 1986).

Additional mechanisms of *Candida*-induced immunosuppression exist. Mouse lymphocytes incubated with formalin-killed *C. albicans* induce a suppressor B lymphocyte, the appearance of which may explain the increased susceptibility of mice treated with *Candida* extracts to infection by a number of micro-organisms (Cuff *et al.*, 1986). Human T lymphocytes incubated with *C. albicans* polysaccharide produce a nonspecific inhibitor of macrophage function which decreases macrophage production of Il-1 and hence lymphocyte production of Il-2, inhibiting lymphocyte proliferation (Lombardi *et al.*, 1985). On the other hand, injection of heat-killed *C. albicans* augments natural killer (NK) cell activity in mice (Marconi *et al.*, 1985; Wojdani and Ghoneum, 1987). Glucan, another yeast-derived polysaccharide, may initiate this effect by stimulating macrophages to release TNF, which raises NK levels (Reynolds *et al.*, 1980). This effect is similar to the immunoenhancing effect of bacterial endotoxin.

Zymosan, an insoluble yeast membrane polysaccharide, activates the APC *in vitro* (Ray and Wuepper 1976); *in vivo*, the inflammation seen in patients with CMC may be mediated by APC. Rosenberg and his colleagues have proposed that psoriasis and Crohn's disease both involve excessive and unregulated activation of the APC and state that various microbial products, including zymosan from *C. albicans*, may be stimulating the APC *in vivo*, causing the appearance of disease in genetically susceptible individuals (Rosenberg *et al.*, 1982, 1983). Having successfully treated scalp psoriasis with ketaconazole (Rosenberg and Belew, 1982b), they proceeded to use oral nystatin for treating psoriasis, with positive results (Crutcher *et al.*, 1984). They postulate that psoriasis is a systemic disease, which can be triggered by *Candida* in the intestine, as well as by other infectious agents.

Iwata *et al.* (1966) first described a high-molecular-weight protein, isolated from a strain of *C. albicans*, with inflammatory and nerve-growth-stimulating effects; they called it canditoxin. They have since discovered several other substances, of low and high molecular weight, which may serve as endo- or exotoxins by activating the classical complement pathway (Iwata, 1977a, 1977b). These substances are not thought to be widely distributed, but rather confined to just a few strains; their role in the pathogenesis of candidiasis is unclear.

In summary, there are numerous and complex immunologic responses to

Candida constituents, both antigenic and non-antigenic, which may follow colonization or infection; these cause release of inflammatory mediators and alterations in CMI. Local infections may have systemic effects.

CMC is known to occur in association with endocrine dysfunction and circulating autoantibodies (Wuepper and Fudenberg, 1967). Although chronic infection and autoimmune disease may result from defective T lymphocyte function, some workers have speculated that polyclonal B cell activation induced by *Candida* components may trigger autoantibody formation (Zouali *et al.*, 1983/1984). Mathur *et al.* (1980) studied 40 women with chronic vaginal candidiasis (CVC). Anti-ovarian and anti-thymocyte antibodies were present at a titer of 1 : 64 or greater in the sera of 27 and 19 patients, respectively. Both autoantibodies were found at significant titers in 16. Mean autoantibody levels of CVC patients were much higher than those of controls. Autoantibody levels were strongly and positively associated with *Candida* antibody levels. Absorption of sera from CVC patients with thymocytes, ovarian follicles or *C. albicans*, significantly lowered antibody titers to all three, suggesting antigenic cross-reactivity. The authors speculated that a high level of multispecific *Candida* antibody produced by chronic yeast infection in these patients cross-reacted with ovarian and T cell antigens, producing autoimmune phenomena.

In 1978, Truss first published six case reports of patients with baffling neurological, psychiatric and inflammatory diseases who were cured following treatment with oral nystatin and injections of *Candida* antigen. A series of papers followed in which he described several cases of multiple sclerosis and one of Crohn's disease which responded to the same therapy (Truss, 1981); he presented a comprehensive treatment program for this condition which included avoidance of dietary carbohydrates, limitation of exposure to food-borne or air-borne fungi, administration of oral antifungal drugs and immunotherapy with *Candida* extract (Truss, 1980a, b). He initially proposed that chronic *Candida* antigenemia may be responsible for this polymorphic illness (Truss, 1981), and later published a theory that acetaldehyde production by intestinal yeast was the cause of metabolic, immunologic and neuroendocrine abnormalities seen in his patients (Truss, 1984). Although direct evidence for Truss' hypopthesis has not been forthcoming, investigations by others since his last paper have demonstrated that *C. albicans* can produce ethanol in infant food formulas (Bivin and Heinen, 1985) and in the human stomach (Bode *et al.*, 1984), and that acetaldehyde, the principal metabolite of ethanol, by conjugating with mammalian protein, induces formation of polyclonal antibodies to acetaldehyde–protein adducts that may mediate tissue damage (Israel *et al.*, 1986).

Truss's concept that systemic illness may be provoked by mucosal *Candida* infection has itself provoked considerable controversy (Crook, 1984; Turner, 1985; Blonz, 1986; American Academy of Allergy and Immunology, 1986).

Although Truss's original case reports primarily described patients with autoimmune or neurological diseases, most patients diagnosed with this *Candida*-related complex (CRC) have symptoms of fatigue, depression, allergy, food intolerance, and a variety of gastrointestinal, gynecologic and musculoskeletal complaints which are generally regarded as 'functional' (Truss, 1982; Zwerling *et al.*, 1984; Crook, 1986; Kroker, 1987; Mabray, 1988).

The first published controlled treatment study to test the CRC hypothesis was done by Schinfeld (1987). He studied 30 patients with premenstrual syndrome (PMS) that had not responded to treatment which included psychotherapy, high-dose vitamin B_6 and, in some cases, psychotropic drugs. Twelve patients had no evidence of vaginal yeast infection, symptomatic or asymptomatic, and the remainder suffered from recent *Candida*, vaginitis. Both *Candida*-free and *Candida*-infected groups were subdivided into active treatment (oral nystatin and yeast-free diet) and contact-only treatment groups. All patients remained symptomatic, with premenstrual depression as their major complaint, but there were significant differences between treatment and non-treatment groups. The worst outcome occurred in *Candida*-infected patients who received no active treatment, and the best outcome occurred in *Candida*-infected patients treated with oral nystatin and a yeast-free diet. The small number of patients limits the number of comparisons that can be made and the interpretation of data.

Another study (Dismukes *et al.*, 1990) reported no significant difference in the effect of oral nystatin or placebo on systemic systems of 42 women with chronic vaginitis. In contrast to Schinfield's study, however, these authors lumped together women with *Candida* vaginitis and women with culture-negative vaginitis, possibly explaining the high inter-patient variability they observed. They also used a cross-over treatment design with no washout period and failed to control for changes in diet and other self-care activities, although all subjects were aware of Truss' treatment regimen, having been selected from his waiting list. Despite these flaws, and the authors' failure to provide any raw data in their report, a careful reading of this highly publicized study indicates some differences in the effect of oral nystatin and placebo that do not support their main conclusion. Oral nystatin significantly reduced somatization scores ('distress arising from perception of bodily functions') ($p = 0.04$). Analysis of other systemic symptoms showed benefits from oral nystatin under conditions where placebo responses appeared to have stabilized. Truss (personal communication) has performed a separate statistical analysis and has prepared a critique of this study which demonstrates a strong effect of nystatin on generalized symptoms, when compared to placebo.

The largest study of CRC reported is that of Jessup, who presented a retrospective analysis of 1100 patients to the First International Conference on Chronic Fatigue Syndrome, San Francisco, California, 15 April 1989.

These patients had been treated over a nine-year period for fatigue, myalgia, headache, dizziness, depression, arthralgias, night sweats, morning stiffness and post-strain malaise. Posterior cervical adenopathy occurred in 35% and neurological examination was abnormal (serial sevens, tandem gait) in 30%. Although 80% reported the sudden onset of their disease following an acute flue-like illness, pre-morbid characteristics of the group revealed a high frequency of chronic or recurrent health problems. About 80% had repeated antibiotic exposures for acne or respiratory or urinary tract infection; 60% of these had developed sensitivity to antibiotics. Alcohol intolerance, irritable bowel syndrome, recurrent vaginitis, migraine headaches, urticaria and pre-menstrual tension were very frequently encountered. Almost all patients had experienced addiction to sugar or alcohol prior to the onset of chronic fatigue. Patients treated between 1980 and 1987 showed little improvement. In September, 1987, 685 patients were unemployed and receiving disability payments. At that point Jessup began treating these patients with ket-aconazole 200 mg a day, combined with a diet free of alcohol, added sugar, fruit or fruit juice. The average length of treatment was five months (range three to 12 months). By April, 1989, 84% of these patients had recovered and only 12 patients remained on disability. Jessup concluded that *Candida* infection was the major cause of disease for those patients who responded to ketaconozole and speculated that intestinal colonization with yeast produced a systemic toxin.

The treatment results do not necessarily support Jessup's conclusion. Although ketaconazole is an effective antifungal agent, it has powerful and complex effects on the function of lymphocytes (Schutt *et al.*, 1987a) and monocytes (Claus *et al.*, 1988) which are consistent with inhibition of certain cytokine effects (Schutt *et al.*, 1987b, 1988). Ketaconazole eliminates the spontaneous lymphocyte proliferation of patients with dermatophytoses (Schutt *et al.*, 1988). Elevated levels of Il-2 (Cheney *et al.*, 1989), increased production of alpha-interferon (Lever *et al.*, 1988) and spontaneous lymphocyte blastogenic activity (Olson *et al.*, 1986) have been described in some patients with CFS. It is possible that Jessup's success resulted from alteration of aberrant immune responses by ketaconazole rather than an antifungal effect. The large number of patients treated and the extraordinarily good outcome in this report, however, mandate a prospective controlled study of imidazole therapy for CFS.

SUMMARY AND CONCLUSIONS

This chapter has reviewed the systemic effects of immune responses to organisms inhabiting the gut lumen and adhering to the intestinal mucosal surface. Type I and type III allergic responses to yeasts and protozoa occur:

the former may precipitate asthma, urticaria, vaginitis and irritable bowel syndrome; the latter may cause arthritis. Type I allergic reactions may also produce local immunosuppression. Cross-reactivity between human and microbial antigens occurs for several strains of Enterobacteriaciae and for *C. albicans*. Enterobacteriaceae are implicated in the pathogenesis of some spondyloarthropathies; *C. albicans* and *Entamoeba histolytica* infections may contribute to autoimmune phenomena. Nonspecific activation of immune responses by microbial components is common and may be necessary for normal maturation of the immune system. Bacterial endotoxin, yeast zymosan and protozoan lectins express non-antigenic immune stimulatory activity, which may be undesirable, eliciting inflammatory reactions, such as psoriasis, in susceptible individuals, or inducing replication of lympho-trophic viruses. Yeast-derived glyoproteins can cause immune suppression *in vitro* and *in vivo*. Chronic *G. lamblia* infection can produce fatigue, myalgia, asthenia and malnutrition without serious gastrointestinal symptoms.

Our results demonstrate that some patients with CFS have *Giardia lamblia* infection as their primary, and unexpected, diagnosis. The excellent response to ketoconazole reported by Jessup suggests that fungal infection may play an important etiologic role in many CFS patients. Mowbray's group has found chronic enteroviral antigenemia in the majority of patients with post-viral fatigue syndrome (Yousef *et al.*, 1988). It is possible that bacterial dysbiosis, enteric protozoan or yeast infection, or intestinal allergy may alter normal immune responses of the gut, allowing persistence of viral replication. The probable importance of enteric factors in the pathogenesis of ME should guide diagnostic and treatment strategies.

REFERENCES

Akiyama, K., Yui, Y., Shida, T. and Miyamoto, T. (1981) Relationship between the result of skin, conjunctival and bronchial tests and RAST with *Candida albicans* in patients with asthma. *Clinical Allergy*, **11**, 323–351.
Alexander, J. G. (1975) Allergy in the gastrointestinal tract. *Lancet*, **2**, 1264.
Allason-Jones, E., Mindel, A., Sargeaunt, P. and Williams, P. (1986) *Entamoeba histolytica* as a commensal intestinal parasite in homosexual men. *New England Journal of Medicine*, **315**, 353–356.
American Academy of Allergy and Immunology (1986) Candidiasis hypersensitivity syndrome. *Journal of Allergy and Clinical Immunology*, **78**, 271–272.
American Medical Association Council on Scientific Affairs (1987) In vivo diagnostic testing and immunotherapy for allergy. Report I, part II, of the allergy panel. *Journal of the American Medical Association*, **258**, 1505–1508.
Archer, D. L. and Glinsman, W. H. (1985) Enteric infections and other co-factors in AIDS. *Immunology Today*, **6**, 292–294.

Beaumont, D. M. and James, O. F. W. (1986) Unsuspected giardiasis as a cause of malnutrition and diarrhoea in the elderly. *British Medical Journal*, **293**, 554–555.

Belosevic, M., Faubert, G. M. and MacLean, J. D. (1984) Susceptibility and resistance of inbred mice to *Giardia muris. Infection and Immunity*, **44**, 282.

Belosevic, M., Faubert, G. M. and MacLean, J. D. (1985a) Suppression of primary antibody response to sheep erythrocytes in susceptible and resistant mice infected with *Giardia muris. Infection and Immunity*, **47**, 21.

Belosevic, M., Faubert, G. M. and MacLean, J. D. (1985b) *Giardia muris*-induced depression of the primary immune response in spleen and mesenteric lymph node cell cultures to sheep red blood cells. *Parasite Immunology*, **7**, 467–478.

Bivin, W. S. and Heinen, B. M. (1985) Production of ethanol from infant food formulas by common yeasts. *Journal of Applied Bacteriology*, **58**, 355–357.

Blonz, E. R. (1986) Is there an epidemic of candidiasis in our midst? *Journal of the American Medical Association*, **256**, 3138–3139.

Bocanegra, T. S. (1988) Rheumatic manifestation of parasitic diseases. In L. Espinoza, D. Goldenburg, F. Arnett and G. Alarcon (eds) *Infections in the Rheumatic Diseases*, pp. 243–265. Grune and Stratton, Orlando.

Bocanegra, T. S., Espinoza, L. R., Bridgeford, P. H., Vasey, F. B. and Germani, B. F. (1981) Reactive arthritis induced by parasitic infestation. *Annals of Internal Medicine*, **94**, 207–209.

Bode, J. C., Rust, S. and Bode, C. (1984) The effect of cimetidine treatment on ethanol formation in the human stomach. *Scandinavian Journal of Gastroenterology*, **19**, 853–856.

Bode, J. and Rinvik, R. (1943) Infection with *Lamblia intestinalis* in children: its clinical significance and treatment. *Acta Pediatrica Scandinavia*, **31**, 125–146.

Brasitus, T. A. (1983) Parasites and malabsorption. *Clinics in Gastroenterology*, **12**, 495–511.

Burkitt, D. P. (1983) The discovery of Burkitt's lymphoma. *Cancer*, **51**, 1777–1786.

Burnstein, S. L. and Liakos, S. (1983) Parasitic rheumatism presenting as rheumatoid arthritis. *Journal of Rheumatology*, **10**, 514–515.

Carroll, M. E., Anast, B. P. and Birch, C. L. (1961) Giardiasis and uveitis. *Archives of Ophthalmology*, **65**, 775–778.

Carrow, E. W. and Domer, J. E. (1985) Immunoregulation in experimental murine candidiasis: Specific suppression induced by *Candida albicans* cell wall glycoprotein. *Infection and Immunity*, **49**, 172–181.

Chadee, K., Meerovitch, E. and Moreau, F. (1985) *In vitro* and *in vivo* interaction between trophozoites of *Entamoeba histolytica* and gerbil lymphoid cells. *Infection and Immunity*, **49**, 828–832.

Charpin, J. (1958) Allergie gegen *Candida albicans. Journal Unterricht Mitarbeiten*, **4**, 189–197.

Chen, Z. C., Herrmann, F., Koleski, F. and Diamantstein, T. (1985) Mitogenic factor for T inducer/helper cells in *Entamoeba histolytica* extracts. *Acta Academiae Medicina Wuhan*, **5** (4), 213–216.

Cheney, P. R., Dorman, S. E. and Bell, D. S. (1989) Interleukin-2 and the chronic fatigue syndrome. *Annals of Internal Medicine*, **110**, 321.

Chester, C. A., Macmurray, F. G., Restifo, M. D. and Mann, O. (1985) Giardiasis as a chronic disease. *Digestive Disease and Sciences*, **30**, 215–218.

Claus, R., Nausch, M., Ringel, B., Zingler, C., Schulze, H. A. and Kaben, V. (1988) *Myloses*. Effects of ketaconazole on the immune system IV. In vitro effects on monocyte functions. **31**, 303–312.

Cowan, A. E. and Campbell, C. B. (1973) Giardiasis—a cause of vitamin B12 malabsorption. *American Journal of Digestive Disease*, **18**, 384–386.

Crook, W. G. (1984) Depression associated with *Candida albicans* in human illness. *Journal of the American Medical Association*, **251**, 2928–2929.

Crook, W. G. (1986) *The Yeast Connection*. Vintage Books, New York.

Croxson, S., Mildran, D., Mathews, H. and Poiez, B. J. (1988) *Entamoeba histolytica* antigen-specific induction of Human Immunodeficiency Virus replication. *Journal of Clinical Microbiology*, **26**, 292–294.

Crutcher, N., Rosenberg, E. W., Belew, P. W., Skinner, R. B., Eaglestein, N. F. and Baker, S. M. (1984) Oral nystatin in the treatment of psoriasis. *Archives of Dermatology*, **120**, 435.

Cuff, C. F., Robers, C. M., Lamb, B. J. and Rogers, T. J. (1986) Induction of suppressor cells in vitro by *Candida albicans*. *Cellular Immunology*, **100**, 47–56.

Dellamonica, P., Le Fichoux, X., Monnier, B. and Duplay, H. (1976) Syndrome dysenterigue et urticaire, au cours d'une giardiase. *Nouvelle Presse Medicale*, **5**, 1913.

denHollander, N., Riley, D. and Befus, D. (1988) Immunology of *Giardia*. *Parasitology Today*, **4**, 124–133.

Dismukes, W. E., Wade, J. S., Lee, J. Y., Dockery, B. K. and Hain, J. D. (1990) A randomized, double-blind trial of nystatin therapy for candidiasis hypersensitivity syndrome. *New England Journal of Medicine*, **323**, 1717–1723.

Dwyer, W. (1984) Anergy, the mysterious loss of immunological energy. *Progress in Allergy*, **35**, 15–92.

El-Hefny, A. M. (1968a) *Candida albicans* as an important respiratory allergen in the United Arabic Republic. *Acta Allergelogica*, **23**, 297–302.

El-Hefny, A. M. (1968b) The Arthus reaction to *Candida albicans* in asthma patients. *Acta Allergologica*, **23**, 303–311.

Farthing, M. J. G., Chong, S. K. F. and Walker-Smith, J. A. (1983) Acute allergic phenomena in giardiasis. *Lancet*, **2**, 1428.

Felman, J. M. and Nikitas, J. A. (1985) Giardiasis. *Cutis*, 305–306.

Fischer, A., Ballet, J. J. and Griscelli, C. L. (1978) Specific inhibition of *in vitro Candida* induced lymphocyte proliferation by polysaccharide antigens present in the serum of patients with chronic mucocutaneous candidiasis. *Journal of Clinical Investigation*, **62**, 1005–1013.

Fischer, A., Pichat, L., Audinot, H. and Griscelli, C. (1982) Defective handling of mannan by monocytes in patients with chronic mucocutaneous candidiasis resulting in a specific cellular unresponsiveness. *Clinical and Experimental Immunology*, **47**, 653–660.

Fossati, C. (1971) Manifestazioni broncopulmonari in corso di infestazione da *Giardia lamblia*. *Revista Iberica de Parisitologia*, **31**, 283–298.

Galland, L. (1986) Increased requirements for essential fatty acids in atopic individuals. *Journal of the American College of Nutrition*, **5**, 213–228.

Galland, L. (1989) Intestinal protozoan infection is a common unsuspected cause of chronic illness. *Journal of Advancement in Medicine*, **2**, 529–552.

Galland, L. and Bueno, H. (1989) Advances in laboratory diagnosis of intestinal parasites. *American Clinical Laboratory*, 18–19.

Galland, L., Lee, M., Bueno, H. and Heimowitz, C. (1990) Giardia lamblia infection as a cause of chronic fatigue. *Journal of Nutritional Medicine*, **2**, 27–32.

Ganguly, N. K., Mahajan, R. C., Radhakrishna, V., Ghosh, S. S., Kanwar, S. S. and Garg, S. K. (1984a) Effect of *Giardia lamblia* infection on the intestinal cyclic AMP level in mice. *Journal of Diarrhoeal Disease Research*, **2**, 69–72.

Ganguly, N. K., Garg, S. K., Vasudev, V., Radhakrishna, V., Anand, B. S. and Maha-jan, R. C. (1984b) Prostaglandins E & F levels in mice infected with *Giardia lamblia*. *Indian Journal of Medical Research*, **79**, 755–759.

Gibb, A. P. (1989) Identification of unsuspected cases of giardiasis by wet-film micro-scopy. *Lancet*, **2**, 216–217.

Gillon, J. (1984) Giardiasis: Review of epidemiology, pathogenetic mechanisms and host responses. *Quarterly Journal of Medicine*, **53**, 29–39.

Gillon, J., Althamery, D. and Ferguson, A. (1982) Features of small intestinal path-ology (epithelial cell kinetics, intraepithelial lymphocytes, disaccharidases) in a primary *Giardia muris* infection. *Gut*, **23**, 498–506.

Gitler, C. and Mirelman, D. (1986) Factors contributing to the pathogenic behavior of *Entamoeba histolytica*. *Annual Reviews of Microbiology*, **40**, 237–261.

Goldin, B. R. and Gorbach, S. L. (1984) Alterations of the intestinal microflora by diet, oral antibiotics, and lactobacillus: Decreased production of free amines from aro-matic nitro compounds, azo dyes, and glucuronides. *Journal of the National Cancer Institute*, **73**, 689–695.

Goobar, J. P. (1977) Joint symptoms in giardiasis. *Lancet*, **1**, 1010–1011.

Gorbach, S. (1982) The role of intestinal flora in the metabolism of drugs, hormones and carcinogens. *Infectious Diseases*, **12**, 4–30.

Gordon, E. H. and Klaustermeyer, W. B. (1986) Hypersensitivity to *Candida albicans*. *Immunology and Allergy Practice*, **8**, 29–34.

Guerrant, R. L. (1986) The global problem of amebiasis: current status, research needs, and opportunities for progress. *Reviews of Infectious Diseases*, **8**, 218–227.

Guerrant, R. L., Brush, J., Ravdin, J. I., Sullivan, J. A. and Mandell, G. L. (1981) Interaction between Entamoeba histolytica and human polymorphonuclear neu-trophils. *Journal of Infectology*, **143**, 83–93.

Gumowski, P., Lech, B. and Chaves, I. (1987) Chronic asthma and rhinitis due to *Candida albicans, Epidermophyton* and *Trichophyton*. *Annals of Allergy*, **59**, 48–51.

Hageage, G. J. and Harrington, B. J. (1984) Use of calcoflour white in clinical mycol-ogy. *Laboratory Medicine*, **15**, 109–112.

Harris, R. H. and Mitchell, J. H. (1949) Chronic urticaria due to *Giardia lamblia*. *Archives of Dermatology and Syphilology*, **59**, 587–589.

Heyworth, M. F., Kung, J. E. and Eriksson, E. C. (1986) Clearance of *Giardia muris* infection in mice deficient in natural killer cells. *Infection and Immunity*, **54**, 903–904.

Heyworth, M. F., Carlson, J. R. and Emark, T. H. (1987) Clearance of *Giardia muris* infection requires helper/inducer T-lymphocytes. *Journal of Experimental Medicine*, **12** (165), 1743–1748.

Hill, D. R. and Pearson, R. D. (1987) Ingestion of *Giardia lamblia* trophozoites by human mononuclear phagocytes. *Infection and Immunity*, **55**, 3155–3161.

Holti, G. (1966) *Candida* allergy. In H. I. Winner and R. Hurley (eds) *Symposium on Candida Infections*, pp. 73–81. E. & S. Livingstone Ltd, London.

Inman, R. D. (1988) Reactive arthritis, Reiter's Syndrome, and enteric pathogens. In L. Espinoza, D. Goldenburg, F. Arnett and G. Alarcon (eds) *Infections in the Rheumatic Diseases*, pp. 273–279. Grune and Stratton, Orlando.

Ionescu, G., Radovicic, D., Schuler, R., Hilpert, R., Negoescu, A., Preda, I., Jurthi, E., Itze, W. and Itze, L. (1986) Changes in fecal microflora and malabsorption phenomena suggesting a contaminated small bowel syndrome in atopic eczema patients. *Microecology and Therapy*, **16**, 273.

Israel, Y., Hurwitz, E., Niemela, O. and Arnon, R. (1986) Monoclonal and polyclonal antibodies against acetaldehyde-containing epitopes in acetaldehyde–protein ad-ducts. *Proceedings of the National Academy of Sciences*, **83**, 7923–7927.

Itkin, I. H. and Dennis, M. (1966) Bronchial hypersensitivity to extract of *Candida albicans*. *Journal of Allergy*, **37**, 187–194.

Iwata, K. (1977a) Toxins reproduced by Candida albicans. *Controversies in Microbiology and Immunology*, **4**, 77–85.

Iwata, K. (1977b) Fungal toxins and their role in the etiopathology of fungal infections. In S. Takima (ed.) *Recent Advances in Medical and Veterinary Mycology*, pp. 15–34. University of Tokyo Press, Tokyo.

Iwata, K., Uchida, K. and Endo, H. (1966) 'Canditoxin' a new toxic substance isolated from a strain of *Candida albicans*. *Medicine and Biology*, **74**, 345–355.

James, J. and Warin, R. P. (1971) An assessment of the role of *Candida albicans* and food yeast in chronic urticaria. *British Journal of Dermatology*, **84**, 227–237.

Juhlin, L. and Michaelsson, G. (1984) Fibrin microclot in patients with acne. *Acta Dermatologia et Venereologia*, **63**, 538–540.

Kabe, J., Aoiki, Y., Ishizaki, T., Miyamoto, T., Nakazawe, H. and Tomaru, M. (1971) Relationship of dermal and pulmonary sensitivity to extracts of *Candida albicans*. *American Review of Respiratory Disease*, **104**, 348–357.

Kamath, K. R. and Murugasu, R. (1974) A comparative study of four methods for detecting *Giardia lamblia* in children with diarrheal disease and malabsorption. *Gastroenterology*, **66**, 16–21.

Kanwar, S. S., Walia, B. N. S., Ganguly, N. K. and Mahajan, R. C. (1987) The macrophage as an effector cell in Giardia lamblia infections. *Medical Microbiology and Immunology*, **176**, 83–88.

Kasliwal, R. M. (1970) Correlation between amoebic colitis and rheumatoid arthritis. *Journal of the Association of Physicians of India*, **18**, 739–743.

Keefer, C. S. (1951) Alterations in normal bacterial flora of man and secondary infections during antibiotic therapy. *American Journal of Medicine*, **11**, 665–666.

Kennou, M. F. (1980) Skin manifestation of giardiasis. Some clinical cases. *Archives de Institut Pasteur de Tunis*, **51**, 257–260.

Kinsella, T. D. (1988) Ankylosing spondylitis and infectious agents. In L. Espinoza, D. Goldenburg, F. Arnett and G. Alarcon (eds) *Infections in the Rheumatic Disease*, pp. 353–360. Grune and Stratton, Orlando.

Kirkpatrick, C. H. (1984) Host factors in defense against fungal infections. *American Journal of Medicine*, **77** (4D), 1–12.

Korman, S. H., Le Blancq, S. M., Spira, D. T., El On, J., Reifen, R. M. and Deckelbaum, R. J. (1986) *Giardia lamblia*: Identification of different strains for man. *Zeitschrift fur Parasitenkunde*, **72**, 173–180.

Kretschmer, R. R. (1886) Immune consequences iof amebiasis. *Pediatric Infectious Disease*, **5**, 5109–5116.

Krogstad, D. J. (1986) Isoenzyme patterns and pathogenicity in amebic infection. *New England Journal of Medicine*, **315**, 390–391.

Kroker, G. (1987) Chronic candidiasis and allergy. In J. Brostoff and S. J. Challacombe (eds) *Food Allergy and Intolerance*, pp. 850–872. Balliere-Tindall, London.

Kurimoto, Y. (1975) Relationship among skin tests, bronchial challenge and serology in house dust and *Candida albicans* allergic asthma. *Annals of Allergy*, **35**, 131–141.

Kuvaeva, B., Orlova, N. G., Veselova, O. L. Kuznezova, G. G. and Borovick, T. E. (1984) Microecology of the gastrointestinal tract and the immunological status under food allergy. *Die Nahrung*, **28** (6/7), 689–693.

Lee, W. M., Holley, H. P., Stewart, J. and Galbraith, G. M. P. (1986) Case report: Refractory esophageal candidiasis associated with a low molecular weight plasma inhibitor of T-lymphocyte function. *American Journal of the Medical Sciences*, **292**, 47–49.

Lever, A. M. L., Lewis, D. M., Bannister, B. A., Fry, M. and Berry, N. (1988) Interferon production in postviral fatigue syndrome. *Lancet*, **2**, 101.

Liebeskind, A. (1962) *Candida albicans* as an allergenic factor. *Annals of Allergy*, **20**, 394–396.

Lindenbaum, J., Rund, D. G. and Butler, V. P. Jr (1981) Inactivation of digoxin by gut flora: reversal by antibiotic therapy. *New England Journal of Medicine*, **305**, 789–794.

Lombardi, G., Vismara, D., Piccolella, E., Colizzi, V. and Asherson, G. L. (1985) A non-specific inhibitor produced by *Candida albicans* activated T cells impairs cell proliferation by inhibiting Interleukin-1 production. *Clinical and Experimental Immunology*, **60**, 303–310.

Lopez-Brea, M., Sain, Z. T., Camarero, C. and Baquero, M. (1979) *Giardia lamblia* associated with bronchial asthma and serum antibodies, and chronic diarrhoea in a child with giardiasis. *Transactions of the Royal Society of Tropical Medicine and Hygiene*, **73**, 600.

Lyon, B. B. V. and Swalm, W. A. (1952) Giardiasis: its frequency, recognition, treatment and certain clinical factors. *American Journal of the Medical Sciences*, **170**, 348–364.

Mabray, C. R. (1988) Chronic candidiasis and polysystemic disorders: Study explores common features. *The Female Patient*, **13**, 34–62.

Mackowiak, P. A. (1982) The normal microbial flora. *New England Journal of Medicine*, **307**, 83–93.

Mahmoud, A. A. F. and Warren, K. S. (1975) Algorithms in the diagnosis and management of exotic diseases. II. Giardiasis. *Journal of Infectious Diseases*, **131**, 621–624.

Marconi, P., Scaring, L., Tissi, L., Boccaniera, M., Bistoni, F., Bonmassat, E. and Cassone, A. (1985) Induction of natural killer cell activity by inactivated *Candida albicans* in mice. *Infections and Immunity*, **50**, 297–303.

Mathur, S., Goust, J. M., Horger, E. O. and Fudenberg, H. H. (1977) Immunoglobulin E anti-*Candida* antibodies and candidiasis. *Infection and Immunity*, **18**, 257–259.

Mathur, S., Melchers, J. T., Ades, E. W., Williamson, H. O. and Fundenberg, H. (1980) Anti-ovarian and anti-lymphocyte antibodies in patients with chronic vaginal candidiasis. *Journal of Reproductive Immunology*, **2**, 247–262.

Mayrhofer, G. (1984) Physiology of the intestinal immune system. In T. J. Newby and C. R. Stokes (eds) *Local Immune Responses of the Gut*, pp. 1–96. CRC Press, Boca Raton.

McGuignan, L. E., Prendergast, J. K., Geczy, A. F., Edmonds, J. P. and Bashi, H. V. (1986) Significance of non-pathogenic cross reactive bowel flora in patients with ankylosing spondylitis. *Annals of the Rheumatic Diseases*, **45**, 566–571.

McNeil, N. I. (1984) The contribution of the large intestine to energy supplies in man. *American Journal of Clinical Nutrition*, **39**, 338–342.

Mirelman, D. (1987) Effect of culture condition and bacterial associates on the zymodemes of *Entamoeba histolytica*. *Parasitology Today*, **3**, 37–40.

Mirelman, D., Bracha, R., Chayen, A., Anst-Kettis, A. and Diamond, L. S. (1986) *Entamoeba histolytica*: effect of growth conditions and bacterial associates on isoenzyme patterns and virulence. *Experimental Parasitology*, **62**, 142–148.

Mogyoros, M., Calef, E. and Gitler, C. (1986) Virulence of *Entamoeba histolytica* correlates with the capacity to develop complement resistance. *Israel Journal of Medical Sciences*, **22**, 915–917.

Morrison, D. C. and Ryan, J. L. (1979) Bacterial endotoxins and host immune responses. *Advances in Immunology*, **28**, 293–299.

Myer, E. A. and Jarroll, E. L. (1980) Giardiasis. *American Journal of Epidemiology*, **111**, 1–12.

Naik, S. R., Rau, N. R., Vinajak, V. K., Narayanna, V. A., Zunzurwade, S., Sehgal, S. C. and Talwar, P. (1978) Presence of *Candida albicans* in normal and in *Giardia lamblia* infected human jejunum. *Annals of Tropical Medicine and Parasitology*, **72**, 493–494.

Nash, T. E., Herrington, D. A., Losonsky, G. A. and Levine, M. M. (1987) Experimental human infections with *Giardia lamblia*. *Journal of Infectious Diseases*, **156**, 974–984.

Nelson, R. D., Herron, M. J., McCormack, R. T. and Gehrz, R. C. (1984) Two mechanisms of inhibition of human lymphocyte proliferation by soluble yeast mannan polysaccharide. *Infection and Immunity*, **43**, 1041–1046.

Nosal, R., Novotny, J. and Sikl, D. (1973) The effect of glycoprotein from *Candida albicans* on isolated rat mast cells. *Toxicon*, **12**, 103–108.

Odds, F. C. (1988) *Candida and Candidosis, a Review and Bibliography*. Balliere-Tindall, London.

Olhagen, B. and Mannson, I. (1968) Intestinal *Clostridium perfringens* in rheumatoid arthritis and other collagen diseases. *Acta Medica Scandinavica*, **184**, 395–402.

Olson, G. B., Kanaan, M. N., Gersuk, G. M., Kelley, L. M. and Jones, J. F. (1986) Correlation between allergy and persistent Epstein–Barr virus infections in chronic-active Epstein-Barr virus-infected patients. *Journal of Allergy and Clinical Immunology*, **78**, 308–314.

Palacios, H. J. (1976) Hypersensitivity as a cause of dermatologic and vaginal moniliasis resistant to topical therapy. *Annals of Allergy*, **37**, 110–113.

Paterson, P. Y., Semo, R., Blumenschein, G. and Swelstad, J. (1971) Mucocutaneous candidiasis, anergy and a plasma inhibitor of cellular immunity: reversal after amphotericin B therapy. *Clinical and Experimental Immunology*, **9**, 595–602.

Pearce, R. B. (1983) Intestinal protozoal infection and AIDS. *Lancet*, **2**, 51.

Pearce, R. B. and Abrams, D. I. (1984) AIDS and parasitism. *Lancet*, **1**, 1411.

Pearce, R. B. and Abrams, D. (1987) *Entamoeba histolytica* in homosexual men. *New England Journal of Medicine*, **316**, 690–691.

Pepys, J., Faux, J. A., Longbottom, J. F., McCarthy, D. S. and Hargreave, F. E. (1968) *Candida albicans* precipitins in respiratory disease in man. *Journal of Allergy*, **41**, 306–318.

Petri, W. A. and Ravdin, J. I. (1986) Treatment of homosexual men infected with *Entamoeba histolytica*. *New England Journal of Medicine*, **315**, 393.

Planes, M., Brunet, D., Dalayenn, H., Paupe, G., Charlas, J., Raupe, J. and Vialette, J. (1972) Allergie e *Candida albicans* chez l'enfant. *Revue Francaise d'Allergologie*, **12**, 115–123.

Rappaport, E. M., Rossieu, A. X. and Rosenblum, L. A. (1951) Arthritis due to intestinal amebiasis. *Annals of Internal Medicine*, **34**, 1224–1231.

Ray, T. L. and Wuepper, K. D. (1976) Activation of the alternative (properdin) pathway of complement by *Candida albicans* and related species. *Journal of Investigative Dermatology*, **67**, 700–703.

Reed, S. L. Curd, J. G., Gigli, I., Gillin, F. D. and Braude, A. I. (1986) Activation of complement by pathogenic and nonpathogenic *Entamoeba histolytica*. *Journal of Immunology*, **136**, 2265–2270.

Rentdorff, R. C. (1954) The experimental transmission of human intestinal protozoan parasites. II. *Giardia lamblia* cysts given in capsules. *American Journal of Hygiene*, **59**, 209–220.

Rentdorff, R. C. and Holt, C. J. (1954) The experimental transmission of human intestinal protozoal parasites IV. Attempts to transmit *Entamoeba coli* and *Giardia lamblia* cysts by water. *American Journal of Hygiene*, **60**, 327–338.

Reynolds, J. A., Kastello, M. D., Harrington, D. H., Crobbs, C. L., Peters, C. J., Jeniski, J. V., Scott, G. H. and Diluzio, N. R. (1980) Glucan-induced enhancement of host resistance to selected infectious diseases. *Infection and Immunity*, **30**, 51–57.

Ridley, M. J. and Ridley, D. S. (1976) Serum antibodies and jejunal histology in giardiasis associated with malabsorption. *Journal of Clinical Pathology*, **29**, 30–34.

Roberts, S. H., James, O. and Jarvis, E. H. (1977) Bacterial overgrowth syndrome without 'blind loop', a cause for malnutrition in the elderly. *Lancet*, **2**, 1193–1195.

Roberts-Thompson, I. C. and Mitchell, G. F. (1978) Giardiasis in mice 1. Prolonged infections in certain mouse strains and hypothymic (nude) mice. *Gastroenterology*, **75**, 42–46.

Rogers, A. (1979) Giardia and steatorrhea. *Gastroenterology*, **76**, 224–227.

Rolsten, V. I., Hoy, J. and Mansell, P. W. A. (1986) Diarrhea caused by non-pathogenic amoebae in patients with AIDS. *New England Journal of Medicine*, **315**, 192.

Rosedale, N. and Browne, M. B. (1979) Hyposensitisation in the management of recurring vaginal candidiasis. *Annals of Allergy*, **43**, 250–253.

Rosenberg, E. and Belew, P. (1982a) Microbial factors in psoriasis. *Archives of Dermatology*, **118**, 143–144.

Rosenberg, E. W. and Belew, P. W. (1982b) Improvement of psoriasis of the scalp with ketaconazole. *Archives of Dermatology*, **118**, 370–371.

Rosenberg, E. W., Spitzer, R. E., Marley, W. M. and Belew, P. W. (1982) Inflammatory bowel disease, psoriasis and complement. *New England Journal of Medicine*, **307**, 685–686.

Rosenberg, E. W., Belew, P. W., Skinner, R. B. Jr and Crutcher, N. (1983) Crohn's disease and psoriasis. *New England Journal of Medicine*, **308**, 101.

Rosenthal, P. and Liebman, W. M. (1980) Comparative study of stool examinations, duodenal aspiration, and pediatric Entero-Test for giardiasis in children. *Journal of Pediatrics*, **96**, 278–279.

Rowland, I. R., Robinson, R. D. and Doherty, R. A. (1984) Effects of diet on mercury metabolism and excretion in mice given methylmercury: Role of gut flora. *Archives of Environmental Health*, **39**, 401–408.

Salata, R. A. and Ravdin, J. I. (1985) N-acetyl-D-galactosamine-inhibitable adherence lectin of *Entamoeba histolytica* II. Mitogenic activity for human lymphocytes. *Journal of Infectious Diseases*, **151**, 816–822.

Salem, E., Zaki, S. A., Moneim, W. A., Kadry, S., Eisa, H. and Ezz, F. A. (1973) Antoantibodies in amoebic colitis. *Journal of the Egyptian Medical Association*, **56**, 113–118.

Savage, D. C. (1980) Colonization by and survival of pathogenic bacteria on intestinal mucosal surfaces. In G. Britton and K. Marshall (eds) *Adsorption of Microorganisms to Surfaces*, pp. 175–206. Wiley, New York.

Schinfeld, J. S. (1987) PMS and candidiasis: study explores possible link. *The Female Patient*, **12**, 66–74.

Schutt, C., Koop, J., Volk, D. H., Jahn, S. and Potzsch, S. (1987a) Effects of ketaconazole on the immune system II. Mechanism of action. *Mycoses*, **30**, 559–573.

Schutt, C., Werner, H., Goan, S. R., Erdmann, D., Potzsch, M., Claus, R., Schulze, H. A. and Kaben, V. (1987b) Effects of Ketaconazole on the immune system I. In-vitro effects on lymphocyte functions. *Mycoses*, **30**, 412–418.

Schutt, C., Westphal, H. J., Kaben, V., Goan, S. R. Holzheidt, G., Nausch, M. and Schulze, H. A. (1988) Effects of ketaconazole on the immune system III. In vitro drug testing and follow-up studies in chronic dermatophytoses. *Mycoses*, **31**, 52–58.

Sclafer, J. (1951) Brulures gastriques par allergie mycosique. In *Proceedings of First International Congress for Allergy*, pp. 961–964. Karger, Basel.

Sclafer, J. (1957) L'allergie a *Candida albicans*. *La Semaine Hopitaux de Paris*, **33**, 1–10.

Sears, H. J., Brownlee, J. and Uchiyama, J. M. (1950) Persistence of individual strains of *Escherichia coli* in the intestinal tract of man. *Journal of Bacteriology*, **59**, 293–297.

Sears, H. J., Janes, H., Saloum, R., Brownlee, I. and Lamoureaux, L. F. (1956) Persistence of strains of *Escherichia coli* in man and dogs under various conditions. *Journal of Bacteriology*, **71**, 370–375.

Seelig, M. S. (1966) Mechanisms by which antibiotics increase the incidence and severity of candidiasis and alter the immunological defenses. *Bacteriological Reviews*, **30**, 442–459.

Shaw, R. A. and Stevens, M. B. (1987) The reactive arthritis of giardiasis. A case report. *Journal of the American Medical Association*, **258**, 2734–2735.

Sherman, P. and Liebman, W. L. (1980) Apparent protein-losing enteropathy associated with giardiasis. *American Journal of Diseases of Children*, **134**, 893–894.

Singh, I. P., Das, S. K., Sharma, P., Dutta, G. P. and Agarwal, S. S. (1985) Antibodies to *Entamoeba histolytica* in patients with rheumatoid arthritis. *Tropical Gastroenterology*, **6**, 141–144.

Smith, P. D., Gillin, F. D., Spira, W. M. and Nash, T. E. (1982) Chronic giardiasis: Studies on drug sensitivity, toxin production, and host immune response. *Gastroenterology*, **83**, 797–803.

Solomons, N. W. (1982) Giardiasis: nutritional implications. *Reviews of Infectious Diseases*, **4**, 859–869.

Sprunt, K. and Redman, W. (1968) Evidence suggesting importance of role of interbacterial inhibition in maintaining balance of normal flora. *Annals of Internal Medicine*, **68**, 579–590.

Stevens, D. P. (1985) Selective primary health care: strategies for control of disease in the developing world, XIX. Giardiasis. *Reviews of Infectious Disease*, **7**, 530–535.

Stokes, C. R. (1984) Induction and control of intestinal immune response. In T. J. Newby and C. R. Stokes (eds) *Local Immune Responses of the Gut*, pp. 97–142. CRC Press, Boca Raton.

Sullam, P. M. (1987) Entamoeba histolytica in homosexual men. *New England Journal of Medicine*, **316**, 690.

Sullam, P. M., Slutkin, G., Gottlieb, A. B. and Mills, J. (1986) Paromomycin therapy of endemic emebiasis in homosexual men. *Sexually Transmitted Diseases*, **13**, 151–155.

Svec, P. (1974) On the mechanism of action of glycoprotein from *Candida albicans*. *Journal of Hygiene, Epidemiology, Microbiology and Immunology*, **18**, 373–376.

Tajima, K., Tominaga, S., Shimizu, H. and Suchi, T. (1981) A hypothesis on the etiology of adult T-cell leukemia/lymphoma. *Gann*, **72**, 684–691.

Tandon, B. M., Tandon, R. K. and Satpathy, B. K. (1977) A study of bacterial flora and bile salt deconjugation in upper jejunum. *Gut*, **18**, 176–181.

Targan, R. S., Kagnoff, F. M., Brogan, M. D. and Shanahan, F. (1987) Immunologic mechanisms in intestinal disease. *Annals of Internal Medicine*, **106**, 854–870.

Tompkins, A. M., Wright, S. G., Draser, B. S. and James, W. P. T. (1978) Bacterial colonization of jejunal mucosa in giardiasis. *Transactions of the Royal Society of Tropical Medicine and Hygiene*, **72**, 33–36.

Tomsikova, A., Tomaierova, V., Kotal, L. and Novackova, D. (1977) An immunologic study of vaginal candidiasis. *Infections and Immunity*, **18**, 398–403.

Truss, C. O. (1978) Tissue injury induced by *Candida albicans*: Mental and neurologic manifestations. *Journal of Orthomolecular Psychiatry*, **7**, 17–36.

Truss, C. O. (1980a) Restoration of immunologic competence to *Candida albicans*. *Journal of Orthomolecular Psychiatry*, **9**, 1–15.

Truss, C. O. (1980b) Restoration of immunologic competence to *Candida albicans*. *Journal of Orthomolecular Psychiatry*, **9**, 287–301.

Truss, C. O. (1981) The role of *Candida albicans* in human illness. *Journal of Orthomolecular Psychiatry*, **10**, 228–238.

Truss, C. O. (1982) *The Missing Diagnosis*. Truss, Birmingham, Alabama.

Truss, C. O. (1984) Metabolic abnormalities in patients with chronic candidiasis: The acetaldehyde hypothesis. *Journal of Orthomolecular Psychiatry*, **13**, 66–93.

Turner, W. J. (1985) Is remote disease associated with *Candida* infection a tomato? *Journal of the American Medical Association*, **254**, 2891.

Valdimarsson, H., Higs, J., Wells, R. S., Yamamura, M., Hobbs, J. R. and Holt, P. J. L. (1973) Immune abnormalities associated with chronic mucocutaneous candidiasis. *Cellular Immunology*, **6**, 348–361.

Vinayak, V. K., Kij, K., Venkateswarlu, K., Khanna, R. and Mehta, S. (1987) Hypo-gammaglobulinaemia in children with persistent giardiasis. *Journal of Tropical Pediatrics*, **33**, 140–142.

Virk, K. J., Mahajan, R. C., Dilawari, J. B. and Ganguly, N. K. (1988) Role of beta-glucuronidase, a lysosomal enzyme, in the pathogenesis of intestinal amoebiasis: an experimental study. *Transactions of the Royal Society of Tropical Medicine and Hygiene*, **82**, 422–425.

Walsh, J. A. (1986a) Amebiasis in the world. *Archivos de Investigacion Medica*, **17**, 385–389.

Walsh, J. A. (1986b) Problems in recognition and diagnosis of amebiasis: estimation of the global magnitude of morbidity and mortality. *Reviews of Infectious Diseases*, **8**, 228–238.

Wannemuehler, M. J., Kicyone, H., Babb, J. L., Michalek, S. M. and McGhee, J. R. (1982) Lipopolysaccharide (LPS) regulation of the immune response: LPS converts germ-free mice to sensitivity to oral tolerance induction. *Journal of Immunology*, **129**, 959–964.

Webster, B. H. (1958) Human infection with *Giardia lamblia*. *American Journal of Digestive Diseases*, **3**, 64–71.

Weinbach, E. C., Costa, J. L. and Wieder, S. C. (1985) Antidepressant drugs suppress growth of the human pathogenic protozoan *Giardia lamblia*. *Research Communications in Chemical Pathology and Pharmacology*, **47**, 145–148.

Weisman, B. L. (1979) Urticaria and *Giardia lamblia* infections. *Annals of Allergy*, **49**, 91.

Welch, P. B. (1944) Giardiasis with unusual findings. *Gastroenterology*, **3**, 98–102.

Wilhelm, R. E. (1958) Urticaria associated with giardiasis lamblia. *Journal of Allergy*, **28**, 351–353.

Witkin, S. S. (1987) Immunology of recurrent vaginitis. *American Journal of Reproductive Immunology*, **15**, 34–37.

Witkin, S. S., Hirsch, J. and Ledger, W. J. (1986) A macrophage defect in women with recurrent *Candida* vaginitis and its reversal *in vitro* by prostaglandin inhibitors. *American Journal of Obstetrics and Gynecology*, **155**, 790–795.

Witkin, S. S., Jeremias, J. and Ledger, W. J. (1988) A localized vaginal allergic response in women with recurrent vaginitis. *Journal of Allergy and Clinical Immunology*, **81**, 412–416.

Witkin, S. S., Roth, D. M. and Ledger, W. J. (1989) Papillomavirus infection and an allergic response to *Candida* in women with recurrent vaginitis. *Journal of the American Medical Association*, **261**, 1584.

Wittner, M. and Rosenbaum, R. M. (1970) Role of bacteria in modifying virulence of *E. histolytica*. Studies of amoebae from axenic cultures. *American Journal of Tropical Medicine and Hygiene*, **19**, 755–761.

Wojdani, A. and Ghoneum, M. (1987) *In vivo* augmentation of natural killer cell activity by *Candida albicans*. *International Journal of Immunopharmacology*, **9**, 827–832.

Woo, P. and Panayi, G. S. (1984) Reactive arthritis due to infestation with *Giardia lamblia*. *Journal of Rheumatology*, **11**, 719.

Wuepper, K. D. and Fudenberg, H. H. (1967) Moniliasis, 'autoimmune' polyendocrinopathy, an immunologic family study. *Clinical and Experimental Immunology*, **2**, 71.

Yardley, J.H., Takano, J. and Hendrix, T. R. (1965) Epithelial and other mucosal lesions of the jejunum in giardiasis. Jejunal biopsy studies. *Bulletin of the Johns Hopkins Hospital*, **115**, 389–395.

Yousef, G. E., Mann, G. F., Smith, D. G., Bell, E. J., Murugesan, V. and McCartney, R. A. M. (1988) Chronic Enterovirus infection in patients with postviral fatigue syndrome. *Lancet*, **2**, 146–148.

Yu, D. T. Y. (1988) Experimental studies of infectious agents in reactive arthritis. In L. Espinoza, D. Goldenburg, F. Arnett and G. Alarcon (eds) *Infections in the Rheumatic Disease*, pp. 287–302. Grune and Stratton, Orlando.

Yu, D. T. Y., Choo, S. Y. and Schaack, T. (1989) Molecular mimicry in HLA-B27-related arthritis. *Annals of Internal Medicine*, **111**, 581–591.

Zinneman, H. H. (1950) Ten cases of amebiasis with arthritic complaints. *American Journal of Digestive Diseases*, **17**, 343–344.

Zouali, M., Drouhet, E. and Eyquem, A. (1983/1984) Evaluation of auto-antibodies in chronic mucocutaneous candidiasis without endocrinopathy. *Mycopathologia*, **84**, 87–93.

Zwerling, M. H. Owens, K. N. and Ruth, M. T. (1984) Think yeast—the expanding spectrum of candidiasis. *Journal of the South Carolina Medical Association*, **9**, 454–456.

Part V

The Future

29

Directions of Future Research

James Mowbray* and Rachel Jenkins†
*St Mary's Hospital Medical School, London, UK
†Institute of Psychiatry, London, UK

Viewpoint of an Immunopathologist

James Mowbray

The current position is that we know many of the factors which are associated with fatigue symptoms, and are able to define some subsets which appear to be coherent. The areas of further investigation which are now opening up are:

(a) Selection of patients for research studies.
(b) Study of natural history of ME in prospective studies.
(c) Study of the chronic infections, particularly viruses, associated with chronic fatigue syndromes.
(d) The hunt for antiviral agents which will cure infections with enteroviruses, and ones which will make active Epstein–Barr virus (EBV) infection dormant.
(e) Investigation of the mediators of the fatigue syndromes, with the aim of producing inhibitors of the mediators, which could be used to ameliorate the condition, even while the precipitating infection is still present.
(f) Animal models of ME, e.g. mice, horses.
(g) Clinical trials of treatments and appropriate controls.

Post-viral Fatigue Syndrome. Edited by R. Jenkins and I. Mowbray
© 1991 John Wiley & Sons Ltd

NATURAL HISTORY OF ME

Because of the delay in presentation of ME and its low incidence, it is very difficult to study patients before onset, and it is rare to find appropriate studies having been carried out early after onset of ME It is less clear why so little in the way of follow-up has been made of established cases. In part this may be due to the rather widespread belief that the syndrome never clears up. This has led to the tautology of a diagnosis of ME being given until recovery, and then a new label being given. Clearly, exactly similar clinical and laboratory findings occur in patients who recover during follow-up and those that do not. Research thus needs to be directed towards continuing follow-up of patients for prolonged periods, with repeated examination of any abnormal findings. In my own case this has led to the recognition of a close relationship between viral protein (VP1) levels in the blood and clinical state, and the associated observation that VP1 disappears from the blood of theenteroviral patients before recovery occurs, and is not found subsequent to that time. Obviously that approach cannot be used for post-viral fatigue syndromes associated with EBV, but the abnormal antibody responses found in EBV-associated ME could be followed to see in which way they change.

Clinical studies of this kind should now also use some measurement of mediator production or levels, and a few centres have started to look at cytokines during the course of disease and recovery. Measurement of blood levels has not proved to date very rewarding, at least when interleukin-1 (IL-1) or interferon (IFN) are concerned. Systematic study of tumour necrosis factor-alpha (TNFα) levels is proving useful in following some other cytokine-mediated events, and this, should be looked at. Unless the investigator has good reason for thinking that an abnormal immune response is responsible for the condition, and I personally have not seen any evidence for this, measurement of IL-2 or granuloyte macrophage colony stimulating factor (GM-CSF) and CSF1 would not be likely to be profitable. Nevertheless it is clear that some systematic studies need to be carried out, and until they are shown not to be relevant, study of any cytokine has a chance of being rewarding.

Detection of abnormal patterns of cytokines or other mediators might be a possible diagnostic aid, in which the presence of elevated production of cytokines might vary across the spectrum of disease, and prove to be a useful way of producing subsets, hopefully with somewhat different clinical patterns.

STUDY OF CHRONIC INFECTIONS ASSOCIATED WITH ME

It appears that ME is largely associated with infection with enteroviruses or EBV. There is a possibility that some other viruses might produce a minority of cases, but until their role is defined, it is impossible to elucidate their mechanisms of disease production. For the main two viruses this can be done. As stated above there is a need to show that chronic persistent infections with these viruses cause the symptoms, and that elimination of the virus is associated with recovery from the disease. There is, in addition, a need to show that persistent infection in the population is associated with ME symptoms, rather than the identification of the infections in patients symptomatic of ME. This may also be associated withh studies of genetically controlled susceptibility to ME. Is there susceptibility to a particularantigenic strain of virus in an individual, or is there susceptibility to persistent infection with any virus of that type? Second, if the persistent infection occurs, is there a genetically controlled susceptibility to ME symptoms in some of those chronically infected?

With enteroviruses it is possible to answer these questions. Identification of persistent infection by cultural, immunological and molecular biological methods has been used by several groups, and enteroviruses have been shown to persist in ME. Much further work is needed to study the chronic persistent state to determine both why the patient did not eliminate the infection early, like the great majority of the population, and whether the persisting virus is a down-regulated mutant which may escape host responses. These questions are being asked in at least two departments, namely my own and Dr Archard's group at Charing Cross.

Where is the virus in persistent infections? In the case of EBV the answer would appear to be trivial, but we need to know if it is actually in cells other than B lymphocytes. With enteroviruses, which are known to be myotropic and cardiotropic, their identification in muscle, myocardium and CNS tissues in persistent infection is not surprising. What is not clear is in which sites of infections the mediators of ME are produced. In other infectious fatigue syndromes it may be that nearly all the CNS symptoms may be produced by substances such as cytokines, carried to the brain from infection and immune responses in other tissues. Thus the central symptoms of flu or a cold without the blocked nose, produced by administration of recombinant interferon, shows that for these infection of the brain is not necessary. In the case of ME, is there any symptom generation from the scattered infected muscle seen with *in situ* hybridisation with enteroviral probes? Much more work needs to be done on the contribution of local infection to systemic or remote disease.

The present view is that the muscle in ME performs normally, apart from some effects of disuse. The predominant fatigue and fatiguability of skeletal muscle may be provoked by earlier production of pain/discomfort signals from muscles which are infected. Techniques are needed to measure the sensory output from exercising normal and ME muscle to see if there is a normal production of pain signals, or if these are generated abnormally

severely or early in ME. I think everyone now appreciates that the interpretation of these signals centrally results in premature cessation of exercise,
and that progress to the point of exhaustion results in a long period of
fatiguability of muscle. It is likely that the resetting of fatiguability of exercise is central, as it affects any muscle groups used, not just those whose
exercise produced the exhaustion and subsequent fatiguability.

Studies are needed of the mediators of fatiguability, and their relation to
the continuation of such a state. This is easier to investigate than the proposition that alteration in the amount of virus in the brain may, more directly,
produce a resetting of brain function.

SELECTION OF PATIENTS FOR CLINICAL STUDIES

The consensus meeting in Oxford (Sharpe et al., 1990) attempted to set out
the minimal set of findings which should be recorded in future studies of
chronic fatigue syndromes. Many of these are of a very general nature, and
are not applicable specifically to a particular fatigue syndrome with a well-
defined set of symptoms, such as ME. Nevertheless there must be specific
criteria for patient selection, for measurement of associated laboratory findings, and for assessment of disease severity. Whether the effect of a possible
treatment is being studied, or the natural history of the condition followed,
the basic epidemiological data are necessary.

For some studies there must be appropriate controls, and for most purposes such controls mean not only normals, but also patient groups with
related, or overlapping, conditions. Where viral studies are involved, because of the geographical nature of exposure to enteroviruses, controls must
be matched for area as well as sex, age, etc.

It is important to recognise, as was done in Oxford, that studies of the
incidence of ME cannot be carried out on patients presenting with the diagnosis. Instead it is essential to find them in the population. With an annual
incidence of about 1/1000 population per year this is a difficult but not
impossible task. For some attempts to split fatigue syndromes, including
ME, into subsets, the same approach is required. There are obviously very
considerable differences in the groups of patients with ME or related conditions when collected by physicians in hospitals, GPs or psychiatrists. There
have been a few studies of patients presenting to rheumatologists, where the
description of the conditions they see is quite different rom that of other
physicians.

There is a clear need to study ME in the population, to determine its
demography, its duration, and the groups who are at risk, rather than for the
statements made by different specialities to be taken at face value. For example, it is widely believed that the condition is *much* commoner in women

than in men. The evidence for this is very poor, and is very considerably biased by ascertainment artefacts associated with the mode of presentation of the patients. Even at this level there is a great need to carry out research on simple epidemiological lines, using appropriate epidemiological and statistical tools.

Finally, this research is not a task to be undertaken without considerable expertise, and should not be done by patients with the condition, as has unfortunately happened in the past. Such work is not different from any other research work, requiring dedication, application, considerable cognitive ability and hard work. Edison described research as 95% perspiration and 5% inspiration. As ME interferes markedly with both these activities, its presence really precludes the ME sufferer from being a suitable research worker until he or she has recovered.

THE HUNT FOR ANTIVIRAL AGENTS

As it is now clear that 85% of classical ME is associated with persistent infection with enteroviruses or EBV, there arises a need to see if there are ways of terminating the virus infection with antiviral drugs. Although a small fraction of ME may have other viruses as the cause, until these are identified it is not possible to consider antiviral treatment for them. At the present time there are no antiviral agents useful for the common viruses either. What research needs to be done to obtain such antiviral chemotherapy?

There must first be ways of accurately determining the continuing presence of active infection with the virus, and a way of measuring the degree of disease activity or incapacity caused by it. Next is the development of screening models which will allow *in vitro* or *in vivo* models of virus infection to assess the effect of therapy.

For enteroviruses there are quite good models *in vitro* for the down-regulated chronic persistent infection seen in ME. We have worked with these and they are reasonably reliable test systems, as are some of the *in vivo* animal models, especially in mice. The detection of infection with enteroviruses in sensitive, either using the production of capsid protein (VP1) or techniques using cDNA probes or polymerase chain reaction (PCR) to detect the virus genome in tissues or body fluids. These are available today to study antiviral agents as they appear.

There has been some impetus from ME, but also from some of the acute enteroviral diseases to look for agents which would interfere with those viruses, and there are now a few worthy of testing. The aim of antiviral chemotherapy would be to eliminate both the disastrous and often lethal acute infections, and the chronic ones which produce less obvious CNS and muscle disease. The acute infection damages cells, and causes acute inflammatory changes in the tissue. Some of the chronic infections may produce cellular damage, such as viral myocarditis and cardiomyopathy or viral polymyositis. The extreme is ME where functional changes are apparent without cellular destruction, in a state in which there is considerable down-regulation of virus replication, and a long-term chronic infection.

Agents which may interfere with one kind of infection may not be as effective in another, so that appropriate models must be available, and are, for the different kinds of enteroviral infection. For EBV the position is much less satisfactory, and better models need to become available for assessing antiviral agents active against reactivation or chronic active infection with this virus.

In the case of enteroviruses, where there is an enzyme unique to picornaviruses, and not part ofthe mammalian genome, there is a possibility of nucleic acid analogues which may interfere with viral RNA synthesis by blocking enzyme activity. There is also a possibility that the specific RNA synthetic pathway might be used to incorporate the wrong nucleotides into the virus, so that the virus infection fails. Similar attempts have been made with the unique reverse transcriptase of retroviruses with some success, and may be tried with the RNA-dependent RNA polymerase of enteroviruses.

Unlike larger viruses, the enteroviruses make only one messenger strand which produces a single protein, the polyprotein. This is cleaved into smaller proteins required for virus replication by proteases in the cell, including that encoded by the virus itself. Agents which can interfere with the proteolytic cleavage of the polyprotein would also potentially be very useful antiviral agents, and again there has been some interest in these for other viruses as well as for enteroviruses.

The scene is set for the development of antiviral agents, the techniques for assessment are available, and the possible first approaches are clear. It is to be hoped that some testing of agents in the clinical situation may be possible before too long. For the most part, that will require collaboration between those scientists and clinicians following the disease in patients with the pharmaceutical industry, which is the only likely source of research agents worth testing.

MEDIATORS OF FATIGUE SYNDROMES

While the basic cause of ME is a virus infection, the ways that the infection produces all the modalities of ME require further study. As discussed elsewhere there is a possibility that a large part of the symptoms of some postinfectious fatigue syndromes may be caused by the cytokines produced as a result of the virus infection itself (INF) and those produced as a result of macrophage stimulation (Il-1 and TNFα), or as a result of the lymphocytic response (IL-2). Further study of these is very important, and although measurement of levels in the blood may be unhelpful for some, for example the interferons, with others it is possible to find elevated levels in conditions other than ME where the changes observed could be produced by the cytokine. There are mediators other than cytokines which would merit study in ME, and these would include any of the CNS neurotransmitter substances such as 5-hydroxytryptamine (5-HT) and its receptors, histamine, dopamine and the neuropeptides. At present one could make only a very vague guess as to which might be mediators of symptoms in ME, so the field is wide open to look at any of them.

If one knows more of the mediators of symptoms in ME one may be in a better position to design chemicals which may interfere with their action and ameliorate symptoms while the virus is still present. There have been a large number of treatments, largely without any particular basis for their use, which have been suggested in ME. The desperate ME patient is prey to anyone offering a nostrum, whether of any use or not. It is essential that research be directed to the study of the efficacy or otherwise of *any* therapy suggested for the condition. The present situation where a variety of fringe treatments, usually very expensive, are offered to ME patients without any clinical trial is a situation which cannot be allowed to continue. We must ensure that all treatments are tested, and those shown in properly conducted trials to be efficacious given the appropriate publicity, and recommended for use. The author took these words to heart some time ago, and is still in the midst of a protracted trial of the efficacy of pooled human IgC (gammaglobulin) in the treatment of enteroviral-induced ME. Until such time as the trial is complete, I cannot recommend this treatment to doctors, nor have I done so. Double-blind trials are an accepted way of seeing if the action of a drug or treatment is placebo, or specifically effective, and this is as true of IgG treatment as of acupuncture, although perhaps both will be shown to be truly effective in due course.

Research in ME must, then, include appropriately designed trials for all therapies suggested, and if those who recommended a treatment are not prepared to conduct properly designed trials, medicine must reply by trying to prevent the advertising and sale of untested treatments of unknown efficacy or indeed hazard. The withdrawal of germanium compounds is a good example of this policy, although there was no need to test their potency, as their toxicity was known to be unacceptable. It is of interest to note that the symptoms of moderate germanium toxicity are myalgia, fatiguability and cognitive difficulties which could be mistaken for the condition that they were supposed to treat.

ANIMAL MODELS OF ME

Although it would be very difficult to study the psychological changes of laboratory animals with a variety of virus infections, or to know if they experienced muscle fatigue, it is profitable to consider chronic virus infections in experimental animals. It appears from some work recently conducted in my department in collaboration with an equine veterinary surgeon (Dr S. Ricketts) that there is a syndrome in horses following a fluelike illness, in which, when on training runs, or when racing, they 'pull up', although initially they perform apparently quite well. We have studied samples from a number of these horses, and somewhat surprisingly the affected animals, but not the controls, show a high incidence of detectable VP1 antigen of enteroiruses in their serum. Obviously this condition, and the virology of it, deserves further study as a possible analogue of human ME.

We, and other groups, have studied chronic enterovirus infection in mice. Unlike the onset of ME in man, there is an initial severe viral myositis, leading to considerable death of myofibres, and permanent scarring and fibrosis. At that time virusis present in large amounts, cellular infiltration is prominent in the muscles, and there is acute inflammation. This settles within weeks to give a pathological and virological picture in the muscle similar to that seen in biopsies of ME. There appears to be down-regulation of virus replication in the affected cells, there is no inflammation, and cytopathic effects of the infection are absent. Nevertheless the mice show considerable difficulty in prolonged exercise, and on walking tend to allow their limb girdles to collapse laterally so that they eventually waddle like alligators, and 'row' themselves along rather than walk with their limbs beneath them. Both of these animal models may merit further use, not so much to determine the nature of production of symptoms, which would be difficult, or impossible, but rather to study the interaction between host and virus. Additionally, the nature of the apparent muscle problem might be studied, as it would be possible to study afferent muscle signals on exercise to see if they were different in infected compared with normal animals.

Viewpoint of a Psychiatrist

Rachel Jenkins

DIRECT AND ANTECEDENT PREDISPOSING CAUSES

Using the multiaxial framework given in Chapter 1, we can map out a coherent research programme from here. We need to build on the discovery that a proportion of people with ME have chronic active Coxsackie infections, and find out what other organisms are implicated in ME, including echoviruses, EBV, and others. We need to find out what characteristics of the virus enable it to persist in the human body instead of being swiftly eradicated by the immune system. We need to find out why most infections are swiftly eradicated, and only a tiny proportion become chronic. Is chronicity related to a characteristic of that particular strain of virus or to some inadequacy of the host immunological response or both? If both, are both necessary conditions or only sufficient conditions for ME? Are there two distinct populations of ME—those previously completely healthy, who are then struck down by a malignant persistent variant of a common or garden type of virus such as Coxsackie, and those who were previously 'run down' physically and psychologically, who then provide a fertile soil for a virus to retain its grip, and, if so, what are the relative sizes of each population? It would seem logical that if such malignant variants of viruses occasionally arise, capable of producing chronic infections in previously healthy people, then they are going to be even more likely to produce chronic infections in unhealthy people. Are bacterial or amoebic infections also implicated in the syndrome of ME? Many people, with identical histories of ME to those of the population positive for VP1, are not positive for VP1. What does this mean?

Would those who are negative for VP1 score positively at another time— does the antibody–antigen response fluctuate over time? Or is another aetiological agent, other than enterovirus, implicated in these patients?

What sort of personality, if any, is predisposed to get ME? Is it true that doctors, nurses and teachers are over-represented? If so, is this because their job brings them into more contact with enteroviruses? Does depression predispose to ME? Do deficiency disorders such as anaemia predispose to ME? Do other debilitating infections such as amoebiasis predispose to ME?

TO INCLUDE OR EXCLUDE THOSE WITH PSYCHIATRIC HISTORIES?

This question has obvious implications for the choice of research subjects. While it may make much sense to exclude previously unhealthy people, including those with psychiatric histories, in order to demonstrate that ME can and does occur in previously healthy people, it does not make sense to exclude previously unhealthy people from all studies since they may be an important subgroup of ME, and only by their inclusion can we study the interaction between the direct aetiological agent, the viral infection, and the indirect predisposing causes such as previous physical and psychological illness, social stresses and lack of support etc. Indirect predisposing causes are relevant to most illnesses, whether infectious, malignant, degenerative or autoimmune, to varying degrees,and we need research to establish their role in ME.

Many have expressed concern that the lack of diagnostic precision and the protean symptomatology make the label attractive to a large number of psychiatrically disturbed patients who seek the status of an organic illness. Of course, the fact that this phenomenon is at all likely is a strong indication of the stigma which psychiatrically disturbed people experience at the hands of both lay people and medical personnel. But the crucial point, from the research angle, is that there is not an a priori reason why people with ME should not have an organic illness *and* be psychiatrically disturbed, either antecedent to the ME, or as a primary or secondary consequence of it. Indeed, antecedent illness is likely to affect immunity, and hence to increase the risk of ME. Thus those patients with antecedent illness are an important subpopulation for research—what is crucial is that their clinical characteristics are carefully documented, so that control groups may be appropriately chosen and studies may be replicated.

INTERPRETATION OF CAUSALITY

We need clearer thinking about causality in the interpretation of research findings. An association is not necessarily aetiological. Some authors have been at pains to point out the frequency of psychological symptoms in ME, and the fact that some of the physical symptoms are also found in depression (although not all, e.g. recurrent fevers, lymphadenopathy, muscle pains only relieved by opiates, muscle fasciculations, positive Romberg's, chronic paraesthesiae in the absence of overbreathing), and that patients with ME often fulfil DSM III criteria for major depression. However, these facts do not prove anything about aetiology. A patient with thyrotoxicosis might fulfil the criteria for DSM III major depression but nonetheless the psychiatric symptoms originate from a primary organic disorder. Similarly, a patient with rheumatoid arthritis may be very depressed as a secondary consequence of a painful and disabling disease. These arguments are carefully set out in Chapter 5 and have considerable significance for the causal interpretation of current research. Are patients with ME more depressed than those with severe rheumatoid arthritis? If so, this would indicate a prevalence of depression over and above what would be expected as a normal secondary consequence of a chronic painful and disabling disease that is not life-threatening.

EXPERIMENTAL DESIGN, INTERNAL AND EXTERNAL VALIDITY

True experiments

What research strategies are open to us to investigate causality? The strongest study design is the experiment, which allows for the manipulation of the study's independent variable and the subsequent assessment of the impact, if any, that such manipulation has had on the study's dependent variable. This strategy has been used in research on the common cold. Healthy volunteers are infected with the common cold, and then monitored to watch the effects. Care is taken (by using sufficient numbers and by keeping them in a controlled environment) to ensure that nothing else happened to the volunteers which would explain the changes. A control population is used to ensure that observed differences between the volunteers before and after infection are not simply a function of being exposed to the same measure at two periods in time. If control and treatment populations are not randomly assigned, then the equality on postinfection measures may be due to initial differences that existed between the two groups, and not to the effects of the treatment. Furthermore, individuals may drop out part of the way through the study, with the resulting effect of biasing the remaining postinfection measures. These problems are known as threats to the internal validity of an experiment. An experiment is internally valid when we as researchers are able to conclude that an experimental treatment has indeed had an effect. To research such a conclusion we must have an experimental design that allows us to rule out the effects of the numerous confounding factors including those mentioned above (see Cook and Campbell (1976) for a detailed discussion). One design that allows us to rule out all threats to internal validity is the Solomon Four Group design, of four randomly assigned groups, two of which receive the pretest measures, two of which receive experimental manipulation, and all four of which receive the post-rest measures. The Solomon Four Group design is a highly effective means for demonstrating that an experimental variable has had a hypothesised effect and that a number of rival hypotheses (e.g. selection bias) are not plausible explanations of the observed effect.

Unfortunately, there are many factors which militate against the use of pure experimental designs in research on causality in medicine in general, and particularly in ME. Firstly, ME is a serious, chronic illness, and to carry out a manipulation which may cause the illness in volunteers has serious ethical implications. Secondly, ME only seems to happen to a tiny percentage of people infected with enterovirus, compared to the high proportion of people who develop the common cold after contact with the relevant virus. Thus, we would need to study populations numbering thousands to produce a handful of people with ME. Thirdly, randomisation procedures are not always effective, particularly if numbers are relatively small, in ensuring the pretreatment equality of groups on the study's dependent variable(s). Fourthly, there may be refusals to participate in the experiment, and attenuation from the experiment which biases the results. Fifthly, there may be contamination between the two groups by individuals in experimental and control conditions interacting with each other.

For these reasons, true experiments are difficult to successfully carry out in field settings, but this does not doom the researcher to performing studies that are totally devoid of internal validity, since a number of quasi-experimental designs can often be used.

Quasi-experiments

Quasi-experimental designs allow the researcher to control who gets measured and when such measurement takes place, but they offer a lesser degree of control than experimental designs which also allow the researcher to control who gets the experimental manipulation and whem. There are a number of quasi-experimental designs, two of which will be mentioned here, including the nonequivalent control group design, and the time series design. In the nonequivalent control group design, pre-experimental measures are needed to determine the equivalent of the two groups, since subjects are not allocated to each group at random. The nonequivalent control group design leaves a number of threats to validity uncontrolled.

The time series design uses a number of periodic observations before and after the experimental manipulation, and is an example of what is commonly called longitudinal research. It controls for some but not all threats to internal validity. These study designs could be used, for example, to study major enterovirus epidemics in which a number of people might be expected to develop ME.

NON-EXPERIMENTAL DESIGNS

These are the designs that have been used to date in research on ME. In non-experimental or *ex post facto* research, the investigator has virtually no control over the study's independent variable, for two possible reasons. Firstly, the independent variable may act upon a study's subjects before the investigator is in a position to determine who will get it and when. For example, a researcher studying people with ME has no control over who will get it or when they will get it. Furthermore, the researcher will have little or no relevant pre-ME data on those who subsequently get ME.

Secondly, the study's independent variable may not be manipulable. This, to all intents and purposes, is true of ME at present. Researchers can manipulate infection with Coxsackie, but such a tiny proportion would go on to develop ME that thousands of subjects would be required.

In non-experimental studies, the investigator concomitantly measures both the independent and the dependent variables. If the two are found to be related to one another, the conclusion that the 'independent' variable is responsible for changes in the 'dependent' variable is often advanced. Since the researcher often knows little or nothing about numerous other variables that may be impacting upon either or both of the study's 'independent' and 'dependent' variables, the conclusion of a causal relationship between the two is totally unjustified.

Non-experimental research generally takes two forms: (a) the cross-sectional study; and (b) the correlational study. In cross-sectional research the investigator compares scores on the study's dependent variables for groups that the researcher assumes have been differentially exposed to the study's independent variables. Because of the lack of control over independent variables, statements of causality cannot be safely made.

In correlational research, the investigation obtains data on the study's independent and dependent variables. These data are then used to assess the strength of relationship between the two variables. However, just because two variables can be shown to be related to one another, the argument that one causes the other is not justified. If, for example, we are dealing with an observed correlation between variables x and y, it is possible that:

(a) x causes y.
(b) y causes x.
(c)   Both x and y are determined by z.
(d) x and y reciprocally influence each other.

Thus not only does an observed relationship between x and y allow us no basis for making statements about causality; we also do not know if the relationship is real, and not simply resulting from the effects of other unknown or unidentified variables. In view of these weaknesses that acompany *ex post facto* research designs, it is recommended that stronger, more experimentally oriented, designs are used whenever possible. If the constraints facing the researcher preclude the use of an experimental or quasi-experimental design, then the researcher should plan to collect data not only on what he considers to be the study's independent and dependent variables, but also on numerous other, possibly confounding, variables as well. The researcher who uses an *ex post facto* or non-experimental design must be in a position to rule out numerous rival hypotheses for any relationship he or she uncovers. Data on potential confounding or nuisance variables are critical in ruling out such competing hypotheses. Such data allow us to hold constant, through various means, the effects of measured potentially confounding variables. However, we are only able to rule out competing hypotheses associated with potentially confounding variables that we have measured. We have no idea of how numerous other unmeasured variables may be influencing our results. So, non-experimental studies leave us in the uncomfortable position of not being able to state with any degree of certainty whether two variables are causally related to one another or whether an observed relationship between two variables is a legitimate one and not spurious.

In spite of the weakness of non-experimental research, this type of study strategy has been and continues to be widely used in most medical research, including research on ME, because of the inherent difficulties outlined earlier in carrying out experimental and quasi-experimental medical research on human populations. However, non-experimental research is nonetheless very helpful to us in that it may result in hypotheses that can be tested in a more rigorous fashion (i.e. by quasi-experimental and experimental research). Secondly, if we relied exclusively on experimental and quasi-experimental research for generating knowledge, numerous important relationships uncovered in the clinical sciences would not be a part of the current body of medical knowledge.

EXTERNAL VALIDITY

A study has external validity to the extent that its results are generalisable beyond the measures, subjects and other conditions associated with the study. If a study has external validity, its findings should be obtained if different measures of the variables under study are used. Secondly, the results demonstrated for one set of subjects should be generalisable to other sets of subjects. Thirdly, the results should be reproducible in various settings. Fourthly, the strength and range of the variables associated with the study should approximate the strength and range of variables in other 'situations' to which the study's results are to be generalised.

RESEARCH ON TREATMENT

While experimental research on the causation of ME is ethically unjustifiable and in any event far too costly in terms of the numbers of subjects required, experimental research on treatment is ethically possible and is not numerically costly. Randomised controlled trials of different treatments are urgently required to evaluate treatments. Medicines can be evaluated in a double-blind fashion by the use of placebo. It is more difficult to arrange double blindness in relation to a behavioural intervention.

In the absence of proven antiviral treatments, and in the face of frightening, painful and disabling disease, it is not surprising that many patients turn to 'alternative' treatments. Such alternative treatments are often based on attempts to boost the body's own powers of immunity to fight the viral infection, and include such treatments as nutritional replacement of vitamins and mineral deficiencies, treatment of co-existing food allergies, and treatment of co-existing candidiasis, as well as homeopathy. It is undoubtedly true that, at an anecdotal level, some patients have done well on such treatments, while others have derived little or no benefit. Against this must be put the fact that the general tendency for patients with ME is to get better anyway. What is urgently needed are carefully controlled trials of different forms of therapy so that patients and their doctors can make rational, informed decisions.

REFERENCES

Cook, T. D. and Campbell, D. T. (1976) The design and conduct of quasi experiments and true experiments in field setups. In Dunnette, M. D. (ed.) *Handbook of Industrial and Organisational Psychology*, pp. 223–326. Rand McNally, Chicago.

Sharpe, M. C. *et al.* (1990) Guidelines for the conduct of research into the chronic fatigue syndrome. Report of a consensus meeting held at Green College, Oxford, 23 March.

Index

Index compiled by June Morrison